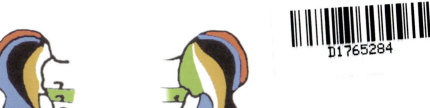

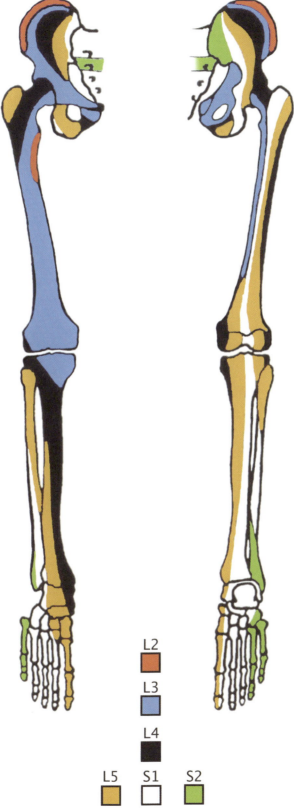

L2

L3

L4

L5 S1 S2

Beyond Thalidomide

Birth Defects Explained

Beyond Thalidomide

Birth Defects Explained

Janet McCredie, AM, MD, FRCR, FRANZCR

Adjunct Associate Professor of Radiology
Faculty of Medicine, University of Sydney
Camperdown, NSW 2006, Australia

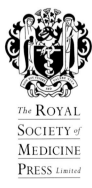

The ROYAL
SOCIETY of
MEDICINE
PRESS Limited

Published by the Royal Society of Medicine Press Ltd
1 Wimpole Street, London W1G 0AE, UK
Tel: +44 (0)20 7290 2921
Fax: +44 (0)20 7290 2929
Email: publishing@rsm.ac.uk
Website: www.rsmpress.co.uk

British Library Cataloguing in Publication Data
A catalogue record for this book is available from the British Library

ISBN 978-1-85315-741-7

Distribution in Europe and Rest of World:
Marston Book Services Ltd
PO Box 269
Abingdon
Oxon OX14 4YN, UK
Tel: +44 (0)1235 465500
Fax: +44 (0)1235 465555
Email: direct.order@marston.co.uk

Distribution in the USA and Canada:
Royal Society of Medicine Press Ltd
c/o BookMasters Inc
30 Amberwood Parkway
Ashland, OH 44805, USA
Tel: +1 800 247 6553/+1 800 266 5564
Fax: +1 419 281 6883
Email: orders@bookmasters.com

Distribution in Australia and New Zealand:
Elsevier Australia
30-52 Smidmore Street
Marrickville NSW 2204, Australia
Tel: +61 2 9517 8999
Fax: +61 2 9517 2249
Email: service@elsevier.com.au

Cover picture: *Une Mère Montrant à Deux Femmes un Enfant Monstrueux* by Francisco
José de Goya y Lucientes (1746-1828). Reproduced with permission from Musée du
Louvre, Paris

Typeset by Phoenix Photosetting, Chatham, Kent
Printed and bound by Krips b.v., Meppel, The Netherlands

Contents

Foreword *Lord Walton of Detchant*   vii
Preface   ix
Dedication   x

1	The thalidomide epidemic	1
2	Pharmacology of thalidomide: Interaction with the human embryo	11
3	Animal studies	23
4	Thalidomide polyneuropathy	39
5	Clinical radiology	57
6	Terminology, classification and the rejection of authority	63
7	The pattern of the disease: First radiological analysis (Sydney)	69
8	Verification of the disease pattern: Second radiological analysis (London)	87
9	Congenital reductions of the radius	91
10	Congenital dislocation	101
11	Congenital synostosis	115
12	The hypothesis of neural crest injury	125
13	The neural crest	139
14	Neurotrophism	157
15	Nerve in limb bud	169
16	Regeneration and embryogenesis	185
17	Neural crest ablation and limb morphogenesis	197
18	Thalidomide deformities and their nerve supply: First morphometric study in rabbits	211
19	Thalidomide deformities and their nerve supply: Second morphometric study in rabbits	229
20	The sensory nerve supply of bone	237
21	The sclerotomes	245
22	Sclerotome aplasia/subtraction	257
23	Sclerotome aplasia/subtraction in 203 cases	269
24	Radial/tibial dysmelia: Limb reductions typical of thalidomide	281
25	Associated internal malformations and their embryology	295
26	Neurotomes and multiple malformation syndromes	317
27	Hands and feet in thalidomide embryopathy: Histology and sclerotomes in the digits	333
28	Other disorders of similar sclerotomes	351
29	Segmental and truncal neuropathies in sclerotomes not affected by thalidomide	365

30   Review of actions of thalidomide   387
31   Conclusion: Beyond thalidomide   399

Index   411

FOREWORD

I can clearly remember when, in 1958, a new sedative, thalidomide (trade name Distaval), was launched on the UK market; it was hailed as being the safest remedy yet introduced for inducing sleep, as huge doses had been shown to be non-fatal, in distinct contrast to the effects of other major sedative drugs then available on the market. Indeed, the drug was used regularly for inducing sleep for EEG recordings in many departments in the UK, including my own in Newcastle upon Tyne. However, soon after its introduction it became clear, first in Germany but also in the UK and Australia, that administration of thalidomide in early pregnancy was followed in many instances with children being born with major congenital defects, usually affecting the limb buds, with partial or virtually complete absence of one or more limbs, a syndrome generally called phocomelia. Many other serious congenital anomalies were also identified in some affected infants. Almost simultaneously, it emerged that many habitual users of thalidomide developed a painful sensory neuropathy, often irreversible, with burning sensations and tingling in the extremities, and with progressive sensory loss, but with little or no evidence of motor nerve involvement. I clearly recall, in my clinical practice, seeing many such individuals; and one hallmark was that the sensory impairment found on examination often ended in a relatively sharp upper border on each limb. Worldwide evidence that the drug not only caused serious defects of embryogenesis but was also neurotoxic, led to its withdrawal from the UK market in 1961. It was widely assumed that the teratogenic effect of thalidomide resulted from abnormalities in the development of mesoderm, but no clear histological supportive evidence emerged.

The author of this fascinating and scholarly volume, Professor Janet McCredie, a diagnostic radiologist working in Sydney, Australia, concluded from her personal studies that the character and distribution of skeletal defects was inconsistent with primary bone disease, but was more likely to be due to damage to embryonic sensory nerves arising in the neural crest, giving rise to secondary failure of bone and joint formation. While the clear clinical evidence of neurotoxicity would seem to support this hypothesis, her view was not generally accepted by embryologists when first proposed. In this well-referenced volume, based not only upon a thorough and comprehensive analysis of the relevant world literature, but also upon much carefully-designed experimental work carried out by the author in collaboration with Professor Jim McLeod and other colleagues in the department of neurology in Sydney, the evidence does, in my opinion, give ample support to her early conclusions, and must surely compel the revision of theories previously advanced to explain many human developmental abnormalities. As the author says in her preface, her views were initially thought to be out of step with received scientific opinion. The evidence presented here is in my view compelling, indicating not only that neural crest injury was the most likely cause of the congenital abnormalities resulting from thalidomide, but also supporting the view that non-genetic birth defects anatomically similar to those caused by the drug, but hitherto unexplained, may well be the result of a similar mechanism.

Professor McCredie has done the profession a singular service in providing this outstanding, scholarly and well-illustrated work. Now that thalidomide has had something of a revival as an agent effective in treating various forms of lepromatous leprosy, for example, it would be timely for further research to be undertaken along the lines of that so skilfully conducted by Professor McCredie and her colleagues, so as to confirm the neural crest origin of these serious anomalies.

John Walton
Lord Walton of Detchant, Kt TD, MA, MD, MSc, FRCP, FMedSci
Former Professor of Neurology and Dean of Medicine, University of
Newcastle upon Tyne; former President of the British Medical Association,
General Medical Council, Royal Society of Mediicne and World Federation
of Neurology Detchant, Northumberland, UK

PREFACE

A major question in modern biology is 'How do birth defects happen?' or 'What goes wrong in the embryo?'

This book presents an answer, supported by evidence drawn from 35 years of research. Although based upon studies of thalidomide embryopathy, the solution reaches far beyond thalidomide. The thalidomide epidemic provided a model of the majority of birth defects that have plagued humanity throughout history. Goya's sketch of a phocomelic baby on the cover captures the horror and bewilderment of a new mother with a tetraphocomelic baby. In Goya's day, the aetiology, pathogenesis and pathology of all birth defects were unknowns. In our own lifetime, the aetiology of a series of similar embryopathies was shown to be thalidomide, a proven neurotoxin. But its mechanism of pathogenesis and pathology has eluded many investigators. Yet thalidomide is the key to understanding the mechanism of Goya's infant – what causes similar, non-thalidomide birth defects? Our generation was given clues to crack the code of thalidomide and perhaps to solve the age-old riddle.

Because of my personal involvement in all stages of the research project, it was difficult to write this book without some intrusion of personal details, opinions and experiences. I have tried to minimize such intrusions into what I intend to be an instructive scientific publication, not a book about myself. Lapses into first-person singular are sometimes unavoidable to explain a point, but I trust that they amplify rather than distract from the main theme.

I would like to acknowledge the personal support I have received from friends, colleagues and family, without which this project would have foundered. Much of the initial work was carried out in the Radiology Department of the Royal Prince Alfred Hospital, Sydney, and I thank all my colleagues there for their early support, particularly the Director, Dr David Stephen for his advice on radiology, and Superintendents Drs Trevor King and Don Child. Many Australasian paediatricians and radiologists, particularly paediatric radiologists, followed this research as it evolved. Radiologists in the UK, particularly Professors Middlemiss and Davies of Bristol and Dr Oscar Craig of St Mary's Hospital, Paddington, have been valuable sounding boards throughout. Dr Craig kindly invited me to give the Harveian Lecture to that Society in London in 2002.

Four medical knights became my mentors. Sir John Loewenthal, Professor of Surgery at The University of Sydney, having fully examined and cross-questioned my initial data, housed the research within his department and promoted my theory among national and international surgeons. Our Emeritus Professor of Paediatrics, Sir Lorimer Dods, when walking his dog, posted papers through my letterbox and called later to discuss them. Sir William Morrow, Chairman of Australia's Drug Evaluation Committee, gave me wise counsel. Sir Howard Middlemiss, Professor of Radiology, University of Bristol, UK, scrutinized my initial X-ray material and compared my films with his X-rays of leprosy. I was very aware that the neural crest theory contradicted entrenched dogma and current orthodoxy in embryology. Sir Howard allayed my fears of being burnt at the stake for heresy. He concluded that the embryology was wrong and the radiology was right, and he steered me towards my first publication and an MD thesis.

Three professors of orthopaedics strongly supported my research: Professors William Marsden, University of Queensland, Rodney Beals, University of Oregon, Portland, Oregon, and Hans-Georg Willert, Georg-August University, Göttingen, Germany. All had very extensive experience in the surgery of skeletal malformations.

The largest collections of thalidomide children were in Germany. At the International Skeletal Society in 1980, I met Professor Willert, to whom I am deeply indebted for sharing his material, ideas and expertise, and for his generous encouragement and helpful comments during preparation of this and other manuscripts.

My laboratory research at the University of Sydney was carried out in the Neurology Laboratory of the Department of Medicine, headed by Professor James G McLeod, whose lifelong interest has been peripheral neuropathy. Was it serendipity or divine intervention that provided this neurologist and his super-specialized facility on campus just when I needed it? The postgraduate neurology researchers in that laboratory submitted our seminar papers to rigorous criticism.

I was blessed with a team of excellent researchers: Drs John Cameron, Jane Elliott, Jill Forrest, Kathryn North, Gillian Dunlop and Kit Lam did the medical research. Anne Kricker, Rose Shoobridge, Robbert de Iongh, Virginia Best, Damaras Velkou, Joy Mahant and Elsa Imber contributed statistics, biology and radiography.

The long and erratic process of writing this book has followed the rollercoaster course of fluctuating public interest in thalidomide. I drafted 16 chapters during study leave from Sydney University in 1986 while a Visiting Fellow at New College, Oxford for Hilary Term, thanks to the Warden, Dr Harvey McGregor. New College allowed me to mine rich seams of information in the libraries of Oxford University, to write undisturbed and to consolidate the neural crest theory. But scientific interest in thalidomide was already waning. The drug was long since off the market and there was decreasing interest in its mode of action. The direction of research into birth defects was swinging away from drugs and extrinsic factors towards organic chemistry, genetics and molecular biology, subsidized by the Human Genome Project. I believed that the tissue or organ targeted by the drug had to be identified at the gross anatomic level before its mode of action was pursued to the molecular level. But, as Jacqueline Géraudie, Professor of Biology in Paris, said to me in the late 1980s, gross anatomy was no longer 'à la mode'. I was out of step with scientific fashion. In this negative climate, I laid the book aside and pursued other commitments. I continued to attend conferences and to observe from the sidelines the impact of various forces on thalidomide research as time passed.

The waxing and waning of interest in thalidomide can be shown by counting the number of papers on thalidomide published per year. From near zero in 1960, a bell curve peaks in the late 1960s and slumps towards the mid 1980s. Later, the internet complicated progress; if used as the only source of references, the net did not retrieve many of the major papers from the bell curve. Paradoxically, such use of the internet created a barrier to information retrieval. Facts have been lost and/or invented. There has followed a wave of historical revisionism in thalidomide research. One publication in *Nature* (1998) sought to present a new molecular theory of the mode of teratogenic action of thalidomide, illustrated by the sketch of a defect that never occurred in thalidomide embryopathy! The real world of deformed babies and distressed parents now seemed to be completely detached from the abstract and highly theoretical world of molecular biology.

I have deliberately quoted many references from the literature 1960-1980, thus inviting criticism for being out of date and politically incorrect. Yet their inclusion is essential. These papers and books record primary data. They were written by professionals who had first-hand experience of many facets of the epidemic, the drug, the malformations and their surgical anatomy, and the public storm and the private anguish generated at the time. Over 40 years later, many of those attending physicians, obstetricians, paediatricians, orthopaedic surgeons, other clinical specialists and laboratory scientists are retired or dead. Their papers, if extant, are archived. Many of their books are out of print. Their accrued wisdom deserves to be translated to the present day, whence it can be retrieved by a new generation of doctors and research scientists who may never have set eyes on a case of thalidomide embryopathy.

In USA, the FDA's Dr Frances Kelsey had refused to license the drug in 1960, thereby saving the American population from the thalidomide catastrophe. The drug was finally licensed in the USA in 1998, accompanied by a record number of caveats to ensure public safety. An exponential rise in the number of publications thereafter reflects the current revival of interest in thalidomide as a therapeutic agent for terminal AIDS, certain malignancies, and a range of autoimmune, inflammatory and dermatological conditions. Thalidomide has been resurrected as a therapeutic agent, albeit for an uncertain target. Some experts see the recent revival as a drug in search of a disease. At the time of the recent US licence application, media presentations sought public acceptance for the infamous drug in a new role. Together with other medical colleagues old enough to remember the thalidomide epidemic, I was concerned at blatant factual errors conveyed by the media, the pharmaceutical companies' pamphlets, and even in subsequent scientific presentations and papers. In particular, the important fact that thalidomide targets sensory nerves and causes profound sensory neuropathy in adults was frequently minimized or even completely ignored. An increasing trend towards historical revisionism and an alarming spread of misinformation prompted me to dust off and finish the book. Professor Margaret Burgess and Dr David Stephen are thanked for advice on final draft chapters. Mrs Janet Flint and Mr Alexander Sussman were invaluable guides in the library.

I am deeply grateful to Mr Peter Richardson and the editorial staff of the Royal Society of Medicine Press for their help, encouragement and commitment to publish my book. Particular thanks are due to Mr Mac Clarke, Ms Alison Campbell, Ms Hannah Wessely, Mr Jamie Oliver (cover designer), Mrs June Morrison (indexer) and Mr Peter Freeman (illustrator) for shaping my original rambling manuscript into this book.

I anticipate that the thalidomide sufferers and their families may gain from this book some insights into the nature of their condition. It will explain what they were born with, or without, and why, and, in some cases, what they have experienced since. This book should reassure them that they will not pass on their legacy of suffering to future generations. Acquired toxic neuropathies cannot be inherited.

I hope that scientists and doctors in the field will read this book. It was necessary to deal in some depth with a few essential principles of clinical neurology for the benefit of readers who have never studied normal and abnormal sensation – part of clinical neurology in the medical course, but not part of a science degree. Similarly, a review of the principles of neurotrophism in amphibia has been added for the benefit of medical readers who may not have come across this important and highly relevant area of biology that does not feature in most medical courses. Without the purposeful exchange of such knowledge between two diverging branches of science – medicine and biology – the pathogenetic mechanism of congenital malformations will remain forever hidden in the chasm that lies between.

Janet McCredie
Sydney

Dedication

To the thalidomiders and their families.
Because they deserve to know.

CHAPTER 1

The thalidomide epidemic

The epidemic unfolds

Between 1958 and 1961, a sudden increase in rare congenital limb deformities occurred in several countries. The phenomenon was most severe in West Germany, where it reached epidemic proportions. At the annual meeting of paediatricians in Kassel in 1960, Kosenow and Pfeiffer, of the Institute of Human Genetics in Münster, presented two infants with multiple gross deformities.[1] The long bones of the arms were so shortened that fingers appeared to arise almost directly from the shoulders. The legs were distorted, but less severely than the arms. Both children had large facial haemangiomas and one had stenosis of the duodenum.

This complex of defects was thought to represent a new syndrome. In September 1961, Wiedemann presented a series of 27 such cases from the Kiel district and suggested that this syndrome might be due to ingestion of one of the many new drugs becoming available to the public.[1]

Meanwhile, Lenz, a paediatrician in Hamburg, was concerned about the increasing number of local referrals of babies with similar severe but hitherto rare reduction deformities of the limbs of phocomelic type.[1,2] Lenz, like Wiedemann, suspected some freely available chemical such as a new detergent. Then one mother told Lenz that she had taken the sedative Contergan (thalidomide). Interrogation of the other mothers revealed that 41 out of 46 had taken Contergan in early pregnancy. Lenz presented his findings to a meeting of paediatricians in Dusseldorf on 18 November 1961, and published the data in the *Deutsche medizinische Wochenschrift* on 22 November 1961.[2] The drug was withdrawn from sale in Germany on 26 November 1961.[1,3] On 16 December 1961, McBride, an obstetrician in Sydney, Australia, reported in a letter to *The Lancet* that he had observed deformities in nearly 20% of babies whose mothers had

Chapter Summary
- **The epidemic unfolds**
- **Geographical distribution of the epidemic**
- **Anatomical distribution of the disease**
- **Problems for the thalidomiders**
- **Legal and insurance issues**
- **Public media, politics and legal responsibility**
- **Compensation and some of its problems**
- **Scientific issues: causal mechanism**
- **References**

been given thalidomide during early pregnancy, noting that the organs affected were those of mesodermal origin.[4] McBride had been conducting a clinical study on thalidomide as a drug for treating morning sickness in early pregnancy.[5] As a result of information received from Germany and Australia, the Distillers Company withdrew thalidomide from the British market on 27 November 1961.[1] Nine months later, the epidemic ceased in these countries.

During 1961, Spiers, a paediatrician in Stirlingshire, Scotland, had seen 10 infants with gross limb malformations.[6] He also had sought a common aetiological factor in the maternal histories without success. After the November announcement of the withdrawal of thalidomide, he again questioned the mothers and their family doctors. When several mothers and their doctors denied using the drug, Spiers instituted a search by the local council of recent prescription forms for that locality:

> 'Evidence was obtained that of these ten mothers, eight took thalidomide during pregnancy. One had a sedative, the nature of which is unknown, and in one case there is no evidence that the mother had any drug at all. However, it became apparent early in the investigation that statements by the patient or doctor that no thalidomide had been taken could not necessarily be accepted. In view of this, it remains quite possible that the two mothers for whom there was no proof did in fact have this drug.'

The connection between deformities and maternal thalidomide was soon confirmed by clinicians in several parts of the world where the drug had been available.[7-9] Somers[10] in the UK in 1962 was the first scientist to produce experimental confirmation, using thalidomide in New Zealand white rabbits to induce phocomelic offspring.

Geographical distribution of the epidemic

The total number of victims throughout the world has never been accurately recorded, but has been guessed to be around 10 000. There were at least 4000 cases in West Germany. Over 400 cases are on record in the UK, and nearly 40 cases occurred in Australia. There were scores of cases in other countries in Europe and the British Commonwealth where the drug was marketed. Accurate estimates were impossible in retrospect because in many instances the prescription, the bottle of tablets and other medical records had been discarded. The high incidence in West Germany is explained by the fact that thalidomide had been invented by the German drug firm Chemie Grünenthal and introduced onto the West German market in 1957, first as an antihistamine for influenza and at least a dozen other indications. Later, after numerous reports of its association with peripheral sensory neuropathy, the marketing policy was redirected into use for the morning sickness of pregnancy.[5]

Two geographical border phenomena appeared as the epidemic unfolded. The West German epidemic stopped at the Iron Curtain. No epidemic appeared in East Germany. The drug was never marketed there. This enabled Lenz to exclude influences such as radiation, infections with insect vectors or aerial transmission. The other striking geographical border was between Canada (where the drug was marketed along whisky trade routes from the UK) and the USA (where it was not licensed by the Food and Drug Administration, (FDA)). Both border phenomena reflected marketing strategies.

The epidemic was prolonged in Japan by delayed withdrawal of the drug there.[11] A low-grade epidemic has rumbled on in Brazil because thalidomide was never withdrawn from the market. It continued to be used there to treat leprosy, and it leaked into the general market because of less stringent regulation of the Brazilian pharmaceutical industry.

Anatomical distribution of the disease

In addition to the obvious dysmelic or longitudinal reduction deformities of the limbs, thalidomide caused a wide range of visceral, facial and other birth defects. The typical manifestations were described by Lenz in the *Deutsche medizinische Wochenschrift* and summarized in *The Lancet*[12] as follows:

> 'defects of the arms, amelia, atypical phocomelia with absence of the thumbs and sometimes of other fingers as well, aplasia of the radius, defects of the long bones of the legs, especially the femora and tibia, absence of the auricles, haemangiomata of the nose and upper lip (wine spot variety), atresia of the oesophagus, the duodenum or anus, cardiac anomalies and aplasia of the gall bladder and of the appendix.'

Lenz estimated that in half of his cases only the arms and in one-quarter both arms and legs were affected. In one-sixth of his cases, the ears were virtually absent (anotia).

Pfeiffer and Kosenow,[8] in a series of 170 cases, noted:

> 'a preponderance of defects of the upper limb, mostly symmetrical. Both sexes are equally affected. Malformations of other organs are often associated, but not of the nervous system or of the skull or spine.'

A subsequent paper from a group of orthopaedic surgeons in Oxford, UK, described spinal deformities due to thalidomide.[13] These included hemivertebrae, fused and cross-fused vertebrae, spina bifida operta and occulta, and scoliosis.

Smithells[9] reported 7 cases of anotia, 5 of them without any limb deformity, as well as 30 cases of limb reductions, from the Liverpool register of congenital abnormalities. He established that non-limb defects can occur without limb defects. Thus longitudinal reduction defects in the limbs, the commonly accepted hallmark of thalidomide embryopathy, were not an essential component.

The unexpectedly wide range of thalidomide-induced deformities has been reviewed in the British literature by Smithells,[14] Quibell,[15] Newman,[16] and Smithells and Newman.[17] Two German authors, Henkel and Willert, published an analysis of the pattern of the defects in the skeleton in 1969, in English,[18] as well as a monograph in German[19] (now out of print). There were many papers in German and other languages in European medical journals.

The most severely damaged babies died in the perinatal period, when the mortality rate was of the order of 40%. Survivors, who provided the basis for further studies, therefore represent (at most) 60% of the total spectrum of the disease. This is an important point to keep in mind. Those who perished succumbed to lethal malformations of internal organs or to complications of early heroic surgery. All notified British thalidomide infants, dead or alive, were annotated and recorded by the British Ministry of Health in a report that is now out of print.[1]

A series of autopsies on 14 thalidomide infants from Hamburg (1959–62) was reported by Pleiss[7] in *The Lancet*. This paper provides an index of the major defects encountered in the lethal cases:

- Hypogenesis or agenesis of long bones   5
- Phocomelia   4
- Defects of metacarpals and phalanges   3
- Anomalies of the outer ear   7
- Microphthalmia   2
- Naevus of the face   1
- Anomalies of the heart and arteries   10
  (tetralogy of Fallot 5
  ventricular septal defect 4)
- Bilobed right lung   5
- Duodenal atresia   4

- Imperforate anus   1
- Absence of the gallbladder   8
- Atresia of the common bile duct   3
- Agenesis of the appendix and caecum   5
- Malrotation   7
- Bicornuate uterus (out of 8 females)   5
- Urinary tract anomalies   10
- Atresia or absence of the vagina   3
- Abnormal liver lobation   5

Knapp,[20] a radiologist working with Lenz in Hamburg, stated that:

'Almost every organ of the body – arms, legs, ears, eyes, heart, cranial nerves, digestive tract, urinary tract and uterus – may be affected in thalidomide embryopathy.'

The numbers of aborted embryos will never be known.

Not only at the most severe end of the embryopathy but also at the least severe extreme, cases were not counted. Knapp[20] drew attention to the difficulty of diagnosis in cases with mild manifestations, and to the crucial role of diagnostic radiology:

> 'Detection of malformations of the limbs presents great difficulties, for without X-ray documentation, one cannot be certain of the bony defect. Mild manifestations of the fingers are much more frequent than severe arm malformations. These minor malformations in a large number of cases of thalidomide embryopathy led to failure to recognise the defect as related to thalidomide. I am sure that even today many of these children are not correctly diagnosed by physicians who have insufficient knowledge of this specific type of malformation.'

Problems for the thalidomiders

I was aware of the parents' anxiety for the future of their children, aged 9–11 years at the time I became involved. As well as concern about the future, almost all parents expressed concern about the past. How did the drug disrupt an otherwise-normal pregnancy?

The babies grew into children of normal intelligence, happy, sensitive, alert, and with the capacity to enjoy life, yet inhibited by their physical deformities. Adolescence was just ahead, and complex problems would have to be faced as they grew to adulthood. Ordinary daily routines and normal living skills were often difficult. Education, social acceptance, employment, marriage and child-bearing would present major obstacles. The future seemed particularly formidable for badly afflicted children, whose gross disabilities meant reliance upon another person at all times for simple daily activities such as eating, dressing, mobility and toiletry. The blind and deaf often lived in institutions. In birth defects of other causes, associated mental deficiency may serve to buffer the individual from some of the 'slings and arrows of outrageous fortune'. For these children, with their normal intellects, no such buffer was present.

Medical costs and upkeep were ultimately subsidized by drug companies, benevolent trusts and some governments, varying with public health policies in different countries. Limb deficiency clinics were set up in some paediatric and orthopaedic hospitals. In other countries, thalidomide victims were left to fend for themselves.

For thousands of victims worldwide and their families, the consequences are still being worked out at the present time, with variable success. They have already tackled multiple challenges of living with the complex burden of physical deformity. Now middle-aged, they grapple with degenerative changes of early onset provoked by and complicating their malformations.

Legal and insurance issues

There were significant repercussions in the law courts and parliaments of the nations affected (Europe and the British Commonwealth). This was the first time a drug had crossed the placental barrier and inflicted damage on the fetus. It opened a new chapter in medicolegal insurance and compensation law.

In the longest and most expensive German lawsuit since the Nuremburg Trials, a court at Aachen took 9 years to establish that the drug company was culpable and should compensate the victims. This litigation was a marathon for the German families, their lawyers and expert witnesses, as documented by Sjöström and Nilsson, who sat through the case. Their 1972 book, a Penguin Special *Thalidomide and the Power of the Drug Companies,*[5] is now out of print.

Public media, politics and legal responsibility

In the UK, the history of the epidemic and its aftermath was closely followed and publicized by the *Sunday Times* from 1967 and in a subsequent (1979) book *Suffer the Children.*[21] The *Sunday Times* set out to generate public support for increasing the compensation payments offered to the children by the drug company. The sympathetic British were roused to boycott whiskies manufactured by the Distillers Company. The campaign evolved into a challenge to freedom of the press and freedom of speech. Issues of current laws, contempt of court and moral responsibility for the disaster were pursued through the House of Commons to the House of Lords. The impact of the thalidomide epidemic upon the law was reported in 1973 by the *Sunday Times* in another book, *The Thalidomide Children and the Law.*[22]

Compensation and some of its problems

After the Aachen verdict in Germany, the process of compensation began worldwide. Thalidomide victims were reviewed by panels of medical experts in order to make the compensation payments relative to the degree of disability. The ability of thalidomide to mimic a wide spectrum of naturally occurring malformations presented new and difficult practical problems for the medicolegal assessors. From the queue of children being presented for compensation, they had to decide who should be compensated and who should not, i.e. which claimants were the responsibility of the drug companies. The large sums of money involved attracted families with no history of thalidomide exposure. The claims of some parents of notified children altered at this time. Some who had previously denied thalidomide exposure now claimed to have taken it. In UK, a shift to the left was recorded between the four categories used by the Ministry of Health (definitely exposed, probably exposed, possibly exposed and definitely not exposed).[1]

Some of the children were obviously too old or too young to be victims of thalidomide, yet their malformations were clinically indistinguishable from those with proven thalidomide exposure. Such claimants could be excluded, relatively easily, by date of birth. But when the birthdate of such a child fell within the era of thalidomide availability, the decision was sometimes impossible. The Canadian assessors accepted all those born when the drug was available. The British assessors also adopted a policy to give such a child the benefit of the doubt and to award compensation, despite absence of proof of thalidomide exposure.[23] It was impossible to prove the negative, i.e. to *prove* that thalidomide had *not* been taken. The child obviously needed money. This 'benefit of the doubt' decision caused the unintentional inclusion of a number of children of possibly genetic or other cause within the 'thalidomide' group in the UK – at least 10% of the total group, according to Dr Claus Newman, one of the assessors. As a result, the 'thalidomide children' in UK were, as a group, what epidemiologists would call a contaminated cohort. There were to be later repercussions as a result of this mixture of cases, but at the time it was impossible to exclude these 'thalidomide lookalikes' on any scientific grounds.

My own introduction to thalidomide embryopathy was in this context. I was asked by McBride to review the radiographs of some Australian children who were under consideration for compensation, in order to determine radiologically, if possible, which defects were caused by thalidomide and which were of non-thalidomide aetiology. I found little or no distinction possible in most cases, for the radiological signs in proven thalidomide cases were duplicated in other cases born before or after the short, four-year, thalidomide era (1958–62). A review of the sparse radiological literature on this topic did not provide an answer. I had to admit that it was impossible to answer the question asked of me. But I was fascinated by the range and the nature of the malformations. The ability to mimic naturally occurring malformations gave this drug a unique significance, for if the mode of action of thalidomide could be established, the pathogenesis of other sporadic malformations (such as those that were causing medicolegal confusion) might also be revealed.[24,25]

Scientific issues: causal mechanism

As a result of the thalidomide disaster, there was an upsurge of interest in teratology – the study of congenital malformations and their causes. Teratologists used thalidomide to induce malformations in many animals. In the decade following the epidemic, it had generally been assumed that the drug acted upon the mesoderm or mesenchyme,[4,7,26] in order to explain the presence of multiple defects in different organ systems of mesodermal origin. However, no histological lesion could be demonstrated, and the teratogenic mechanism of thalidomide eluded investigators. The underlying pathology remained to be established.[26]

How did thalidomide do this? What had gone wrong in an apparently normal embryo? These unanswered questions resonated through the scientific world. By what mechanism did this drug exert its devastating effects upon the embryo? That thalidomide mimics many birth defects of unknown cause complicated the puzzle for scientists. The drug had inadvertently provided, in our generation, a model for study of the pathogenesis of many common congenital malformations.

References

1. Ministry of Health Reports on Public Health and Medical Subjects No. 112. *Deformities Caused by Thalidomide*. London: HMSO, 1964.

2. Lenz W. Kindliche Missbildungen nach Medikament-Einnahme während der Gravidität. Fragen aus der Praxis. *Dtsch Med Wsch* 1961; **86**: 2555.

3. Taussig H. Thalidomide and phocomelia. *Pediatrics* 1962; **30**: 654–9.

4. McBride WG. Thalidomide and congenital abnormalities. *Lancet* 1961; **i**: 45.

5. Sjöström H, Nilsson R. *Thalidomide and the Power of the Drug Companies*. Harmondsworth: Penguin, 1972.

6. Spiers AL. Thalidomide and congenital abnormalities. *Lancet* 1962; **i**: 303–5.

7. Pleiss G. Thalidomide and congenital abnormalities. Lancet 1962; **i**: 1128–9.

8. Pfeiffer RA, Kosenow W. Thalidomide and congenital abnormalities. *Lancet* 1962; **i**: 45–6.

9. Smithells RW. Thalidomide and malformations in Liverpool. *Lancet* 1962; **i**: 1270–3.

10. Somers GF. Thalidomide and congenital abnormalities. *Lancet* 1962; **ii**: 912.

11. Kida M. *Thalidomide Embryopathy in Japan*. Tokyo: Kodansha, 1987.

12. Lenz W. Thalidomide and congenital abnormalities. *Lancet* 1962; **i**: 45; *ibid* 271; *ibid* **ii**: 1358.

13. Nichols PJ, Boldero JL, Goodfellow JW, Hamilton A. Abnormalities of the vertebral column with thalidomide-induced limb deformities. *Orthopaedics Oxford* 1967; **1**(1): 71–90.

14. Smithells RW. Defects and disabilities of thalidomide children. *BMJ* 1973; **i**: 269–72.

15. Quibell EP. The thalidomide embryopathy: an analysis from the UK. *Practitioner* 1981; **225**: 721–6.

16. Newman CGH. Teratogen update: clinical aspects of thalidomide embryopathy – a continuing preoccupation. *Teratology* 1985; **32**: 133–44.

17. Smithells RW, Newman CGH. Recognition of thalidomide defects. *J Med Genet* 1992; **29**: 716–23.

18. Henkel H-L, Willert H-G. Dysmelia: a classification and pattern of malformations in a group of congenital defects of the limbs. *J Bone Joint Surg* 1969; **51B**: 399–414.

19. Willert H-G, Henkel H-L. *Klinik und Pathologie der Dysmelie: Die Fehlbildungen an den oberen Extremitäten bei der Thalidomid-Embryopathie.* Berlin: Springer-Verlag, 1969.

20. Knapp K. Radiological aspects of thalidomide embryopathy. In: Swinyard C, ed. *Limb Development and Deformity: Problems of Evaluation and Rehabilitation.* Springfield, IL: CC Thomas, 1969.

21. The *Sunday Times* Insight Team. *Suffer the Children: The Story of Thalidomide.* London: Andre Deutsch, 1979.

22. The *Sunday Times. The Thalidomide Children and the Law: A Report by The Sunday Times.* London: Andre Deutsch, 1973.

23. Smithells RW. Thalidomide might be a mutagen. *BMJ* 1994; **309**: 477.

24. Gordon G. The mechanism of thalidomide deformities correlated with the pathogenetic effects of prolonged dosage in adults. *Develop Med Child Neurol* 1966; **8**: 761–7.

25. Brent RL. Implications of experimental teratology. *Excerpta Medica ICS* 1970; **204**: 187–95.

26. Woollam DHM. Principles of teratogenesis: mode of action of thalidomide. *Proc R Soc Med* 1965; **58**: 497–501.

27. Tuchmann-Duplessis H. *Drug Effects on the Fetus: Monographs on Drugs,* Vol 2. Hong Kong: Adis Press, 1975.

CHAPTER 2

Pharmacology of thalidomide: Interaction with the human embryo

Advent of thalidomide

Thalidomide is the approved name given by the British Pharmacopoeia Commission of the General Medical Council to the substance α-phthalimidoglutarimide. Synthesized by Kunz and Mückter in 1954, it was marketed in Germany from 1957 as a light sedative under the proprietary name of Contergan.[1]

Later, it was marketed in Britain under licence to the Distillers Company with the proprietary name of Distaval, and in mixtures as Asmaval, Tensival, Valgis and Valgraine.[1] It is not chemically related to the barbiturates or to the narcotic alkaloids, and, unlike these, it allegedly had no lethal dose.

It was finally a component of 37 preparations worldwide.

Indications for use

'In August 1956, a leaflet was printed enumerating the following indications: irritability, weak concentration, stage fright, ejaculatio praecox, menstrual tension, postmenopausal symptoms, fear of examination, functional disorders of the stomach and gall bladder, febrile infectious diseases, mild depression, anxiety, hyperthyroidism, and tuberculosis. The claim was raised and maintained for several years that such a multipotent drug was virtually free from side effects.'[2]

Safety

Unlike other sedatives, thalidomide had the remarkable feature that very high doses are not lethal. This made it a 'safe sedative', and as such it was welcomed by prescribing doctors and the lay public.

Chapter Summary
- Advent of thalidomide
- Indications for use
- Safety
- Structure and metabolism
- Hydrolysis in solution
- Teratogenicity: molecular questions
- Teratogenicity: questions about its target in the embryo
- Pharmacokinetics of thalidomide in vivo
- The human embryo: clinical considerations
- Thalidomide-sensitive period and risk of malformations
- Zero-time: LMP or date of conception?
- Sensitive days for particular malformations
- Sequence of malformations following exposure in the sensitive period
- Impact of thalidomide upon the pharmaceutical industry
- References

Experimental animals tolerated 1000 times the sedative dose of 50 mg without ill-effect, and several reported cases of overdosage in humans proved that up to 160 times the ordinary sedative dose is tolerated with complete recovery.[1] The explanation was possibly its limited absorption based upon the relative insolubility of the substance. Kunz et al[3] described it as a non-toxic, sedative hypnotic drug with a quietening effect upon the central nervous system, reducing the voluntary activity of laboratory animals and promoting sleep.

'Its ability to promote sleep in man was shown by Jung in 1956, and by 1960, there was apparently convincing evidence of its sedative effect in man and of its non-toxicity.'[4]

Subsequently, the editor of *Arzneimittelförschung* (which had published the papers by Kunz et al[3] and by Jung[5]) was rebuked by Lenz[6] for accepting papers when certain details of controls and experimental methods were incomplete or inadequately described. Publication by a prestigious medical journal gave the green light to the manufacturers, and as a result, this

'highly effective sleeping pill with amazing absence of acute toxicity even in high doses, triumphantly conquered the market.'[6]

Structure and metabolism

The thalidomide molecule is made up of two parts: the phthalimide structure on the left in Figure 2.1 and the glutarimide ring on the right. It is a white, tasteless, crystalline powder, melting point 271°C, sparingly soluble in water, dilute hydrochloric acid, benzene, methanol, ethanol and ether, but highly soluble in chloroform, dimethylformamide and dioxane. Its low solubility in water suggests that its concentration in body fluids would be small at any time. Attempts to make stronger aqueous solutions by dissolving it in dilute alkali and then neutralizing the solution failed because the drug is immediately decomposed by dissolution in alkali.[4] Such solutions contain by-products, but not the original thalidomide molecule.

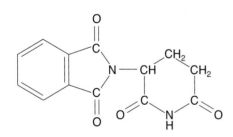

Figure 2.1 *Structure of thalidomide.*

Hydrolysis in solution

Thalidomide is unstable in aqueous solution, where it rapidly undergoes spontaneous hydrolysis at its amide bonds.[7] After storage of an aqueous solution of the drug at physiological pH values, it broke down spontaneously into 12 products of hydrolysis. Solutions in the laboratory must be freshly prepared for each experiment because of this short half-life in solution of 2–5 hours at pH 7.4.[8]

When the drug was fed to rabbits, the 12 hydrolysis products were found in plasma and urine. These compounds are also found in human, rat and dog urine after thalidomide ingestion. Thus the behaviour of the drug in vivo is similar to that in vitro, and, because of this instability, it was necessary to consider thalidomide and all 12 hydrolysis products as possible teratogens – i.e. 13 compounds.

No enzymes or complex metabolic pathways are involved in this simple hydrolysis.

Teratogenicity: molecular questions

Which of the 13 molecules was or were teratogenic?

All hydrolysis products have been separately tested in pregnant rabbits, and not one of them has been found to be teratogenic.[7] This may be because they are polar, and less able to cross membranes, whereas the intact thalidomide molecule is non-polar and can readily cross membranes. For further details of the relationship between chemical structure and teratogenicity, the reader is referred to Keberle et al,[9] Williams[4] and Jonsson.[10] The accrued evidence indicates that the thalidomide molecule itself is the teratogenic agent.

What specific property of the thalidomide molecule confers upon it the teratogenic property? This has remained one of the major unanswered questions of teratology. Several suggestions have been made, but none has been proved.

Teratogenicity: questions about its target in the embryo

Does thalidomide interfere with some aspect of embryonic glutamate metabolism?[11] Glutamine and glutamate do not protect the embryo, however.

Does thalidomide act as a phthalylating agent, reacting with spermine, spermidine or putrescine? All three diamines stimulate RNA synthesis.[12] Spermine and spermidine are present in the chick embryo after 2–3 days of incubation. Williams has speculated that thalidomide phthalylates polyamines in the embryo, and thus indirectly interferes with messenger RNA concerned with enzymes involved in the initiation of growth of certain structures during morphogenesis.

Another hypothesis has been proposed by Jonsson:[10]

1. Thalidomide is similar in structure to nucleic acid bases.
2. It may therefore intercalate between base pairs, and cause depurination of nucleic acids similar to that produced by radiomimetic alkylating agents.
3. Three structural elements of the thalidomide molecule are involved in this hypothetical reaction: the flat phthalimide ring system, one reactive carbonyl group of this system, and the ionizable glutarimide.

4. It is hypothesized that the nucleic acids affected are involved in the synthesis or function of some factor(s) with regulatory activities in skeletal tissue formation.

Pending proof of any such hypotheses at the molecular level, however, much remains to be understood concerning the normal mechanisms involved in the initiation of growth and morphogenesis in the embryo, at the grosser levels of cells, tissues and organ structures. All biological information concerning thalidomide needs to be studied in the search for the ultimate site of its teratogenic reaction. The target organ must be identified before molecular targets are explored.

Pharmacokinetics of thalidomide in vivo

Since intact thalidomide appears to be the main teratogen, it is important to study its fate in vivo. Schumacher et al[13] studied the pharmacokinetics of the intact molecule in rabbits and rats. After absorption through the gastric mucosa, it enters the plasma at normal pH, and undergoes rapid breakdown by hydrolysis.

The plasma level of intact thalidomide rises rapidly to a peak at 1 hour after ingestion (Figure 2.2).[13] Then hydrolysis overtakes absorption, and the plasma level of intact drug falls rapidly by 3 hours to half the initial peak level. Thereafter, the level subsides further, and approaches zero at 12 hours after ingestion. Schumacher et al[13] showed that this curve was modified by the presence of food in the stomach, which reduced absorption and decreased the amplitude of the initial peak. Schumacher et al[13] graphed the levels of thalidomide

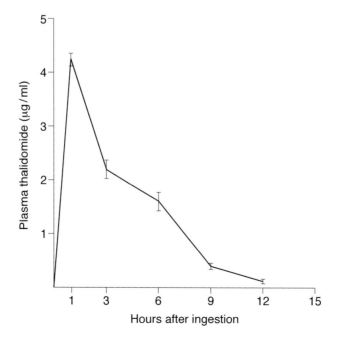

Figure 2.2 *Plasma levels of intact thalidomide in an adult rabbit with an empty stomach. The drug (10 mg/kg) was ingested at zero time. Plasma levels were measured at intervals of 1, 3, 6, 9 and 12 hours. (From Schumacher H et al.* J Pharmacol Exp Ther *1968; 160: 189–200.[13])*

in plasma of rats and rabbits, on full and on empty stomachs (Figure 2.2 is for a rabbit with an empty stomach at the time of thalidomide ingestion).

The human embryo: clinical considerations

Such information is relevant to the pregnant woman who has been prescribed the drug for morning sickness in doses from 50 to 200 mg (1 mg/kg body weight). In the presence of nausea and vomiting, the stomach would probably be empty. Within 3 hours following ingestion of a tablet, there is an abrupt rise and fall of the teratogen in the woman's plasma. This transmits across the placenta into the embryonic blood, so that the embryo receives a short, sharp insult.

A woman would have received a bottle of tablets on prescription and was likely to take a series of tablets on several mornings. The embryo would therefore be subjected to a series of single-pulse injuries, following each dose of thalidomide.

The pattern of attack of the teratogen upon the embryo would be a function of the timing of administration of medication, and would be modified by other factors, such as whether it was taken before or after meals and alterations in pH (e.g. due to vomiting). Each short teratogenic dose would damage the embryonic development taking place at that time. Between episodes, with thalidomide cleared from the blood, embryonic growth and development would proceed normally. Such a pattern could explain many of the multiple, scattered malformations observed in thalidomide embryopathy.

Thalidomide-sensitive period and risk of malformation

That thalidomide acted upon the embryo during a specific phase of its development (which became known as the thalidomide-sensitive period) was an observation recorded by Lenz in his original paper in *Deutsche medizinische Wochenschrift*.[14] He stated that 41 out of 46 mothers of deformed infants in his own practice had definitely taken thalidomide preparations within the first 2 months of pregnancy. Similar findings in 40 more cases were reported to him by colleagues. On the other hand, systematic questioning of more than 300 mothers of normal infants did not reveal a single instance where a pregnant woman had taken this drug between the 4th and 9th weeks following the last menstrual period. This comparison of cases with controls indicated a very high risk of deformity attached to thalidomide ingestion within that period, which, as Lenz[15] and Pleiss[16] pointed out, coincided with the period of major organogenesis.

Lenz stated in *The Lancet*[15] that he believed that the risk to the fetus, if exposed within 4–8 weeks post menstruation, was 'definitely higher than 20%'. He estimated that there were 2000–3000 Contergan babies in Germany. Burley,[17] arguing the case for the Distillers Company, claimed that the malformation risk from thalidomide, as it had been used in pregnancy in Britain, was of the order of 2%. Lenz countered strongly by emphasizing the critical importance of assessing the risk within the sensitive period, rather than within other stages of pregnancy.[18,19] Lenz reiterated that he had found:

- no case in which the mother of a *normal* infant had taken thalidomide between the 3rd and 8th weeks after conception, and
- no case of this type of malformation in which the mother had *not* taken the drug.

Lenz cited 55 cases in which the exact date of prescription and/or intake of thalidomide was known and coincided with the time of development of the malformed organs. Dose was not critical, but timing was.

In a subsequent paper that year, Lenz and Knapp[20] gave further evidence for a critical period in thalidomide embryopathy. Within their rapidly expanding collection of cases, the exact date of prescription was known by 86 women. Of 32 mothers who also knew the dates of conception, none had taken thalidomide only before the 27th day or only after the 40th day post conception. Thus the sensitive period was at least between the 27th and 40th days of embryonic age.

By 1963, Nowack, Knapp and Lenz were able to ascertain a timetable for thalidomide embryopathy.[21] The sensitive period of the embryo commences at day 35 after the last menstrual period, at which time anotia and facial and ocular palsies result. Ear defects and duplication of the thumb result from exposure commencing 3 days later. Upper amelia follows exposure around the 39th to the 44th post-menstrual days, mainly on the 40th day. Lower amelia results from taking the drug between 41st and 44th post-menstrual days.

Heart defects and duodenal atresia, and also dislocation of the hips, follow drug ingestion between the 39th and 45th post-menstrual days. The most severe malformations derive from taking thalidomide between the 35th and 45th post-menstrual days. Triphalangeal thumbs and anorectal problems occur from exposure about the 50th post-menstrual day. Anal atresia was often, but not always, of similarly late date.

Zero-time: LMP or date of conception?

Lenz chose to date events from the recorded date of the first day of the last menstrual period (LMP), rather than from the date of conception. His reasons were as follows:

'A certain temporal scattering can be expected partly through differing intervals between menstruation and conception, and partly through the differing speed of development of the embryos. Therefore the sensitive phase for organ malformations, based on my material, is primarily valid for the collective group. In the individual case it may well be shorter.'[22]

The post-menstrual day can be converted into the day of embryonic age (day post conception, or day of gestation) by subtracting 14 days, as is routine in obstetric practice. This conversion is necessary in order to date the age of the embryo from the day of conception, which is an approximate date for the reasons given by Lenz. But it is essential at this point to make this conversion from post-menstrual days to *post-conceptional or gestational days*, because all data on embryonic development are given in 'gestational days', not 'post-menstrual days'. Gestational days (days post conception) are the true age of the embryo – as close as we can establish in the circumstances.

The two sets of dates have led to some confusion in the literature. Two current textbooks on congenital malformations have mistakenly quoted post-menstrual days as gestational days.

Sensitive days for particular malformations

An important 1965 paper by Nowack from Lenz's Human Genetics Institute at the University of Hamburg, entitled 'The sensitive phase for thalidomide embryopathy',[23] dealt in detail with the fully documented histories of 82 mothers and established the sensitive period for the following defects (the equivalent gestational day is also given):

- anotia was associated with administration of thalidomide between the 34th and 38th days after the last menstrual period (pm) (equivalent to 20–24 gestational days)
- aplasia of the thumb: 38th–40th days pm (24–26 gestational days)
- amelia of the arms: 38th–43rd days pm (24–29 gestational days)
- dislocation of hip: 38th–48th days pm (24–34 gestational days)
- phocomelia of arms: 38th–47th days pm (24–33 gestational days)
- deformities of the ears: 39th–43rd days pm (25–29 gestational days)
- ectromelia of the arms: 39th–45th days pm (25–31 gestational days)
- amelia of the legs: 41st–45th days pm (27–31 gestational days)
- phocomelia of the legs: 42nd–47th days pm (28–33 gestational days)
- ectromelia of the legs: 45th–47th days pm (31–33 gestational days)
- triphalangism of thumbs: 46th–50th days pm (32–36 gestational days)

Nowack[23] comments that their data agree with those reported by investigators of 30 other cases.

The gestational day has been substituted for post-menstrual day in a diagram of the thalidomide-sensitive period based on the observations by Nowack, Knapp and Lenz and published in Saxén and Rapola's textbook on congenital malformations[24] (Figure 2.3).

Figure 2.3 *Thalidomide-sensitive periods. (From Saxēn L, Rapola J.* Congenital Defects. *New York: Holt, Rinehart and Winston, 1969: 202.*[24]*)*

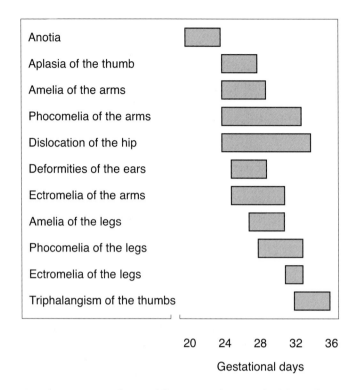

Anotia

Aplasia of the thumb

Amelia of the arms

Phocomelia of the arms

Dislocation of the hip

Deformities of the ears

Ectromelia of the arms

Amelia of the legs

Phocomelia of the legs

Ectromelia of the legs

Triphalangism of the thumbs

20   24   28   32   36

Gestational days

Sequence of malformations following exposure in the sensitive period

In the few infants referred to him by 1963 in which thalidomide had been taken in the sensitive period without obvious ill-effect, Lenz discovered minor anomalies on physical examination:

> 'I have been accused of wanting to deny the existence of cases of thalidomide intake during the sensitive stage without harm to the embryo. Nothing is further from my intentions. On the contrary, I would very much like to become acquainted with such cases. So far as I know, there is no well documented case where a woman has taken thalidomide during the sensitive phase without damage to the embryo.'[22]

As his clinical experience of these cases grew with referrals in the aftermath of his statements in the medical press, Lenz became even stronger on this point.[25] By 1965, he had collected 869 cases. In 1966, he stated that the risk of a malformation if thalidomide had been taken between 35 and 50 days after menstruation (21–36 gestational days) was probably higher than 50%. Even a risk of 100% had not been strictly excluded, and estimates lower than 50% were, he believed, due to inaccuracies in the time data, or to erroneously equating early pregnancy and the sensitive period. The epidemic subsided in parallel with the collapse of the drug's sales figures (Figure 2.4).

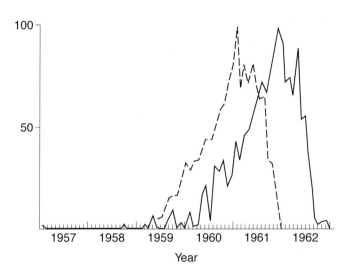

Figure 2.4 *Record of epidemic compared with sales figures. The dashed line shows thalidomide sales, with January 1961 as 100 on the scale. The solid line shows 845 deformed births, with October 1961 as 100 on the scale. (From Sjöström H, Nilsson R. Thalidomide and the Power of the Drug Companies. Harmondsworth: Penguin, 1972: 156.[19])*

Observations on twins demonstrated the possible time differences in the development of two individual embryos, for discordance of affected twin pairs was not uncommon. Lenz and colleagues stated that if, as exceptionally occurs, only one twin is affected, its malformations are of a type attributable to thalidomide action at the very beginning or the very end of the sensitive period.[26] If organ development in the other twin were a few days retarded or accelerated in comparison with the affected twin, malformations would not be expected, because it would not have been exposed to thalidomide in the sensitive period of organ development, which is sharply limited.

Lenz became convinced that the *morphological type of the malformation was essentially a function of the time of intake*, with the proviso that variations in rate of maturation of individual embryos allowed for fluctuations within this timetable. His experience was greater than that of anyone else in the world, and his scientific integrity, sorely tested in the witness box at Aachen, never faltered. The court case in Aachen was the attempt to claim compensation for the children from the drug company. It was the first time in industrial/compensation law that litigation against a product was based on exposure before birth. The plaintiffs were successful after a protracted hearing of 9 years.[19]

Lenz's careful and lucid science was crucial to the case. The mapping of the thalidomide-sensitive period by Nowack and Lenz has been totally accepted by scientists and clinicians in this field, and remains the gold standard to this day.

Impact of thalidomide upon the pharmaceutical industry

One major outcome of the thalidomide catastrophe has been the institution of improved procedures for screening of new drugs. In

1974, US Food and Drug Administration (FDA) issued guidelines on good laboratory practice in order to standardize drug-testing procedures for safety in pregnancy.[27] These require teratological screening of new drugs in at least two animal species, with any equivocal results being checked in a third animal, preferably a non-human primate. Thus the pre-marketing requirements have been made more thorough, safer and also more costly to conduct, as a direct result of thalidomide.[27]

References

1. Ministry of Health Reports on Public Health and Medical Subjects No. 112. *Deformities Caused by Thalidomide*. London: HMSO, 1964.

2. Lenz W. A short history of thalidomide embryopathy. *Teratology* 1988; **38**: 203–215.

3. Kunz W, Keller H, Mückter H. *Arzneimittelforschung* 1956; **6**: 426–30.

4. Williams RT. Thalidomide. *Arch Environ Health* 1968; **16**: 493–502.

5. Jung H. Klinische Erfahrungen mit einen neuen Sedativen. *Arzneimittelforschung* 1956; **6**: 430–2.

6. Lenz W. Malformations caused by drugs in pregnancy. *Am J Dis Child* 1966; **112**: 99–106.

7. Schumacher HJ, Smith RL, Williams RT. The metabolism of thalidomide: the spontaneous hydrolysis of thalidomide in solution. *Br J Pharmacol* 1965; **25**: 324–337.

8. Williams RT, Schumacher H, Fabro S, Smith RL. The chemistry and metabolism of thalidomide. In: Robson JM, Sullivan F, Smith RL, eds. *A Symposium on Embryonic Activity of Drugs*. London: Churchill, 1965: 167–93.

9. Keberle H, Faigle JW, Fritz H et al. Theories on the mechanism of action of thalidomide. In: Robson JM, Sullivan F, Smith RL, eds. *A Symposium on Embryopathic Activity of Drugs*. London: Churchill, 1965: 210–33.

10. Jonsson BG. Teratological studies on thalidomide in rabbits. *Acta Pharmacol (Kbh)* 1972; **31**: 17–23.

11. Fabro S, Schumacher H, Smith RL, Williams RT. The chemistry and metabolism of thalidomide. In: Robson JM, Sullivan F, Smith RL, eds. *A Symposium on Embryopathic Activity of Drugs*. London: Churchill, 1965: 167–93.

12. Krakow JS. Ribonucleic acid polymerase of *Azotobacter vinelandii* III. Effect of polyamines. *Biochim Biophys Acta* 1963; **72**: 566–71.

13. Schumacher H, Blake DA, Gurian JM, Gillette JR. A comparison of teratogenic activity of thalidomide in rabbits and rats. *J Pharmacol Exp Ther* 1968; **160**: 189–200.

14. Lenz W. Kindliche Missbildungen nach Medikament-Einnahme während der Gravidität. Fragen aus der Praxis. *Dtsch Med Wsch* 1961; **86**: 2555.

15. Lenz W. Bone defects of the limbs – an overview. *Birth Defects: Original Article Series V* 1969; **3**: 14–17.

16. Pleiss G. Thalidomide and congenital abnormalities. *Lancet* 1962; **i**: 1128–9.

17. Burley DM. Thalidomide and congenital abnormalities. *Lancet* 1962; **i**: 271.

18. Lenz W. Thalidomide and congenital abnormalities. *Lancet* 1962; **i**: 271–2.

19. Sjöström H, Nilsson R. *Thalidomide and the Power of the Drug Companies.* Harmondsworth: Penguin, 1972.

20. Lenz W, Knapp K. Die Thalidomid Embryopathie. *Dtsch Med Wochenschr* 1962; **87**: 1232.

21. Knapp K, Lenz W, Nowack E. Multiple congenital abnormalities. *Lancet* 1963; **ii**: 725.

22. Lenz W. Das Thalidomid-Syndrom. *Fortschr Med* 1963; **81**: 148–55.

23. Nowack E. Die sensible Phase bei der Thalidomid-Embryopathy. *Humangenetik* 1965; **1**: 516–36.

24. Saxén L, Rapola J. *Congenital Defects.* New York: Holt, Rinehart and Winston, 1969: 202.

25. Lenz W. Epidemiology of congenital malformations. *Ann NY Acad Sci* 1965; **123**: 228–36.

26. Jörgensen G, Lenz W, Pfeiffer RA, Schaafhausen C. Thalidomide embryopathy in twins. *Acta Genet Med Gemellol* 1970; **19**: 203–10.

27. Kelsey FO. Thalidomide update: regulatory aspects. *Teratology* 1988; **38**: 221–6.

CHAPTER 3

Animal studies

The first problem was to see whether or not thalidomide induced the same deformities in animals. If so, could an animal model be established on which to explore other aspects of the drug's action, such as its teratogenic mechanism?

Experimental models

The manufacturers of thalidomide had tested the drug in pregnant rats, and no visible congenital defects were reported. Until 1961, it was standard practice to use the rat for tests of safety in pregnancy. That a tested and apparently harmless drug could cause fetal malformations on a large scale in the human population was soon established beyond question. This property of the drug had not been picked up in the laboratory – a fact that destroyed confidence in the previous system of safety testing. Was this damage peculiar to the human embryo? Was the rat embryo able to resist the drug's action? If so, was the rat an acceptable experimental model for use in routine teratology in the future? What other animal model could be substituted, in order to ensure the safety of human beings exposed to new chemicals? Above all, was it possible to avoid another thalidomide disaster?

Scientists, pharmaceutical manufacturers, drug regulatory authorities and the general public needed answers to these urgent questions. Between 1962 and 1972, many research papers were published, in which the effect of thalidomide on the embryos of many animal species was reported.[1–22] These early investigations sought to establish whether or not thalidomide induced malformations in various laboratory animals, and at what dosage and stage of embryonic development such defects occurred. These animal studies were summarized by Cahen in 1966.[2] Most of them did not search for 'the thalidomide lesion', the point (or tissue) within the embryo at which thalidomide acted.

Chapter Summary
- **Experimental models**
- **The search for the target tissue or cells in animals**
- **Principles of chemotoxicity**
- **Thalidomide in rabbits**
- **Thalidomide in rats**
- **Thalidomide in chicks**
- **Conflict and confusion in animal research**
- **References**

Rats

First, the effect on the rat embryo was checked using different breeds of rat and various dosage regimes. Seven laboratories confirmed absence of birth defects.[2] But in 1962, two groups recorded malformations of limbs and tail of rats, and later of the spine. The rat embryo appeared to be less subject to damage than the human, and the reason for such 'species specificity' was debated. Was it some differential permeability of placental tissues? Or was it due to species variations in the handling of the drug, such as different processes of absorption and breakdown? Somers[1] of the Distillers Company laboratories argued that the rat embryo might be more sensitive than that of humans and other species and that the drug therefore killed the rat embryo, which was then resorbed. The human and rabbit fetuses, being more resistant, might survive the assault, to be born deformed.[23] Biochemical reasons for 'species specificity' were proposed in turn by Keberle et al[24] and Schumacher et al,[25] but no firm conclusion was reached. It was generally agreed that the manufacturers were unfortunate to have produced a compound that indeed appeared to be safe in pregnancy according to standard animal tests at the time but that in retrospect demonstrated the inadequacy of these tests. In the quest for a better model than the rat, a number of laboratories undertook experiments with other animals.

Rabbits

The first laboratory animal to be deformed by thalidomide was the New Zealand White rabbit. Somers[1] published in *The Lancet* in April 1962 the first animal deformed by thalidomide. His photographs and radiographs of rabbit fetuses showed foreshortening of radius, ulna and tibio-fibula. These defects were radiologically similar to those described in humans. By the end of 1962, Somers' results in the rabbit had been confirmed.[5,7,16,17] Numerous different breeds of rabbit were tested in laboratories worldwide, and all responded to thalidomide with the typical embryopathy: positive results were not confined to New Zealand Whites.[2] The rabbit model had the practical appeal of being cheap, widely available and prolific, with a short period of gestation (32 days). The average dose necessary was 150 mg/kg body weight. The sensitive period in the rabbit was approximately 7–10 days post conception, and could be precisely defined for particular experimental purposes as 192–250 hours' gestation.[4]

The human embryopathy was exactly replicated in the rabbit model. In addition to reductions in long bones and absence or duplication of digits, there were defects of orofacial structures and of the cardiac, pulmonary, urinary and digestive systems of the types seen in human infants. The number, type and particulars of deformities differed from fetus to fetus within a litter, and between litters. Some fetuses escaped injury in spite of an exposure that deformed their own littermates. This range of effects was attributed to natural variations in time of implantation and to individual differences in rates of fetal and placental development.

High resorption (embryonic death) rates were universal, which confirmed the embryolethal effect of the drug – a typical feature of any teratogen. Teratogens cause embryos to abort or resorb if affected very early, to survive with deformities if affected a little later, and to survive physically unscathed if the drug is given after the sensitive period has elapsed.

Mice

In the 2 years after the thalidomide disaster, 11 laboratories published studies of thalidomide-exposed pregnant mice.[2] Seven reported no deformities, which meant that mice, like rats, were not reliable indicators of the human reaction. Three papers described club-foot or limb-reduction defects. Others found clefts of midline structures, and head and neck deformities that fitted the thalidomide syndrome.

Chicks

The chick embryo is the classical model used in normal embryology, since it has no placenta, and can be directly observed and manipulated. Seven chick embryological laboratories around the world took up the challenge of thalidomide in 1962–63.[2] All but one reported deformities of various organs, and three reports included limb defects. A major impediment to further investigation in the chick embryo has been the relative insolubility of the drug, and the knowledge that the physical presence of inert particles will provoke defects in chick embryos.[26] This difficulty dissuaded some scientists from the use of the chick model, in spite of its attractions as a cheap and simple screening system.

Cats and dogs

Cats and dogs treated with thalidomide in pregnancy have had offspring with cranial and vertebral defects.[2,12]

Primates

Non-human primates have replicated most closely the human embryopathy. Lucey and Behrman[13] observed fetal resorption in all thalidomide-treated *Macacca irus* monkeys in their series, confirming the drug's embryolethal activity. Delahunt and Lassen[27] gave smaller doses a little later in pregnancy to 14 cynomolgus (*Macacca fascicularis*) monkeys, and produced amelia, phocomelia and facial haemangiomas. Hendrickx, Axelrod and Clayborn[9] gave 5 mg/kg to

10 pregnant baboons at various stages of pregnancy. Four, treated from the time of conception to day 30, resorbed the embryos. Of four treated between 18 and 30 days' gestation, two resorbed, and two gave birth to young with severe dysmelic deformities. One animal treated from days 22 to 30 produced an oedematous fetus with a single umbilical artery. One baboon treated at day 30 produced a normal fetus. This demonstrated a chronological gradient of severity, induced by amounts approximating the human dose (which is from 1 mg/kg) in a species whose reproductive physiology closely resembles that of the human. Wilson and Gavan[21] examined rhesus (*Macaca mulatta*) monkeys, and established the sensitive period to be about 25–30 days. They suggested that there may be a dose–response relationship in primates, and showed a cephalocaudal gradient within the sensitive period. Barrow, Steffek and King[28] produced limb and visceral defects in two rhesus monkeys and made the interesting and important observation that 'to produce the full phocomelic syndrome, thalidomide must be administered *either immediately before or during the appearance of the limb buds*'.

In the UK, Poswillo, Hamilton and Sopher[29] advocated the marmoset monkey as an ideal animal model for teratological research. Teratologists in the USA also advocated primates because of their similarity to humans in terms of reproductive physiology and drug response. But primate breeding colonies are costly and more elaborate in their maintenance requirements than rabbits, chicks and other common animals. The optimum animal model for teratological testing is a matter of opinion, as discussed at the European Teratology Society in 1984. National trends were evident. American teratologists advocated primates, despite their scarcity and high cost. Scientists of other nations favoured animals that were more cheaply and readily available. For example, Danes preferred pigs and Australians preferred rabbits. The French would continue to use the chick model, in which so much basic embryology had already been established. It was resolved at a workshop there that the choice of experimental animal would rest with individual research groups. In the final analysis, all results of tests on all laboratory animals deserve careful and critical attention.

The search for the target tissue or cells in animals

Having reproduced thalidomide malformations in several animal models, scientists turned to the more difficult question of establishing thalidomide's site of action.

It is hard to know where to begin a search for the site of chemical action within a process as remarkably complex as embryogenesis. The processes of cell proliferation, migration, differentiation and organogenesis comprise a rapid, precisely programmed sequence that repeats itself to the last detail in every zygote of the species.[30] Little is known of the essential mechanisms that govern these events, yet there must be specific ways of interfering with the normal mechanisms, at certain times, to result in reproducible complexes of malformations such as those caused by thalidomide. Each step in embryogenesis probably depends upon a previous one, and even a temporary delay in the development of one group of cells may throw it out of phase with the rest of the embryo and thus lead to an eventual malformation.[30] There is immense difficulty in knowing where to look for the primary lesion when so much of the normal process of embryogenesis is not understood.

Principles of chemotoxicity

Additional difficulties arise when pursuing the action of chemical poisons.[31] The following are three general principles of chemotoxicity:

- The toxic chemical injury to a cell is invisible.
- Different cells and tissues have different vulnerability or resistance to chemical attack.
- Biochemical interference precedes morphological change in tissues or organs.

The impact of these principles is as follows.

Toxic chemical injury to a cell is invisible

A toxic substance may injure a cell by a subtle and invisible action, for example by acting upon a particular metabolic pathway, enzyme or gene, so that one reaction is blocked, accelerated or delayed. Such a disturbance may cripple or destroy the cell, tissue or organ, and even perhaps destroy the organism itself. Many toxic chemicals have profound effects that become visible later at a gross level, yet the precise metabolic targets are unknown.[31,32]

Four intracellular systems are particularly vulnerable:

- aerobic respiration
- maintenance of the integrity of cell membranes
- synthesis of enzymes and structural proteins
- preservation of the integrity of the genetic apparatus

Biochemical injuries are *invisible* at the time of the insult and for a period thereafter, but the damage is nevertheless profound, with far-reaching consequences. Different agents may insult the same biochemical pathway. Disruptions to different sites on different occasions may finally overcome the capacity of the cell to adapt and heal, with cell death as a result.[32]

It follows that the chemical injury inflicted by thalidomide may not be visible or identifiable.

Sensitivity and vulnerability of cells, tissues and organs is variable

Some chemicals have a high degree of affinity for certain organs, cells or activities. For example, carbon tetrachloride and dichloromethane target the liver, botulinum toxin targets nerve terminals in muscle, heavy metals are attracted to nerves, while nitrogen mustards damage mitotic spindles and thus injure any rapidly dividing cells.[31,32]

In addition, some cells are inherently more sensitive than others to adverse environmental changes. Neurons are the most sensitive of all cells to fluctuations in the environment, and suffer irreversible damage after 3–5 minutes of oxygen deprivation, whereas nephrons survive for 20 minutes and epithelial cells for 30 minutes. Myocardium, hepatocytes and renal tubular epithelium survive for up to 2 hours, while fibroblasts, epidermis and skeletal muscle survive hypoxia and other adverse environmental changes for many hours.

Biochemical injury precedes morphological changes

It is also a fundamental concept of pathology that biochemical interference precedes morphological changes. Cell injury only becomes apparent microscopically many hours after some critical biochemical system within the cell has been deranged.

Most experimental work in the period immediately after the thalidomide disaster aimed to establish a safe and reliable animal model for tests of chemical teratogenicity in place of the rat. The endpoint of most teratological studies with thalidomide in those days was to record whether or not it caused malformations in the animal in question under the conditions of exposure particular to that experiment.

The amount of detail provided about the deformities was variable in early publications, usually being limited to brief descriptions of gross external dysmorphology. Histopathology was not explored.

A more profound interpretation of animal experiments is handicapped when no member of the team has a background knowledge of pathology – veterinary or medical. The correct interpretation of histopathology is crucial to discovering 'the thalidomide lesion'. Hughes[33] deplored the trend of teratologists prior to the 1970s to investigate animals in vacuo, without integration with other fields of expertise.

Bearing in mind the known metabolic complexities, the differential sensitivities of organ systems, and the many unknown mechanisms of normal embryology, it is not surprising that the primary lesion of thalidomide embryopathy has eluded investigators. Our understanding of mechanisms of action in this field is pitifully deficient. We do not know precisely how any teratogen acts, nor whether chemical teratogens play any significant role in 'spontaneous' human malformations.[30]

Against this background, some progress was made in the search for the timing of cell damage in thalidomide-damaged animals. Rabbits, chicks and monkeys prevailed as models, and the following useful facts were established.

Thalidomide in rabbits

Fabro and Smith's study

Fabro and Smith[4] examined the resorption sites in their series of rabbits, and concluded that the thalidomide lesion was not immediately lethal to the conceptus, but that death occurred *at a later stage*, when, as a result of the initial damage, *further organized development became impossible*.

In liveborn malformed fetuses, the defects induced by thalidomide were not incompatible with survival, but the disturbances in development of particular organs presented as congenital malformations at birth. The rabbit proved to be a good model for thalidomide embryopathy in the series of Fabro and Smith.

Vickers' study

Vickers,[19,20] an Australian pathologist, recognized the importance of using the rabbit to find the thalidomide lesion:

> 'The remarkable similarity between human and rabbit thalidomide dysmelia would be reason enough to consider the morphogenesis of each, even if direct observations in man were possible. That they are not, increases the need for commentary.'

Vickers examined paws of 244 thalidomide-treated rabbit embryos of 10–25 days' gestation, 118 of which had discernible defects.

Positive findings

Reduction defects of rabbit limbs are first recognizable on the 13th day of gestation. Figure 3.1 demonstrates one of the major problems in the search for the thalidomide lesion. *The short period during which the rabbit embryo is sensitive to thalidomide* and in which the thalidomide lesion occurs is 7–11 days' gestation, which *predates the formation of limb buds*. Deformity of limb buds cannot be discerned until day 13. Bearing in mind that some fetuses in the litter will *not* be deformed, it is not possible to identify the deformed ones until at least 2 days after exposure ends, i.e. until some days after the thalidomide lesion has occurred. For this reason, Vickers examined a series of embryos of 10–25 days' gestation in order to encompass all these stages, including the end of the sensitive period. Within those aged 10–13 days, some treated embryos would be destined to be normal and others to be deformed.

Figure 3.1 Sequence of development of the neural crest and upper and lower limbs in the rabbit embryo. The shaded area represents the thalidomide-sensitive period. The arrows at 260 and 290 hours' gestation indicate the ages of embryos to be examined in Chapter 15. (Courtesy of Dr John Cameron PhD.)

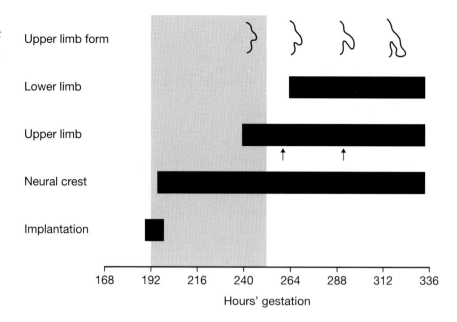

Vickers found that the earliest sign of a future limb-reduction defect was *failure of proliferation and condensation of limb-bud mesenchyme to form digital rays*. The failure of these processes could be transient or complete.

Subsequently, differentiation in deformed bone may be retarded, or may proceed to completion.

A *circumscribed proliferation of mesenchyme* in the preaxial edge of developing hindpaws is the *forerunner of accessory digit formation* (polydactyly).

Important negative findings

- There was *no evidence* in early preparations that defective rays were due to *necrosis or degeneration* in the mesenchyme before, during or after its condensation.
- *No vascular lesion* could be detected in thalidomide-exposed paws before the defect appeared.
- No dead or dying cells were seen to identify a site of damage.

In summary

The thalidomide lesion remained invisible.

Nudelman and Travill's study

Nudelman and Travill[14] examined upper limbs of 21-day-old thalidomide-treated rabbit embryos macroscopically, microscopically and histochemically. The most severely affected limbs contained *atrophic chondrocytes*, undifferentiated mesenchyme, and *absence of primordial centres for the long bones*. There was no detectable difference in the amount or the distribution of acid mucopolysaccharides between abnormal and control limbs. However, calcium deposition in the cartilaginous matrices was reduced or absent in the abnormal limbs. In limbs with reduction of bony tissue, *there was no evidence of histochemical aberration in the deposited bone.*

In other words, *what bone was present was histochemically normal.* Nudelman and Travill[14] found:

'that thalidomide affected mesenchymal derivatives at various stages of development; that it was associated directly or indirectly with the utilisation of glycogen and the production of alkaline phosphatase; and that its influence was expressed by aberrations in the chondrification and calcification processes during later foetal development.'

Thalidomide in rats

Globus and Gibson's study

Globus and Gibson[34] reported a histological and histochemical study of the development of the sternum in thalidomide-treated rats. Thalidomide induced either abnormal fusion of sternum and ribs or failure of fusion between the primordial parts of the sternum (cleft sternum). There was delay in onset of chondrification and inhibition of glycogen utilization within the chondrocytes at the sites of cartilage hypertrophy, and an atypical, reduced pattern of alkaline phosphatase activity in the zones of endochondral bone formation. Periosteal bone formation was normal. They concluded that there was not only a *delay in the onset of development of parts of the sternum, but a continuing retardation of the rate of development of early chondrification.* The abnormalities reflected maldevelopment of the *cartilage model* rather than any upset in the mechanism of ossification. They suggested that thalidomide or one of its metabolites influences glycolysis.

Thalidomide in chicks

Salzgeber and Salaun's study

Salzgeber and Salaun[26] tested various preparations of thalidomide in chick embryo and produced typical limb malformations in approximately 20% of exposed chicks.

Salzgeber[35] had previously examined the effect of nitrogen mustard upon chick limb buds. This compound produced phocomelia in over 90% of treated chick embryos. Histopathologically, rapidly dividing mesenchymal cells in limb buds were shown to be destroyed by nitrogen mustard. Disordered mitotic figures were abundant. This evidence of destruction of rapidly dividing cells in the embryo parallels the antimitotic action of nitrogen mustards in cancer therapy, where rapidly dividing malignant cells are the target of the drug. In a series of elegant experiments, Salzgeber proved that nitrogen mustard affected mesenchyme, but did not affect apical ectoderm. This was important evidence that the role of the apical ectodermal ridge was less vital than had been assumed.

Her meticulous experiments with thalidomide were expected to reveal an effect similar to that of nitrogen mustard. But *no histological damage to mesenchymal cells* was found in limb buds of thalidomide-exposed chicks, and there were *no abnormal mitotic figures* (Salzgeber B, personal communication,1976). Thus the thalidomide lesion (whatever it is) differs from the nitrogen mustard lesion, although both drugs induce malformations. All of Salzgeber's experiments were clearly designed and meticulously recorded, with large numbers in each series.

Jurand's study

Jurand[11] designed a complicated experiment in chick embryos. He injected albumen suspensions of thalidomide plus antibiotics into the egg white or yolk of fowl eggs of 60–64 hours' incubation, and albumen-suspended calcium carbonate plus antibiotics into controls. After a further 24 hours of incubation, surviving embryos were processed and examined by light and electron microscopy. Jurand described dilation of the axial artery of the thalidomide-exposed limb buds, with or without necrotic changes in the surrounding mesoblast, and intracellular changes in the endothelial lining of the artery on electron microscopy. He suggested that the primary cause of thalidomide abnormalities (i.e. the thalidomide lesion) is an injury of the endothelial lining of the axial limb artery. While this suggestion is plausible, and indeed has been accepted by some scientists, there are serious weaknesses in this paper.

There is no mention anywhere in the paper of the number of chick embryos tested. The materials and methods describe four different experimental treatment groups and only one control group. No table of results is presented whereby the reader can see the total numbers of embryos in each group, the numbers examined histologically, and the proportions of each group that displayed the histological changes described. The results may be based on very few chicks, judging from the data provided. The histological abnormalities after thalidomide treatment (which of the four treatments?) are compared with histology of a normal chick wing bud. Normal – correctly defined in the results section – is an untreated chick of 64–68 hours' incubation. But 'normal' is not the same as 'control'. The control group had been subjected to injection of albumen and calcium carbonate and anti-biotics. The light-microscopic findings in the controls are not mentioned. Therefore the reader is unable to ascertain the effect of the albumen and calcium carbonate and antibiotics, i.e. the vehicle. This is the baseline against which the effect of albumen and thalidomide and antibiotics is to be measured, according to the statement in the 'Materials and methods' section of the paper, and therefore it is surprising that no tabulated results are presented. One could also debate the adequacy of the single control group. A correctly designed experiment would require seven control groups to provide scientific baselines for all manipulations.

In the absence of these experimental details, Jurand's results cannot be accepted without serious reservations. Experimental teratology is difficult enough because of the many variables involved. It should be obligatory for authors to provide a clear table of results related to the experimental plan, with the numbers in each box for comparison. Journals should reject papers that omit this basic information.

Conflict and confusion in animal research

In addressing the question of what cells or tissues are injured by thalidomide, the reader is presented with conflicting observations in the chick – on the one hand by Jurand, who found arterial abnormalities and necrosis in mesoblast, and on the other hand by Salzgeber, who did not. Vickers[19,20] in 1967 and Cameron[36] in 1979 both searched for vascular lesions and necrosis in early rabbit embryos exposed to thalidomide, and found none, in support of Salzgeber's findings in chicks. No vascular lesions were found by surgeons operating on limb defects of thalidomide children (Willert H-G, personal communication) or by scientists who examined non-human primates.[37] In spite of this, some people have chosen to accept Jurand's conclusions without criticism, and to further elaborate on the uncertain possibility of a vascular target for thalidomide.

Since publication in reputable scientific journals gives weight to experimental results, conflicting information presented in published papers creates a distressing predicament for those who seek answers to important medical and biological questions through animal experiments. In 1966, the year of publication of Jurand's paper,[11] Cahen[2] attempted to review the state of the art in teratology, and concluded, in despair:

> 'Despite the numerous investigations carried out during the last quarter of a century, the problem of the experimental investigation of the teratogenic potential of drugs is far from being resolved ... From the theoretical point of view, the general impression acquired from a reading of the innumerable publications on this topic is the total lack of cohesion. There is no pharmacological or chemical correlation among the various teratogenic drugs. For the same teratogenic drug there is no correlation of effect among different species or different strains of the same species, even when they are tested with the same

experimental procedure. There is often no correlation between the teratogenic effect observed in laboratory animals and in humans. This may perhaps account for the futility of the efforts of all who are attempting to produce experimental fetal malformations, to study the metabolism of teratogenic drugs and their mechanism of action, and especially to understand what happened in the case of thalidomide.'

A decade later, Hughes reviewed teratology research and concluded thus:[38]

'Any survey of the literature on the biological effects of physiologically active substances reveals an all too sharp distinction between the main bulk which deals with their pharmacology, molecular biology, and so forth, and the far smaller proportion concerned with their teratological properties. Only seldom is the teratological effect of an agent discussed against the background of its general biological actions ... The study of abnormal development is at present a morass of empirical observation, and is not helped by the artificial barriers of disciplinary organisation. One factor retarding progress in the understanding of malformations is the tendency towards the development of teratology in an insufficiently close relationship with other branches of cell biology.'

In a review article for *Developmental Medicine and Child Neurology* in 1975, Hughes[39] commented on the disconnection between malformations and the study of chemical teratogens:

'Some chemical teratogens affect reduplication of the genome, others inhibit enzyme systems, and some are believed to act on the cell membrane. While something is known of the initial mode of action of some agents, almost nothing is understood of the further steps which must lie between cellular injury and the maldevelopment of organs.'

In 1980, the eminent Berlin toxicologist and pharmacologist, Neubert, and colleagues, who, by then, had experimented with thalidomide in primates and other laboratory animals for nearly 20 years, stressed:[40,41]

'Our present inability to piece together from the toxicological and embryological data available a complete and detailed image of the mode of a teratogenic action.'

And, in 1994, Wolpert, a prominent British biologist, uttered a cri du coeur in in his paper entitled 'Do we understand development?'[42] He answers his own rhetorical question in the negative: If normal development is not understood, how can abnormal development be understood?

After four decades of animal experiments, the occult thalidomide lesion had been found, but had not been read, recognized or understood. Over 30 hypotheses of pathogenesis sat in the English literature,[43] not counting those in German and other languages.

As the 20th century ended, argument and confusion reigned in the literature.[37,44–52] Developmental biology had lost its way as far as thalidomide was concerned.

References

1. Somers GF. Thalidomide and congenital abnormalities. *Lancet* 1962; **i**: 912.

2. Cahen RL. Experimental and clinical chemoteratogenesis. *Adv Pharmacol* 1966; **4**: 263–349.

3. DiPaolo JA. Congenital malformation in strain A mice: its experimental production by thalidomide. *JAMA* 1963; **183**: 139–41.

4. Fabro S, Smith RL. The teratogenic activity of thalidomide in the rabbit. *J Pathol Bacteriol* 1966; **91**: 511–19.

5. Felisati S, Nodari R. Effets toxiques et tératogéniques de la thalidomide sur les foetus de lapin. *Schweiz Med Woch* 1963; **44**: 1559–62.

6. Fratta ID, Sigg EB, Maiorana K. Teratogenic effects of thalidomide in rabbits, rats, hamsters and mice. *Toxicol Appl Pharmacol* 1965; **7**: 268–86.

7. Giroud A, Tuchman-Duplessis H, Mercier-Parot L. Thalidomide effect on mice, rabbits and rats. *Lancet* 1962; **ii**: 298.

8. Hay MF. Effects of thalidomide on pregnancy in the rabbit. *J Reprod Fertil* 1964; **8**: 59–76.

9. Hendrickx AG, Axelrod LR, Clayborn LD. Thalidomide syndrome in baboons. *Nature* 1966; **210**: 958–9.

10. Jonsson BG. Teratological studies on thalidomide in rabbits. *Acta Pharmacol Toxicol* 1972; **31**: 17–23.

11. Jurand A. Early changes in limb buds of chick embryos after thalidomide treatment. *J Embryol Exp Morphol* 1966; **16**: 289–300.

12. Khera KS. Fetal cardiovascular and other defects induced by thalidomide in cats. *Teratology* 1975; **11**: 65–9.

13. Lucey JF, Behrman RE. Thalidomide: effect upon pregnancy in Rhesus monkey. *Science* 1963; **139**: 1295–6.

14. Nudelman KL, Travill AA. A morphological and histochemical study of thalidomide-induced upper limb malformations in rabbit fetuses. *Teratology* 1971; **4**: 409–25.

15. Robson JM. Testing drugs for teratogenicity and their effects on fertility. *Br Med Bull* 1970; **26**: 212–16.

16. Seller MJ. Thalidomide and congenital abnormalities. *Lancet* 1962; **ii**: 249.

17. Spencer KEV. Thalidomide and congenital abnormalities. *Lancet* 1962; **ii**: 100.

18. Tennyson V. Electron microscopic study of the developing neuroblasts of the dorsal root ganglion of the rabbit embryo. *J Comp Neurol* 1965; **124**: 267–318.

19. Vickers TH. The thalidomide embryopathy in hybrid rabbits. *Br J Exp Pathol* 1967; **48**: 107–17.

20. Vickers TH. Concerning the morphogenesis of thalidomide dysmelia in rabbits. *Br J Exp Pathol* 1967; **48**: 579–91.

21. Wilson JG, Gavan JA. The thalidomide syndrome of malformations produced in rhesus monkeys. *Anat Rec* 1967; **157**: 342.

22. Wilson JG, Gavan JA. Congenital malformations in non-human primates: spontaneous and experimentally induced. *Anat Rec* 1967; **158**: 99.

23. Williams RT, Schumacher H, Fabro S, Smith RL. The chemistry and metabolism of thalidomide. In: Robson JM, Sullivan F, Smith RL, eds. *A Symposium on Embryopathic Activity of Drugs*. London: Churchill, 1965: 186.

24. Keberle H, Faigle JW, Fritz H et al. Theories on the mechanism of action of thalidomide. In: Robson JM, Sullivan F, Smith RL, eds. *A Symposium on Embryopathic Activity of Drugs*. London: Churchill, 1965: 210–233.

25. Schumacher H, Blake DA, Gurian J, Gillette JR. A comparison of teratogenic activity of thalidomide in rabbits and rats. *J Pharmacol Exp Ther* 1968; **160**: 189–200.

26. Salzgeber B, Salaun J. Action of thalidomide on the chick embryo. *J Embryol Exp Morphol* 1965; **13**: 159–70.

27. Delahunt CS, Lassen LJ. Thalidomide syndrome in monkeys. *Science* 1964; **146**: 1300.

28. Barrow MV, Steffek AJ, King CT. Thalidomide syndrome in rhesus monkeys. *Folia Primatol Basel* 1969; **10**: 195–203.

29. Poswillo DE, Hamilton WJ, Sopher D. The marmoset as an animal model for teratological research. *Nature* 1972; **239**: 460.

30. Goldstein A, Aronow l, Kalman SM. *Principles of Drug Action*, 2nd edn. New York: Wiley, 1974.

31. Prasad K, Vernadakis A. *Mechanisms of Actions of Neurotoxic Substances*. New York: Raven Press, 1982.

32. Robbins SL, Kotran RS, Kumar V. *Pathologic Basis of Disease*, 3rd edn. Philadelphia: WB Saunders, 1984.

33. Hughes AFW. *The American Biologist Through Four Centuries*. Springfield, IL: CC Thomas, 1982.

34. Globus M, Gibson MA. A histological and histochemical study of the development of the sternum in thalidomide-treated rats. *Teratology* 1968; **1**: 235–56.

35. Salzgeber B. Production élective de la phocomélie sous l'influence d'ypérite azotée. *J Embryol Exp Morphol* 1963; **11**: 413–29.

36. Cameron J. A histological study of the effect of thalidomide on the developing peripheral nervous system of the rabbit. PhD thesis, University of Sydney, 1979.

37. Neubert R, Neubert D. Peculiarities and possible mode of action of

thalidomide. In: Kavlock RJ, Daston GP, eds. *Drug Toxicity in Embryonic Development*. Berlin: Springer-Verlag, 1996: 41–119.

38. Hughes AF. Developmental biology and the study of malformations. *Biol Rev Camb Philos Soc* 1976; **51**: 143–79.

39. Hughes A. Teratogenesis and the movement of ions. *Dev Med Child Neurol* 1975; **17**: 111–14.

40. Neubert D. Teratogenicity: Any relationship to carcinogenicity? *IARC Sci Publ* 1980; **27**: 169–78.

41. Barrack HJ, Merker HJ, Neubert D. Drug induced damage to the embryo of fetus (molecular and multilateral approach to prenatal toxicology). *Curr Top Pathol* 1980; **69**: 241–331.

42. Wolpert L. Do we understand development? *Science* 1994: **266**: 571–2.

43. Hill B. Characterization of embryopathy risks. In: *Thalidomide: Potential Benefits and Risks: Open Public Scientific Workshop*. NIH, Bethesda, MD, 9 September 1997. Available at http://www.fda.gov/oashi/patrep/nih99.html#hill.

44. McBride WG. Thalidomide may be a mutagen. *BMJ* 1994; **308**: 1635–6.

45. Smithells RW. Thalidomide may be a mutagen. *BMJ* 1994; **309**: 477.

46. Kida M. Thalidomide may not be a mutagen. *BMJ* 1994, **309**: 741.

47. Tabin CJ. A developmental model for thalidomide defects. *Nature* 1998; **396**: 322–3.

48. Neubert R, Merker HJ, Neubert D. A developmental model for thalidomide defects. *Nature* 1999; **400**: 419–20.

49. D'Amato RJ, Loughnan MS, Flynn E, Folkman J. Thalidomide is an inhibitor of angiogenesis. *Proc Natl Acad Sci USA* 1994; **91**: 4082–5.

50. McCredie J. Segmental embryonic peripheral neuropathy. *Pediatr Radiol* 1975; **3**: 162–8.

51. Strecker TR, Stephens TD. Peripheral nerves do not play a trophic role in limb skeletal morphogenesis. *Teratology* 1983; **27**: 159–67.

52. McCredie J. Skeletal morphogenesis is controlled by the neural crest: an overview of medical and scientific principles which govern skeletal morphogenesis and malformation. *Osteologie* 1997; **6**: 59–69.

CHAPTER 4

Thalidomide polyneuropathy

The first thalidomide epidemic: sensory peripheral neuropathy

Thalidomide had one important and serious action other than teratogenicity. It caused serious sensory nerve damage in adults who used it as a sedative. I purposely avoid the term 'side-effect' with which this action is often labelled. There is a strong case for sensory nerve damage being considered its primary action, not a side-effect.

Thalidomide was introduced into Germany in 1956 as a non-addictive sedative with no lethal dose – unique and very attractive features for any sedative in the era of barbiturates and narcotics. Known as Contergan, it captured a rapidly expanding share (40%) of the West German sedative market,[1] especially in hospitals and institutions for the aged and infirm. Before very long, painful paraesthesia and numbness in hands and feet began to be reported by people who had used the new sedative[1,2]. German neurologists quickly identified Contergan as the common exposure factor in these case histories, named the condition 'Contergan neuritis', and took steps to limit the availability of the drug.[1,2] After 4 years of denial by the manufacturers and a groundswell of reports from neurologists all over Germany, in August 1961, thalidomide was transferred from over-the-counter sales to sale on medical prescription only.[3–6]

Case reports of this serious neurological damage were gathering in the English medical literature.[7–10] Häfstrom[11] reviewed the subject of polyneuropathy after thalidomide and published clinical summaries of 73 Swedish cases. In all accounts, the clinical description was similar. The dose was from 1 mg/kg body weight. After taking 50–200 mg daily for 1 month or more, patients complained of paraesthesia and numbness in the feet or hands, gradually spreading up the limbs. There was frequently pain, hypersensitivity, muscular spasm and a feeling of weakness. In some patients, reflexes such as the ankle jerks were

Chapter Summary
- The first thalidomide epidemic: sensory peripheral neuropathy
- Neuroanatomy
- Sensory neuroanatomy
- Clinical neurology
- Neuropathology
- Toxic neuropathies
- Thalidomide polyneuropathy in animals
- Thalidomide polyneuropathy in humans
- Thalidomide neuropathy disappears
- Thalidomide returns – without the neuropathy
- The second epidemic of sensory peripheral neuropathy
- A clinical balancing act
- References

depressed; in others, reflexes were increased. Most series reported only sensory symptoms, without any motor problems. In all cases, the neurological examination showed sensory disturbances. The longer the patient had been taking the medication, the more widespread were the disturbances. There was evidence of variation in individual resistance to the effect of the preparation. Some cases were recorded where no polyneuropathy occurred, despite regular dosage.

Thus the characteristic features of Contergan neuritis were those of *sensory peripheral neuropathy*, with maximum effects upon the longest nerves to the hands and feet. There was minimal involvement of motor nerves, and little evidence of damage to the central nervous system.[8-14] The shooting pains of thalidomide neuropathy were of an intensity that could drive patients to suicide (O'Sullivan D, personal communication).

Häfstrom[11] reported that practically all his 73 cases continued to suffer persistent sensory disturbances 3–5 years after medication had ceased. Fourteen British cases were studied by Fullerton and Kremer[8] in 1961; these 14 plus 8 more cases were reviewed 6 years later by Fullerton and O'Sullivan.[14] Histological and electrophysiological studies showed that there was little or no remission of symptoms after withdrawal of the drug. This is unusual. Most toxic neuropathies caused by drugs or chemicals disappear in due course once the toxic factor has been removed. In the case of thalidomide neuropathy, however, the sensory neuronal damage was unchanged in 50% of cases 6 years later[14] – an indication of powerful sensory neurotoxicity. Some cases became rapidly worse after withdrawal of the drug.[11]

There have been very few animal studies of thalidomide neuropathy. In fact, the subject of sensory peripheral neuropathy is rarely found in non-medical literature – for obvious reasons. Disorders of sensation are invisible and subjective. Only humans can communicate to one another the subjective symptoms of disorders of sensation such as tingling, numbness and pain – the diagnostic features of sensory neuropathy. In laboratory animals, there is no verbal connection with the researcher, and such symptoms cannot be communicated. Therefore researchers whose knowledge and experience is confined to animal models sometimes find the concept of sensory peripheral neuropathy difficult to grasp.

Physical signs (objective evidence) of sensory neuropathy in humans always surface later than complaints (subjective symptoms). Sensory signs may be observed in animals, but they are infrequent, subtle and very late in the course of the condition, when chronic sensory deficit is complicated by disorders of balance and gait.

What follows is a brief summary of the neurological facts that enable a diagnosis of sensory peripheral neuropathy to be made. Readers who are already familiar with basic neurology should bypass the next two sections on neuroanatomy and neurology. But non-medical scientists are urged to read on, since the principles outlined here are essential to the comprehension of later chapters.

Neuroanatomy

According to Ranson's and Clark's *Anatomy of the Nervous System*:[15]

1. The neuron is the *genetic unit* of the nervous system – each neuron being derived from a single embryonic cell, the neuroblast.
2. The neuron is the *structural unit* of the nervous system, a nerve cell with all its processes. These cellular units remain anatomically separate; i.e. while they come into contact with each other at the synapses, there is no continuity of their substance.
3. The neurons are the *functional units* of the nervous system, with the conduction pathways being formed of chains of such units.
4. The neuron is also a *trophic unit*, as is seen (a) in the degeneration of a portion of an axon severed from its cell of origin, (b) in the phenomenon of chromatolysis or axon reaction, and (c) in the regeneration of the degenerated portion of the axon by an out-growth from that portion of the axon still in contact with its cell of origin.
5. Neurons are the only elements concerned in the conduction of nerve impulses. The nervous system is composed of untold numbers of such units linked together in conduction systems.

Sensory neuroanatomy

This section is summarized from Walton's *Essentials of Neurology*.[16]

The apparatus that conveys sensations from the periphery to the brain consists of a series of two or three nerve cells (neurons) forming a direct chain of communication.

1. The first sensory neuron lies outside the spinal cord, and transmits sensations from the skin or other sense organ to the second sensory neuron.
2. The second neuron lies within the spinal cord and conducts impulses via the spinal cord and brainstem to the thalamus or cortex of the brain.
3. A third set of nerve cells or internuncial neurons in the spinal cord are thought to modulate the sensory input.

Sensory impulses from the viscera are conveyed in a similar manner within the autonomic nervous system, and pass centrally along similar pathways.

The dorsal root ganglion cell

The most important and most vulnerable link in the chain is the first sensory neuron (Figure 4.1). Its cell body containing the nucleus is in the dorsal root ganglion adjacent to the spinal cord. This cell is known as the 'dorsal root ganglion cell'. It is bipolar, meaning that it

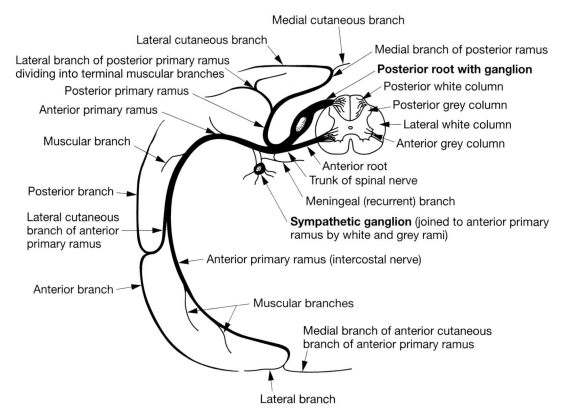

Figure 4.1 *Anatomy of a peripheral nerve segment, including motor and sensory components with link to autonomic ganglia.*

has two long axons or prolongations of cytoplasm. The shorter *central axon* passes medially into the spinal cord, where it synapses with the second cell of the chain. The much longer *peripheral axon* extends peripherally to the skin or other organ, where it connects with special sensory receptors or simply ramifies and ends as fine branches. The remarkable length of this peripheral axon makes the dorsal root ganglion cell one of the largest cells in the body in terms of volume of cytoplasm. It certainly has the most bizarre shape. A neuronal cell body in a dorsal root ganglion of the lumbar region has a finely drawn out filamentous axon of cytoplasm stretching from the waist to the tips of the toes, uninterrupted. The nucleus, the metabolic factory of the cell, is therefore far removed from the cell boundaries. Yet the nucleus is responsible for the nourishment and maintenance of the whole cell, and there is a continuous two-way flow of nutrients and metabolites within the axon itself. This is known as axoplasmic flow (Figure 4.2). This communication and transport system between the nucleus and the periphery is essential for the nerve's normal function and survival.

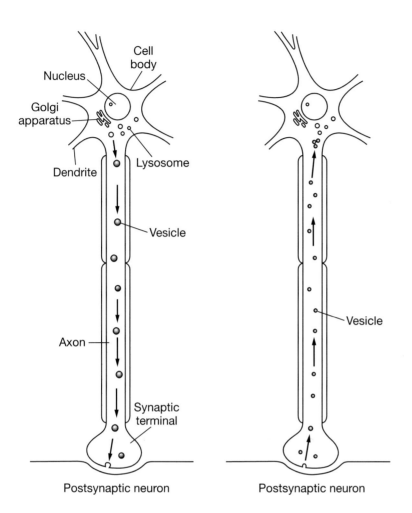

Nucleus

Cell body

Golgi apparatus

Dendrite

Lysosome

Vesicle

Axon

Synaptic terminal

Postsynaptic neuron

Vesicle

Postsynaptic neuron

Figure 4.2 *Directions of flow in the axoplasm. Slow transport of nutrients to the periphery, and of waste products from the periphery, is via cytoplasm. Fast transport of neurotransmitters is via neurotubules, a subcellular conveyor system housed within the cytoplasm.*

Functions of axons

The primary function of a peripheral sensory nerve is to conduct fast electric impulses from the periphery towards the brain, generally with messages about the environment.

The secondary function of the peripheral sensory nerve is to service its own cytoplasmic extensions – to supply nutrients and raw materials and to remove waste products via axoplasmic flow of chemicals. Axoplasmic flow is in two directions and is slower than electrical conduction. There are also two speeds of axoplasmic flow: slow for nutrients in the cytoplasm, and fast through fine neurotubules, which carry neurotransmitters to the periphery.

It is important to understand these separate functions of the axon and the different directions and speeds of each activity.

Form of axons

Sensory fibres (axons) in the peripheral nerves are of several different types. Some have an insulating sheath of myelin. Axons vary in diameter and in their rate of conduction. Large, heavily myelinated, rapidly conducting fibres convey touch, pressure and proprioception (sense of position in space), but some transmit pain and temperature. Small, unmyelinated, slowly conducting fibres also convey touch, but also temperature and pain sensation. There is no exact relationship between size or myelination and function. Nevertheless, some peripheral nerve disorders are characterized by selective effects upon fibres of a particular diameter or degree of myelination. Some diseases cause alterations in particular sensory modalities, for example loss of pain without loss of touch sensation.

Clinical neurology

Examination of the patient

Any patient with neurological symptoms must be analysed clinically in the first instance. A careful clinical history documents the onset, duration and severity of subjective symptoms. The history is combined with a physical examination in which objective signs are elicited. In diseases that cause disorders of sensation, the cooperation of the patient is essential in order to define the symptoms and signs precisely; in fact, in no neurological examination is the patient's cooperation more important.

Symptoms and signs resulting from diseased nerves are positive or negative – too much or too little sensation. Sensory nerves commonly have a biphasic response to injury, i.e. initial irritation with excess activity (positive) followed by subsequent loss of function (negative) if the trauma persists. Loss of function can be temporary or permanent. Minor stimuli induce irritation, while major stimuli induce rapid loss of function.

Positive symptoms are those produced by irritation or stimulation of a part of the nervous system, causing it to behave abnormally, such as focal epileptic fits caused by irritation of part of the motor cortex of the brain. In the sensory peripheral nervous system, irritation provokes a heightened perception of pain or touch, or hypersensitivity. Tingling of the skin, pain, hot and cold sensations, and exquisite sensitivity to sound or bright light, are positive symptoms.

Negative symptoms are those produced by temporary or permanent loss of function, so that an activity or ability, normally present, is lost. Paralysis of a limb is an example of loss of motor function due to disease involving motor neurons. In the sensory peripheral nervous system, loss, reduction or alteration of sensation is described by the patient as numbness, anaesthesia, tingling, loss of pain sensation with painless injuries, or spontaneous unpleasant sensations.

Positive and negative physical signs corresponding to these symptoms are elicited by testing the different modalities of sensation.

The doctor at this stage reviews the data gathered from the history and physical examination. They must decide first, the site, and second, the nature of the pathological changes responsible for the patient's disorder. (First, where is it? Then what is it?) This methodical approach is critical, for it is upon interpretation of the data that the diagnosis is made, and future management depends upon the diagnosis.

Localization of nerve lesions

In localizing the lesion responsible for an abnormality of sensation, it must be asked whether the sensory changes could be due to a lesion of one or more peripheral nerves, of the sensory roots, of the spinal cord, of the brainstem, of the thalamus or of the sensory cortex. A knowledge of the cutaneous (skin) distribution of the various peripheral nerve roots and trunks is essential for correct localization of peripheral nerve lesions (Figure 4.3).

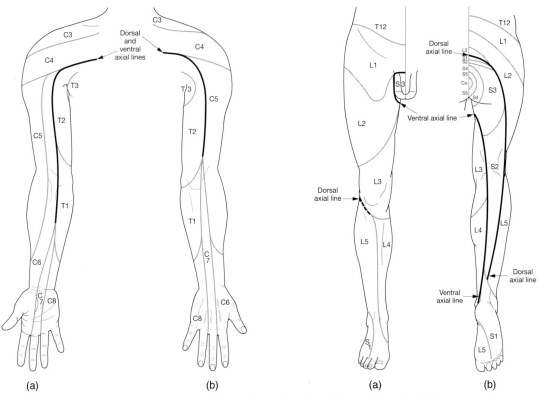

Figure 4.3 *Segmental dermatomes of arms and legs: (a) anterior surface; (b) posterior surface. Each segmental sensory nerve supplies a band of skin called a dermatome. The skin of the thorax and abdomen is encircled by consecutive dermatomes. In the limbs, the dermatomes are attenuated into longitudinal strips that are usually (but not always) consecutive.*

If a nerve is divided and it is one with an extensive cutaneous (skin) distribution, there is a central area of skin with sensory loss of all forms of sensation, and a surrounding zone in which tactile loss (touch) is more extensive than loss of pain and temperature sensation. There is considerable overlap in the cutaneous supply of individual peripheral nerves, so that division or injury of a small cutaneous nerve may produce no definable sensory abnormality. Adjacent branches of the damaged nerve take over the transmission of sensation.

Segments and dermatomes supplied by sensory nerves

Nerves are always loyal to the tissues they supply. A good illustration of this is the constant relationship between the segmental dermatomes innervated by the individual sensory roots. These dermatomes have a strictly segmental distribution (Figure 4.4).

If a single root is divided, it may be impossible to distinguish any area of sensory loss, because of the overlap of neighbouring segmental roots. When more than one root is interrupted, however, there is generally some cutaneous sensory loss, and its segmental distribution clearly indicates the roots involved.

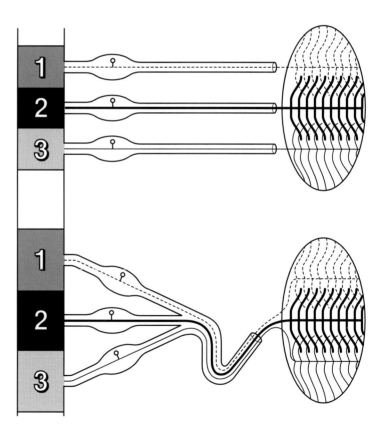

Figure 4.4 *Diagram of peripheral cutaneous nerve fields.*

Sir John Walton said:[16]

'A working knowledge of the dermatome distribution of the individual sensory roots is essential in clinical neurology. With this information it is relatively easy to distinguish on clinical grounds the sensory loss due to a root lesion from that due to a peripheral nerve lesion.'

Other patterns of sensory nerve injury

It is common (but not always the case) in peripheral neuropathy that multiple peripheral nerves are involved bilaterally and symmetrically. The longest sensory fibres are affected first and most severely. Thus symptoms and signs are most severe in the periphery of the limbs, where the nerves are longest.

Sensory impairment usually involves all forms of sensation, but sometimes affects one modality more than the others. The borderline between normal and abnormal areas of sensory perception is not usually abrupt, but there is a gradual transition between them due to overlap of innervation between affected and normal nerves (Figure 4.4).

Compression or irritation of peripheral nerves or nerve roots can cause intolerable and persistent pain. In the case of a lesion of a peripheral nerve, this pain is felt in the skin area from which the nerve receives its afferent sensory fibres. Similarly, root pain (arising from a lesion of the spinal sensory root) radiates throughout the dermatome of the root concerned. Deep muscular pain due to the same cause may be more widespread, corresponding broadly to the muscles supplied by the homologous motor root. Painful lesions of muscles or viscera sometimes cause pain in the overlying skin or even in a comparatively remote area of skin (referred pain). At first sight, these cutaneous areas are not anatomically related to the organ concerned. But the afferent pathways for visceral sensation, initially along afferent fibres accompanying autonomic (especially sympathetic) nerves, enter the posterior nerve roots and travel centrally with somatic afferents. The nerve supply of the heart and the arm converge in the cervical segments of the peripheral nervous system. Thus cardiac pain may be referred to the substernal region, to the left arm or to both arms.

After transection of the spinal cord, the negative symptoms of paraplegia (loss of motor function) and anaesthesia (loss of sensory function) are combined below the level of the injury. Just above the level of the damage, there is a narrow band, like a belt, of cutaneous hypersensitivity (a positive sensory symptom), indicating sensory irritation by the injury at that level. This neurological phenomenon of a band of irritation adjacent to a band of suppression will be important in later discussion (Chapter 27).

The long-term outcomes of a sensory nerve lesion are often more serious than those of a motor nerve lesion. This is especially so if pain fibres are involved. When a part of the body is rendered anaesthetic, an injury to its insensitive skin results in 'indolent' or 'perforating' ulcers of the skin. These persist without healing and penetrate into structures deep to the skin. They are also known as 'trophic ulcers'. Patients with longstanding sensory nerve lesions are also subject to excessive damage to desensitized bones and joints, with painless fractures, sprains and dislocations. The bones become tapered, especially the terminal phalanges. The joints become grossly disorganized, with painless subluxation and dislocation (Charcot's arthropathy). Several diseases characteristically progress to these destructive disturbances of denervated skin and bone: diabetes mellitus, leprosy, syringomyelia, tabes dorsalis, and other conditions with sensory nerve damage.

Thus, over time, a wide variety of patterns of sensory nerve damage can evolve.

Neuropathology

The peripheral neuropathies are a group of clinical syndromes with many causes. Some diseases affect predominantly motor nerves, others affect mainly sensory nerves, and some are mixed sensorimotor.

Two types of neuropathology (nerve cell abnormality) are found in the peripheral neuropathies. Both types are first evident in the axons of the neurons.

Axonal degeneration

The first type – primary axonal degeneration – is damage to the axons with swelling and fragmentation of the column of cytoplasm (axoplasm). Surviving nerve fibres conduct at a normal rate, but the strengths of motor or sensory impulses (action potentials) are reduced. At first, the myelin sheath (the fatty insulation around the axon) is normal, but the process of primary axonal degeneration may go on to secondary demyelination later.

Demyelination

The second type of neuropathy is primary segmental demyelination or destruction of the myelin sheath around a normal axon. Both the sheath and the Schwann cells (which form and maintain the sheath) are abnormal in appearance. Demyelinating neuropathies involve axons secondarily, not in the first instance, and a combination of demyelination and axonal degeneration is the end-result.

Clues as to the predominant process are sought from nerve conduction studies and nerve biopsy.

Toxic neuropathies

Many metabolic disorders seriously impair nerve functions but produce relatively little histopathological change.[16] In disorders due to poisons (toxic neuropathies), it is often difficult – in fact rare – to find an anatomical basis for functional disturbances. Both clinical neurological examination and animal studies may fail to provide confirmation of the nature of the abnormal process. Furthermore, the tissues of the nervous system vary in their susceptibility to many different noxious influences: ischaemia (lack of blood supply and therefore lack of oxygen) affects nerve cell bodies more than fibres; multiple sclerosis affects the myelin sheath of fibres; motor and sensory fibres are affected differently by different agents.[16]

The clinical neurological picture and the underlying neuro-pathology, or cell injury, will be modified by the capacity of the peripheral nerves to regenerate and repair themselves. Regeneration of peripheral axons is characteristic of the healing process of peripheral neuropathy. After the axon has 'died back' from its distal tip, one or more sprouts, smaller in diameter than the original, grow from the cut upper stump, back along the course of the distal damaged axon. The recovery of disordered function, such as loss of sensation, depends partly on the efficiency of this regeneration and partly on the magnitude of the initial damage. The final histological result may be quantitative changes in relative sizes and numbers of nerve fibres in the peripheral nerves, balancing axonal loss against axonal sprouting.

Thalidomide polyneuropathy in animals

Experimental studies of thalidomide polyneuropathy in animals have been limited. The inherent difficulty of achieving an animal model of a subjective human disorder has already been mentioned, and indeed some scientists have been unable to produce peripheral neuropathy in animals.

Staemmler and Lager[17] of Chemie-Grunenthal found no neuro-pathology in chronically exposed rats, hamsters, guinea pigs, rabbits, dogs or chicks. Others, however, have had more success. Diezel[18] gave thalidomide to dogs for 15 months, and found 'ribbon-like dilations' of the sensory peripheral axons, plus balloon-like distended neurons in the dorsal root ganglia and in the posterior horns of the spinal cord. No regression in these changes was observed 2 months after withdrawal of the drug. Axonal dilatation is a sign of peripheral neu-ropathy, and Diezel considered the histological changes in the sensory nerves to be 'a morphological equivalent of thalidomide neuropathy in man'.

Klinghardt[18] reported axonal degeneration and demyelination in rats, hamsters and mice after long-term treatment with high doses of thalidomide.

Thalidomide polyneuropathy in humans

Neurologists agreed unanimously that the human polyneuropathy caused by thalidomide was predominantly sensory, with minor involvement of motor and central nervous systems in some cases. Conduction studies provided unequivocal electrical evidence of involvement of peripheral sensory nerve fibres.[8] Human nerve tissue for microscopy is rarely available. Klinghardt[18] was fortunate to have access to two autopsies where patients with thalidomide neuropathy had died of other diseases. He confirmed the presence of axonal degeneration in posterior columns of the spinal cord, with fat granule masses. There was destruction of spinal ganglion cells, myelin degeneration, and swollen and deformed axons. Klinghardt described 'club-like distensions' of axons in ganglia and posterior roots.

The clinical feature of poor recovery, so typical of thalidomide neuropathy, was thought to be explained by Kinghardt's observation that some entire neurons in the dorsal root ganglia had degenerated and died back, including the cell body. Such neurons are dead, beyond regeneration. It was observed by neurologists that the worst-affected patients with least chance of recovery were generally those with the most prolonged exposure, with probable death of some neurons.

Fullerton and O'Sullivan[14] followed up 22 patients 4–6 years after cessation of the drug. They stated:

> 'Symptoms and signs are unchanged in approximately 50%; have improved in a quarter, and the remainder have recovered. Improvement was usually slow and, in some patients, did not begin for three years.'

In addition to clinical and electrophysiological evidence of persistent neuropathy in 75% of cases, they accessed tissue in six cases from biopsies of the sural nerve (a purely sensory cutaneous nerve). Single nerve fibres were teased free and studied. No segmental demyelination was seen. Transverse sections of the sural nerves were examined quantitatively. That is, the numbers and sizes of axons within the nerves were recorded. Compared with normal values, there was a reduction in total fibre density, a selective loss of large-diameter fibres and, in some cases, an increase in small-diameter fibres. These findings agreed with the electrophysiological evidence of failure of recovery of the peripheral parts of sensory nerve fibres, and with incomplete regeneration reflected in the increased number of small diameter fibres. Fullerton and O'Sullivan concluded that their observations would support the concept of a dying-back process, where the greatest damage is at the peripheral ends of the longest axons, with some neurons being irreversibly damaged and variable regeneration of others.

Krücke et al[19] examined sural nerve biopsies from eight patients, 7–9 years after thalidomide exposure. They found a reduction of fibre density and a loss of large-diameter fibres. On electron microscopy, they confirmed that many of the small-diameter fibres were regenerating, and that there was no disorder of myelination.

Häfstrom's highly significant report[11] of 73 Swedish patients with persistent, often painful, sensory peripheral neuropathy 3–5 years after cessation of thalidomide was supported by Fullerton and O'Sullivan[14] in 1968.

Thus the primary *site* of the thalidomide lesion in the human polyneuropathy has been located within peripheral sensory axons, possibly at the distal end. At least the first visible abnormality is dying back at the distal end of the axon. Its extent varies from mild and distal with regeneration (axonopathy) to total involvement with death of the entire neuron (ganglionopathy).

The *nature* of the lesion is axonal degeneration, late evidence of which can be observed at the cellular level. The nature of the earlier biochemical lesion is unknown.

These findings have been incorporated into subsequent neurology textbooks. The conclusion that thalidomide damaged sensory nerves was perfectly clear clinically, even though the biochemical basis of its toxicity remained unknown.

Thalidomide neuropathy disappears

After the demise of thalidomide in 1961, a new generation has emerged without any experience or even knowledge of the thalidomide disaster, especially if their homeland had not suffered the embryopathy. Many facts seem to have been forgotten, although they were probably never known.

The facts of the neuropathy faded fast during the drug's 30 years in the wilderness.

Some facts were lost in translation. The statement of Fullerton and O'Sullivan[14] is a case in point. Their conclusion is relayed in a major American neurology textbook:[20]

'Improvements of the peripheral neuropathy, however, occurred relatively rapidly and completely over several months in the patients reported by Fullerton and O'Sullivan.'

An official pamphlet[21] later informed the American public that:

'Thalidomide might cause damage to your nerves. It is not known whether this nerve damage is reversible after the drug is stopped.'

In Germany, a promotional circular for thalidomide was shown to me by a worried orthopaedic surgeon. Peripheral neuropathy was not even mentioned.

At a 2002 symposium in Sydney on mesothelioma and its management, a speaker presented results of a local trial of thalidomide for that condition, and startled some of the senior clinicians in the audience by stating that 'apart from its teratogenicity, thalidomide is a harmless drug'.

The sensory peripheral neuropathy had finally vanished.

Thalidomide returns – without the neuropathy

In the late 1970s, the drug was discovered to help in the treatment of a painful lumpy skin complication of leprosy: erythema nodosum leprosum (ENL).[22,23] Thalidomide had never been withdrawn from use for leprosy – itself a disease of nerves. It was a conundrum that a neurotoxic drug helped a neuropathic disease. However, thalidomide reduced both pain and skin masses in erythema nodosum leprosum.

A hypothesis was proposed in 1994 that high doses of thalidomide reduced inflammation by preventing blood vessel formation.[24] This 'anti-angiogenesis hypothesis' is discussed in Chapter 30; it impacted medical practice because it suggested that thalidomide might reduce vascularity in inflammatory and malignant conditions. Clinical interest was kindled in the therapeutic possibilities.

In 1998, the US Food and Drug Administration (FDA) approved thalidomide for restricted use in ENL. In addition to this approved use, by 2004, thalidomide in large doses was used or being investigated for use in other skin, gastrointestinal and malignant diseases, including, among others, discoid lupus erythematosus, aphthous ulcers, prurigo nodularis, chronic inflammatory bowel disease, sarcoidosis, multiple myeloma, some leukaemias, glioma, mesothelioma and prostate cancer.

Based upon the original experiments, large doses of thalidomide were recommended for these treatments – up to 200 mg/kg. Sensory neuropathy occurs at the original (1950s) sedative dose of 1 mg/kg. Therefore its use at very high doses has been limited by peripheral sensory neurotoxicity erupting en route – a surprise to those who had believed the historical revision.

Many case reports and series of cases have been reported in recent years, creating a second monolith of thalidomide literature, too extensive and contradictory to present here. I have selected a few papers that examine the reasons for discrepancies in diagnosis of the neuropathy, to explain claims and counterclaims of its safety.

The second epidemic of sensory peripheral neuropathy

The second outbreak of neuropathy was confined to people enrolled in therapeutic trials for various diseases.

Thalidomide has continued to be used in the treatment of ENL, where it has succeeded in reducing dramatically the bulk of the nodular mass lesions. Because leprosy is itself a neuropathy, there is an assumption that any loss of sensation during treatment is due to the disease itself. This assumption has been attributed to absence, inadequacy or inappropriate choice of neurological tests in patients with leprosy.

'Electrophysiological studies, particularly the recording of sural nerve action potentials, have proved valuable in detecting thalidomide neuropathy at an early stage, but these have not been used in patients with leprosy. When thalidomide has been used to treat non-leprous disorders the frequency of neuropathy is at least 21%.[25] Waters[26] accepts this figure but claims that "the nerves [of patients with lepromatous leprosy] are relatively insusceptible to thalidomide-induced peripheral neuropathy". Without details of the neurological findings, this assertion cannot be sustained. Because of the failure of leprologists to take thalidomide neuropathy seriously the drug has been distributed widely in developing countries, culminating in the disaster in Brazil, where to date 47 children have been born deformed after their mothers took thalidomide during pregnancy.'[27–29]

A debate along these lines has continued in letters to the editors of *The Lancet* and the *BMJ* as the safety of thalidomide is still questioned, and claims are challenged.

By 1985, dermatologists in Europe were testing thalidomide for use in a number of other chronic inflammatory conditions of the skin. Wulff et al,[30] dermatologists from Copenhagen, observed the development of polyneuropathy during thalidomide treatment in seven patients with prurigo nodularis and one with aphthous stomatitis, at 40–115 g total dosage over 1–6 years' duration. Despite dramatic improvement in the dermatological disorder in all cases, treatment had to be discontinued in all because of the severe sensory neuropathy. Neurological test results duplicated those already described in the first outbreak. In discussion, these dermatologists analyse the first accounts of the remarkable therapeutic effect of thalidomide in prurigo nodularis from five different centres.

Wulff et al[30] observed that:

'The neurotoxic side-effects of thalidomide were not mentioned as a major problem in these publications.

'Sheskin and Yaar[23] followed 26 patients on thalidomide for reactional lepromatous leprosy over 6–13 years and found normal or unchanged MOTOR conduction along the ULNAR nerve. On the basis of this they concluded that neurotoxicity was low.

'In contrast to these reports we found that all patients under treatment developed a peripheral neuropathy confirmed by abnormally small and desynchronized SENSORY action potentials from leg nerves. As thalidomide neuropathy is of an axonal type affecting mainly SENSORY fibres in the lower limbs, motor conduction studies are of little value regarding the diagnosis. We found no change of motor conduction along the median or ulnar nerve in any of our patients. The clinical and neurophysiological abnormalities in our patients were not different from those mentioned in earlier reports.[1,7,8,11,14]

'The present study[30] indicates that the incidence of thalidomide neuropathy after long-term treatment is higher than previously estimated. We therefore conclude that thalidomide should be used exclusively in disorders involving only a short-term treatment.'

A clinical balancing act?

The debate continues in the literature, with neurologists advising caution in deployment of thalidomide as a therapeutic agent. Encouraging reports on its 'safety' are often due to failure to do the appropriate neurological tests.

Dermatologists are alert to the dangers of iatrogenic damage to sensory nerves in their patients.[30–35] Oncologists report neuropathy in cancer patients,[36] and neuroradiologists report lesions in their posterior (sensory) columns in the spinal cord on magnetic resonance imaging.[37] Neurologists sound caution,[38] and raise the alarm that the damage is an irreversible ganglionopathy,[39] more serious than axonopathy.

Apfel and Zochodne,[40] neurologists from New York, in an editorial for *Neurology* in 2004, have questioned whether thalidomide neuropathy was due to amount or length of dosage:

'Our recommendation is that . . . the lowest effective dose should be used. Because thalidomide neurotoxicity may be dose related and is often irreversible, care must be taken to avoid high doses wherever possible . . . Regardless of the dose, peripheral nerve function should be closely monitored through review of symptoms, regular neurologic examinations, and periodic screening of sensory nerve electrophysiology.

'When evidence of neuropathy appears, consideration should be given to discontinuing thalidomide.

'The decision to discontinue should be made on an individual basis and should consider the seriousness and severity of the underlying condition and the severity of the neuropathy.'

References

1. Amelung W, Püntmann E. Klinik und Therapie der sog. Contergan-Polyneuropathie. *Nervenarzt* 1966; **37**: 189–99.

2. Sjöström H, Nilsson R. *Thalidomide and the Power of the Drug Companies.* Harmondsworth: Penguin, 1972.

3. Voss R. *Münch Med Wschr* 1961; **103**: 1431–2.

4. Hultsch EG, Hartmann J. *Münch Med Wschr* 1961; **103**: 2141–4.

5. Becker J. *Nervenarzt* 1961; **32**: 321–3.

6. Raffauf HJ. *Dtsch Med Wschr* 1961; **86**: 935–8.

7. Florence AL. Is thalidomide to blame? *BMJ* 1960; **ii**: 1954.

8. Fullerton PM. Kremer M. Neuropathy after intake of thalidomide (Distaval). *BMJ* 1961; **ii**: 855–8.

9. Simpson JA. *BMJ* 1961; **ii**: 1287.

10. Ministry of Health Reports on Public Health and Medical Subjects No. 112. *Deformities Caused by Thalidomide*. London: HMSO, 1964.

11. Häfstrom T. Polyneuropathy after Neurosedyn (thalidomide) and its prognosis. *Acta Neurol Scand* 1967; **43**(Suppl 32): 6–42.

12. Lenz W. Das thalidomid Syndrom. *Fortschr Med* 1963; **81**: 148–55.

13. Lenz W. Epidemiology of congenital malformations. *Ann NY Acad Sci* 1965; **123**: 228–36.

14. Fullerton P, O'Sullivan D. Thalidomide neuropathy – a clinical, electrophysiological and histological follow-up study. *J Neurol Neurosurg Psychiatr* 1968; **31**: 543–51.

15. Ranson SD, Clark SL. *The Anatomy of the Nervous System: Its Development and Function*. Philadelphia: WB Saunders, 1953.

16. Walton J. *Essentials of Neurology*, 5th edn. London: Pitman, 1982.

17. Staemmler M, Lagler F. Tierexperimentelle suchungen zur Frage Thalidomid und Nervenschadigung. *Arzneimittelforschung* 1965; **15**: 504.

18. Diezel PB. Morphological changes in experimental thalidomide neuropathy and thalidomide-induced deformities of the extremities. *MMW Kongresse und Vereine* 1963; **45**: 2265.

18. Klinghardt GW. Ein betrag der experimentellen neuropathology zur toxizitätsprüfung neuer chemotherapeutica. *Mitt Max-Planck Gesell* 1965; **3**: 142–55.

19. Krücke W, von Hartrott H-H, Schröder JM et al. Light and electron microscope studies of late stages of thalidomide polyneuropathy. *Fortschr Neurol Psychiatr Grenzgeb* 1971; **39**: 15–50.

20. Spencer P, Schaumberg HH. Classification of neurotoxic disease: a morphological approach. In: Spencer P, Schaumberg HH, eds. *Experimental and Clinical Neurotoxicology*. Baltimore: Williams and Wilkins, 1980: 92–9.

21. *Thalidomide – Important Patient Information*. DHHS Publication No. (FDA) 96–3222.

22. Sheskin J. The treatment of lepra reaction in lepromatous leprosy. *Int J Dermatol* 1980; **19**: 318–22.

23. Sheskin J, Yaar I. Motor conduction velocity of cubital nerves in patients with leprosy reactions: summary of a 13 year observation of a series during thalidomide therapy. *Hautarzt* 1979; **30**: 376–9.

24. D'Amato RJ, Loughnan MS, Flynn E, Folkman J. Thalidomide is an inhibitor of angiogenesis. *Proc Natl Acad Sci USA* 1994; **91**: 4082–5.

25. Ochonisky S, Verroust J, Bastuji-Garin S et al. Thalidomide neuropathy incidence and clinicoelectrophysiologic findings in 42 patients. *Arch Dermatol* 1994; **130**: 66–9.

26. Waters MF. Use of thalidomide in leprosy. *BMJ* 1991; **303**: 470.

27. Crawford CL. Use of thalidomide in leprosy. *BMJ* 1991; **303**: 1062–3.

28. Crawford CL. Safety of thalidomide. *BMJ* 1994; **308**: 1437–8.

29. Crawford CL. Does thalidomide have a role in leprosy? *Lancet* 2004; **363**: 1911.

30. Wulff CH, Hoyer H, Asboe-Hansen G, Brodthagen H. Development of polyneuropathy during thalidomide therapy. *Br J Dermatol* 1985; **112**: 475–80.

31. Clemmensen OJ, Olsen PZ, Andersen KE. Thalidomide neuro-toxicity. *Arch Dermatol* 1984; **120**: 338–41.

32. Gardner-Medwin JMM, Smith NJ, Powell RJ. Clinical experience with thalidomide in the management of severe oral and genital ulceration in conditions such as Behçet's disease: use of neurophysiological studies to detect thalidomide neuropathy. *Ann Rheum Dis* 1994; **53**: 828–32.

33. Karim MY, Ruiz-Irastorza G, Khamahta MA, Hughes GR. Update on therapy – thalidomide in the treatment of lupus. *Lupus* 2001; **10**: 188–92.

34. Briani C, Zara G, Rondinone R et al. Thalidomide neurotoxicity: prospective study in patients with lupus erythematosus. *Neurology* 2004; **62**: 2288–90.

35. Wines NY, Cooper AJ, Wines MP. Thalidomide in dermatology. *Australas J Dermatol* 2002; **43**: 229–38.

36. Molloy FM, Floeter MK, Seyd NA et al. Thalidomide neuropathy in patients treated for metastatic prostate cancer. *Muscle Nerve* 2001; **24**: 1050–7.

37. Isoardo G, Bergui M, Durelli L et al. Thalidomide neuropathy: clinical, electrophysiological and neuro-radiological features. *Acta Neurol Scand* 2004; **109**: 188–93.

38. Chaudhry V, Cornblath DR, Corse A et al. Thalidomide-induced neuropathy. *Neurology* 2002; **59**: 1872–5.

39. Giannini F, Volpi N, Rossi S et al. Thalidomide-induced neuropathy: a ganglionopathy? *Neurology* 2003: **60**: 877–8.

40. Apfel SC, Zochodne DW. Thalidomide neuropathy: too much or too long? Editorial. *Neurology* 2004; **62**: 2158–9.

CHAPTER 5

Clinical radiology

'One cannot complain of having no clues . . .
There are clues here in abundance'
Agatha Christie, *Murder on the Orient Express*

Because the microscope was invented before Röntgen discovered X-rays, pathology was an established science before radiographic images existed. Diagnostic radiology has been built upon the older science of pathology. It is an axiom in medicine that radiology mirrors macroscopic pathology. The two sciences are complementary in modern clinical diagnosis, and are integrated as powerful diagnostic tools in daily practice. Radiology points to the diseased organ. Histopathology confirms or disproves it.

A place for radiology in the search for the underlying pathology of thalidomide embryopathy

Thalidomide embryopathy presented a peculiar problem – there was grossly abnormal anatomy, but no known pathology.

A unique possibility existed for reversal of the historic roles. That is, the nature of the pathology might be first established by radiological analysis. Could clues in radiology lead to the unknown histopathology in these birth defects?

Absence of radiography and radiology in animal studies

In spite of its established reputation as a reliable and essential contributor to diagnosis in clinical medicine, diagnostic radiology had not been used to advantage in animal research into birth defects. To a radiologist who ventures into the literature of teratology, the absence of radiography and radiology in animal studies of thalidomide embryopathy is quite remarkable.

Radiography of bone defects has apparently been rejected in favour of the *ARAB staining technique*: the whole animal or a part thereof is

Chapter Summary
- A place for radiology in the search for the underlying pathology of thalidomide embryopathy
- Absence of radiography and radiology in animal studies
- Order of investigation in medicine
- Order of investigation in teratology research
- Integration of radiology and pathology
- A place for radiology in the search for the pathogenesis of thalidomide embryopathy
- References

cleared and stained. Bone stains red with *Alizarin Red*, and cartilage stains blue with *Alcian Blue*.[1,2] This process takes 2 weeks and destroys tissues for future microscopy. A simple radiograph takes a few minutes, and all tissues remain available for histological examination.

The only advantage of the ARAB method over radiography is that it shows cartilage, which cannot be imaged by standard radiography unless it is calcified. This makes for pretty illustrations, but does not assist the search for causation.

Diagnostic radiology, a valuable resource, has been overlooked in animal research projects with thalidomide, partly because of adoption of the ARAB technique, but also because of a seemingly illogical order of investigations.

Order of investigations in medicine

This section is included for non-medical readers.

The approach to making a medical diagnosis varies with the disease, but in general the diagnostic process involves three sequential steps:

1. The diagnosis starts with clues provided by the patient's complaints and physical examination. From these, a provisional diagnosis is deduced.
2. In the second phase, a radiologist, haematologist, biochemist or other specialist examines the patient. A radiologist looks for abnormalities of gross anatomy. This often reveals the diagnosis or differential diagnosis.
3. The third phase focuses upon the cells in the suspect organ or tissue. Here, the disease entity is proved by finding abnormal cells via the pathologist's microscope.

This is a time-honoured and logical approach to medical diagnosis. It clearly obeys the rules of scientific method. Furthermore, it works. For instance, in Chapter 4, it was applied to neurological disorders.

Order of investigations in teratology research

A logical progression of investigation is not necessarily followed in animal research into birth defects. There is a tendency to leap from the deformed animal to cell or molecular biology, particularly in laboratories set up for subcellular investigations. Macroscopic assessment of organs and tissues by radiological imaging and gross pathology is usually omitted from the diagnostic sequence. It is not clear whether this approach is a seriously considered policy or a deficiency that has become entrenched with the passage of time.

It is surely unwise to plunge into subcellular and molecular levels of investigation before it has been ascertained which tissue, of the 200 or more different components of the body, is host to the disease process. Furthermore, subcellular data is meaningless unless it relates to the clinical and pathological facts of the disease.

Omission of the tissue or organ level of investigation induces an illogical process of deduction, with erroneous and at times bewildering conclusions. In view of past omission of the 'macro' step, and failure to find the causative mechanism of these birth defects, there was a case for a retrospective review to put the missing part of the analysis in place.

Integration of radiology and pathology

How does diagnostic radiology really work? This section for non-medical readers explains how radiology and pathology interrelate in establishing a diagnosis in medicine.

Pathology (the study of disease) is learnt during the undergraduate medical course and again during postgraduate training for both specialist radiologists and pathologists. It is constantly learnt and revised in everyday practice.

Most diseases have a characteristic pattern of abnormal signs or images on a radiograph that matches the gross pathology. Radiological patterns of disease are memorized by trainee radiologists in order to build in their minds a databank of facts and mental images. By comparing these known disease patterns with the image of the unsolved case in question, the correct diagnosis may be deduced. This so-called 'pattern-matching' exercise is done in the radiologist's mind. It is an intellectual exercise that draws upon a thorough knowledge of medicine, pathology, and the visual memory databank, together with logic and experience.

A pattern of disordered anatomy may be characteristic and therefore diagnostic of one particular disease – in which case the diagnosis is clearly established. Sometimes, the pattern of radiological signs may be common to several different diseases. In this situation, all alternatives (differential diagnoses) are short-listed in the radiologist's report – preferably with some weighting of opinion in order to suggest to the referring doctor the most likely answer in that clinical setting.

Any imaging technique yields only part of the information actually present. Radiologists are aware that not all the information is necessarily recorded by the selected imaging method; a proportion of the evidence is likely to be missing (especially if it is beyond the power of resolution of that imaging method). The limitations of each imaging technique are studied. The sensitivity and specificity of any test in relation to a particular disease is learnt in order to minimize the risk of making false-positive or false-negative diagnoses.

An X-ray report must be accurately worded. Having learnt the limitations of the various methods they use, radiologists express their opinions accordingly. For instance, 'No evidence of cancer is detected' means exactly what it says. It does *not* mean 'no cancer is present'.

Absence of evidence is not evidence of absence in the real world of clinical radiology.

To check or refine the diagnosis, the radiologist may sometimes suggest the next step. A different imaging method may be advisable to clinch the diagnosis. A non-imaging test or a biopsy for histopathology may be more appropriate. The clinician puts this advice together with all the other accrued information and advice about the patient's problem, and decides on the next move.

An awareness of known traps in everyday clinical radiology refines discrimination and sharpens professional appraisal of written reports, diagnostic tests and also of published papers: interpretation and conclusions are critically assessed against materials and methods for claims and accuracy.

There is a profound difference between seeing an image and understanding what that image means. A radiologist is like an interpreter of words written in another language. One has to imagine that one can listen with the eyes to what the image is saying, and translate it into the language of disease entities (pathological diagnosis). The translation may require knowledge of several languages. In the case of thalidomide deformities, one needs to know the languages of anatomy, neurology, embryology, neuropathology and radiology. If one of these is disregarded, the message in radiographic images of these birth defects will remain unheard. If the malformations are not submitted to organ imaging, the clues are not even obtained, let alone analysed.

A radiologist also resembles an archaeologist who works to decipher an ancient inscription from weathered stone in order to understand the writer's message. The lettering is like the observed abnormalities on the radiograph. The message may be compounded of several ancient languages, all of which are known to the archaeologist. The radiologist analyses the image (message) using the sciences of anatomy, pathology and physics, and translates the image into the diagnosis.

This level of perception totally engages eyes and mind, and brings to bear upon the image all the intellectual resources of observation, analysis, logic and memory – prior knowledge of normal and abnormal conditions, and recognition of their patterns. It often requires an ability to make difficult, challenging decisions and finely tuned judgements. Diagnostic radiology is essentially an intellectual exercise, inherently dependant upon but separate from the machinery of capturing the image by pressing a button: the latter is radiography, not radiology.

Medical problems are solved every day by diagnostic radiology, occasionally using controlled intellectual constructs, but always observing the principles of scientific method. Because they understand the language of images, radiologists are responsible for translating the information embedded therein into a diagnosis, i.e. naming the disease entity that is present.

Pasteur's 1854 aphorism that 'where observation is concerned, chance favours only the prepared mind' applies just as much to diagnostic radiology as to any other branch of science. As already explained, 'the prepared mind' of a radiologist is an intellectual library of recognizable patterns of disease in all organs of the body. Patterns of disease in the limb skeleton are but a small part of the total memory bank. Diagnostic radiologists are the ultimate 'limb-patterning experts', and are thus likely to be favoured by chance in any search for the cause of diseased limbs through the medium of imaging.

Some radiologists might have seen one or two cases of thalidomide embryopathy at most – insufficient material to reveal the pattern. It usually requires study of a series of several cases (case reports or small series) for the pattern of a disease to emerge. I was sent a group of cases with positive histories of thalidomide exposure. In that respect, I was favoured by chance.

A place for radiology in the search for the pathogenesis of thalidomide embryopathy

Thalidomide deformities presented yet another unusual scientific problem. Not only was there no demonstrable histopathology, but the pathogenesis was unknown.

It had been established beyond doubt that deformities resulted if a pregnant woman ingested thalidomide in the 'thalidomide-sensitive period' of pregnancy. But how did the drug do this? The *pathogenesis* (i.e. *the mechanism within the embryo whereby thalidomide caused this damage*), remained a mystery.

The undamaged part of the skeleton was composed of regularly structured bone and cartilage. No abnormal histopathology (abnormal cells) had been found in the misshapen bones, nor had any been found in cells of other malformed organs when examined by the light microscope. Gross pathology and microscopic pathology were out of step for reasons unknown. Thalidomide embryopathy was a very gross disease in search of a histopathological identity *and* a mechanism of pathogenesis.

A dearth of information about the pathology and pathogenesis of this disease was at odds with an 'abundance of clues' within the images. In fact, the mismatch was quite spectacular! The bizarre distortions of the bones and joints were among the most extreme in the whole range of skeletal radiology. The images presented ample evidence of very gross abnormality somewhere – but where? It did not seem possible that such grotesque malformations occurred and even recurred, without reason, without an underlying pathological process to match and explain them. Absence of evidence of cellular injury challenged the fundamental tenet that radiology mirrors pathology.

Furthermore, if such defects just happened by chance, as spontaneous haphazard events, then the pattern of distortion within the embryo should be completely random. This was not so. Even within the first five cases in my Sydney collection, certain patterns of deformity (e.g. reduction of radius and thumb) were repeated – not just once, but several times. This strongly favoured a systematic process underlying the defects. It argued against the concept of chance, haphazard disruptions of embryonic development. It implied that a mechanism of pathogenesis was indeed present, but was as yet unrecognized.

Initially, my curiosity about congenital malformations had been aroused by the gross discrepancy between radiology and pathology. A commitment to study the problem more carefully grew during each brief encounter with the children and their parents in radiographic sessions.

Could an analysis of the abundant information displayed in the radiographs provide some clue as to the nature and the mechanism of this disease? To translate an abnormal radiographic image into known pathology is an everyday task for a clinical radiologist. 'Where is it?' and 'What is it?' are the two basic questions that radiologists apply to every case they see. The problem peculiar to the thalidomide cases was the absence of known pathology to which the malformations could be related. The 'What is it?' question was a total blank. In attempting to answer that, I would be groping for a hitherto-unknown disease process. I did not imagine getting that far. At least, I might be able to derive a radiological definition or disease pattern for a thalidomide deformity. At most, I might answer the first question and locate the target organ attacked by the drug. That would presumably help people who research birth defects, in supplying the missing information as to the site of disease and the macroscopic target tissue.

With these ends in view, I examined the radiographs in a systematic fashion, and analysed each radiological feature, always seeking to identify the essential process of which these features were evidence.

Chapters 7–11 document my analyses of the radiological features of thalidomide embryopathy, leading to the derivation and formulation of a hypothesis of pathogenesis (Chapter 12). I had no preconceived hypothesis that I was attempting to prove when I embarked upon this exercise. I deduced the hypothesis from radiological evidence that emerged in case after case during the initial stages of my investigation.

References

1. Green MC. A rapid method for clearing and staining specimens for the demonstration of bone. *Ohio J Sci* 1952; **52**: 31–3.

2. Crary DD. Modified benzyl alcohol clearing of alizarin-stained specimens without loss of flexibility. *Stain Technol* 1962; **37**: 124–5.

CHAPTER 6

Terminology, classification and the rejection of authority

' "Then you should say what you mean," the March Hare went on.
"I do," Alice hastily replied. "At least – at least I mean what I say –
that's the same thing, you know."
"Not the same thing a bit!" said the Hatter.'
Lewis Carroll, *Alice in Wonderland* (Quoted by Dr George Simon[1])

Terminology

Thalidomide's distortions of bone and joint morphology were not
subtle. Rather, the abnormalities were gross: easy to see but difficult to
describe in words. The first problem was that of terminology for
documentation.

The literature revealed a subject surrounded by apparently
intractable confusion. The terminology relating to congenital limb
malformations was complex and mainly derived from Greek or Latin.
This in itself did not pose an insuperable difficulty, as long as the
terms remained consistent. However, inconsistency and ambiguity
seemed to be the rule rather than the exception, because various
definitions existed for any one term. In discussing hand deformities,
Kelikian[2] stated that:

> 'diverse names are assigned to one and the same deformity by
> different authors, and labels which originally were set aside for
> some malformations have come to be tagged on to others.'

Four terms that have been commonly used and are embedded in the
literature are *phocomelia, reduction deformity, thalidomide embryopathy*
and *dysmelia*. Each term has inherent problems as well as advantages.

Phocomelia

Strictly speaking, this means seal limb, indicating that the limbs are
like seal flippers. If you examine the skeleton of a seal in the museum,
you will realize that this is not true. Limb bones of seals are dys-
chondroplastic rather than dysmelic in their size and shape, and there
are no missing bones or digits, no hypoplasia, no aplasia. This term is

Chapter Summary
- Terminology
- Classification
- Rejection of authority
- References

misapplied to longitudinal reduction deformities, but it suffices to convey a superficial impression of the external appearance of short limbs on a normal body.

Lenz[3] drew attention to the inadequacy of the term 'phocomelia' as applied to thalidomide victims:

> 'The concept of phocomelia, in the way in which Geoffrey Saint-Hilaire coined the concept in 1836, cannot be applied to thalidomide embryopathy, as according to Saint-Hilaire,[4] in phocomelia "hands and feet, of normal size and mostly completely normally formed, are borne on extremely short limbs, so that in the majority of cases they appear to originate directly from the shoulders or the hips".'

Lenz was making the point that the upper extremities in thalidomide-induced phocomelia are always incomplete, with missing digits. However, phocomelia and related terms have continued to be 'loosely used' in the literature describing thalidomide embryopathy.[3] 'Ectromelia' is another term with various definitions, of no help in this analysis.

Reduction deformity

Another commonly used term is 'reduction deformity', or 'longitudinal reduction deformity', which indicates in a general fashion the diminished nature and loss of length of the defective limbs. The exact origin of this term could not be ascertained. It recognizes that the missing strips of tissue lie in the long axis of the limb. Longitudinal reduction defects were typical of the thalidomide syndrome. They are totally different from 'amputation-like deformities', or transverse defects, which were not typical of the thalidomide syndrome. As such, the term 'longitudinal reduction deformity' is accurate and useful.

Thalidomide embryopathy

The term 'thalidomide embryopathy' is acceptable in those cases where the aetiology is known to be thalidomide. However, proof of thalidomide intake by the mother was frequently impossible to establish in retrospect. This left a collection of cases of unproven aetiology, but identical morphology, to which the term 'thalidomide embryopathy' should, strictly speaking, not be applied. However, once the aetiological label 'thalidomide' is applied, the belief that thalidomide was to blame for that particular person's birth defects becomes impossible to eradicate. At least 10% of the British children labelled as 'thalidomide embryopathy' lacked any proof of exposure at the time,[5] but were given the benefit of the doubt by assessors and received compensation payments. Now that a small number of them have had children with similar malformations, the original cases are believed to be genetic. But they have carried the thalidomide label, in error, for 40 years. It is almost impossible to correct the mindset, or the consequent belief that thalidomide can damage the second generation. This decision about classification 40 years ago, generous at the time, has caused distress in the families involved, generated bogus support for a 'scientific' case, followed by fruitless claims for additional compensation.

Dysmelia

In an attempt to provide a comprehensive label for the whole collection of limb defects exemplified by thalidomide embryopathy, in 1962 Wiedemann[6] named the group 'dysmelia' – meaning abnormal limbs. This term is widely accepted in the German literature, and is defined as 'a group of malformations in which there is hypoplasia, and partial and total aplasia of the tubular bones of the extremities, ranging from isolated peripheral hypoplasia to complete loss of the extremity'.[7] The term 'dysmelia' is general enough to encompass all morphologically similar cases, yet it is independent of aetiological implications. As such, it is one of the best terms, because it covers the whole array of limb defects expressed in true thalidomide embryopathy.

Application of terminology

Difficulties arise when attempts are made to label particular deformities within the spectrum of dysmelia. My own impression, as my experience of limb malformations increased, was that each term was subject to such a wide range of variation that the categorization of any one defect seemed arbitrary. Such categorization seemed to me to impose artificial divisions upon a single, underlying, confluent natural process. My own objective was to seek out this process if possible – not to subdivide it. Entanglement with dubious terminology did not promise to help me reach my objective.

Classification

Classification was beset by similar problems. A multiplicity of systems, with synonyms, ambiguity and obscurity of definition, caused confusion in the literature. For example, there are 21 different methods of classification of malformations of the forearm and hand,[2] not to mention eponymic syndromes containing forearm and hand defects. Such profusion implies inadequacy. Many of these systems have been criticized for being either artificial or excessively complicated, while others have been considered too narrow.[8,9] None succeeds in incorporating the non-skeletal malformations that can occur in association with limb defects. Proceedings of meetings and their discussions lend insight into the attitudes adopted by protagonists of different systems, and it has been said[9] that one expert would rather use another's toothbrush than his system of classification!

Obsession with nomenclature and classification in the past has deflected attention from the search for pathology and causative mechanisms in the embryo. Classification appeared to have been accepted as the endpoint of investigation by some researchers. The battle with terminology and classification may have exhausted them before the search for pathogenesis had begun!

The obsession with classification has occasionally been questioned. Cohn[10] considered any attempt to classify such deformities as quixotic, 'ridiculous, because there are millions of possible combinations of defects'. Kelikian[2] stated that congenital anomalies of the hand are often too bizarre to be 'corraled into discrete categories', and pleaded for a simplified English terminology. In an attempt to correct the confusion, a working party of the International Society for Prosthetics and Orthotics recommended a new International Terminology for the Classification of Congenital Limb Deficiencies.[11,12] This provides the most practical classification to date, and it includes the recommendation that previous systems of classification should be abandoned!

It must be admitted that a workable classification is essential for the clinician examining patients. It provides a useful, if approximate, labelling system based upon the outward appearance of the limbs. But the radiologist reading the anatomy of the skeleton often finds quite different bony complexes within clinically similar limbs. Many bone malformations of thalidomide victims are so bizarre that clinical terms fail to describe them at all. At best, an approximate label can be applied, yet important morphological details are thereby ignored or discounted. Since my objective was to seek the underlying process, I decided that my collection of radiological data should include all details in the first instance. I decided to side-step all ambiguous terminology, subdivisions and classification systems. From a comprehensive database, I would aim to derive a statement or interpretation that would incorporate all details – a general statement of a process, which could be applied to any patient.

Rejection of authority

I therefore elected to abandon all existing systems of nomenclature and classification. I chose to annotate my initial radiological observations in simple descriptive English. Where words proved inadequate, I added pencil sketches.

References

1. Simon G. *Principles of Chest X-Ray Diagnosis*. London: Butterworths, 1962.
2. Kelikian H. *Congenital Deformities of the Hand and Forearm*. Philadelphia: WB Saunders, 1974.

3. Lenz W. Das Thalidomid Syndrom. *Fortschr Med* 1963; **81:** 148–55.

4. Saint-Hilaire IG. *Histoire generale et particuliere des anomalies de l'organisation chez l'homme et les animaux*. Paris: JB Baillière, 1836; **2:** 206–37.

5. Newman CG. The thalidomide syndrome: risks of exposure and spectrum of malformations. *Clin Perinatol* 1986; **13:** 555–73.

6. Wiedemann HR. *Med Welt* 1962; **1:** 1343–9.

7. Henkel H-L, Willert H-G. Dysmelia. A classification and a pattern of malformation in a group of congenital defects of the limbs. *J Bone Joint Surg [Br]* 1969; 51-B, 399–414.

8. Lenz W. Bone defects of the limbs – an overview. *Birth Defects: Original Article Series V* 1969; **3:** 1–6.

9. O'Rahilly R. Nomenclature and classification of limb anomalies. *Birth Defects: Original Article Series V* 1969; **3:** 14–17.

10. Cohn I. Skeletal disturbances and anomalies. A clinical report and a review of the literature. *Trans South Surg Assoc* 1932; **44:** 485–521.

11. Henkel H-L, Willert H-G, Gressman C. *Acta Orthop Trauma Surg* 1978; **93:** 1–19.

12. Kay, HW. The proposed International Terminology for the Classification of Congenital Limb Deficiencies. *Dev Med Child Neurol* 1975; **34**(Suppl): 1–12.

CHAPTER 7

The pattern of the disease: First radiological analysis (Sydney)

Introduction

Twelve cases of congenital limb malformations were referred to me by McBride in early 1971 at the Royal Prince Alfred Hospital, Sydney, for my radiological opinion as to which were thalidomide-induced and which were not. Compensation from the drug companies was now available, and many children with congenital malformations became claimants. These had to be sorted into those due to thalidomide, and other 'look-alikes', with similar deformities but lacking a thalidomide history.

Five of the twelve cases were known to be caused by thalidomide. Three of these were living children aged between 9 and 11 years, whose parents had produced satisfactory medicolegal evidence, such as the prescription, the tablets, and their medical and other records. They have subsequently been accepted by the Distillers Company for compensation. I also received the radiographs of two newborn infants (dated 1961) who had perished in the neonatal period. Their mothers had documented thalidomide ingestion during early pregnancy. These five cases represented authentic examples of the embryopathy due to thalidomide, and I used their radiographs for my initial study of five cases with proven exposure to thalidomide.

The seven cases where thalidomide aetiology was in doubt were examined and radiographed in the same way as the proven thalidomide cases. My colleagues on the radiographic staff of the Royal Prince Alfred Hospital assisted me in obtaining a set of good-quality films of each child, so that the skeletal defects were thoroughly recorded.

The aim of the first study was to document all abnormal radiological signs in the five known cases of thalidomide embryopathy, and to attempt to define the pattern of the disease process from these observed signs.

Chapter Summary
- **Introduction**
- **Observations and descriptions**
- **Method of analysis of the disease pattern**
- **Results**
- **Analysis of this disease pattern**
- **Discussion**
- **Conclusion**

Observations and descriptions

Case 1

Case 1 was born in 1961 at The Women's Hospital, Crown Street, Sydney, with bilateral radial aplasia and club hands. The right thumb was absent and the left was hypoplastic. The left femur was shorter than the right. A sigmoid, distended gas shadow in the upper abdomen in the supine view (Figure 7.1) altered in the vertical film to form the classical 'double-bubble' sign of duodenal atresia (Figure 7.2).

This baby had been submitted to surgical repair of the duodenal atresia, but had died postoperatively.

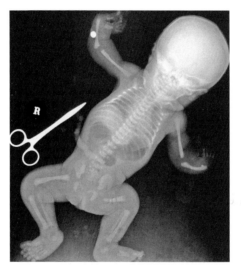

Figure 7.1 *Case 1: supine film of newborn baby with bilateral absent radii, left proximal femoral focal deficiency, and duodenal atresia shown by the sigmoid gas shadow of distended stomach and duodenum.*

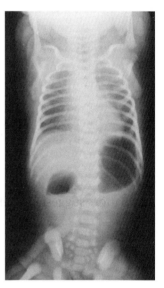

Figure 7.2 *Case 1: a vertical film of the same baby as in Figure 7.1 shows the double-bubble sign, diagnostic of duodenal atresia.*

Case 2

Case 2 was also born in 1961 at The Women's Hospital, Crown Street, Sydney, with multiple limb malformations (Figure 7.3). Radiographs of the arms showed bilateral radial aplasia, partial polydactyly and soft tissue fusion of several digits. Both thumbs were hypoplastic and triphalangeal. The left foot was normal, but there was fusion and partial polydactyly of the right first and second toes. This child's anorectal agenesis was diagnosed on clinical evidence. It died in the nursery without surgery, and without subsequent autopsy.

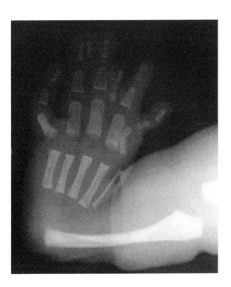

Figure 7.3 *Case 2: newborn baby with radial aplasia, polydactyly, syndactyly and triphalangeal thumb.*

Case 3

Case 3 was born in 1961 with bilateral upper limb phocomelia (Figure 7.4). At the age of 9 years, a radiograph of the right arm showed a grossly hypoplastic shoulder joint, entirely lacking the bony glenoid process, with a small, poorly moulded humeral head.

The three long bones of the arm were replaced by a single long bone shaped like a hunting boomerang or a hockey-stick (Figure 7.5). The angulation suggested itself as the site of the unformed, absent elbow joint. A reasonable interpretation of this bone was that the short proximal component represented residual humerus, much reduced in length, and that its associated epiphyses were absent. The long distal component had ulnar characteristics. The radius and thumb were absent.

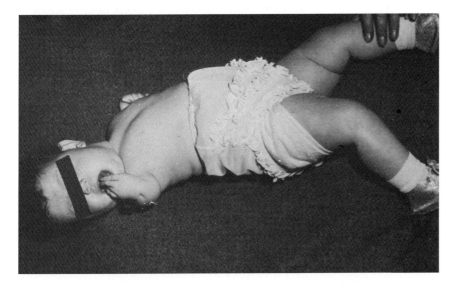

Figure 7.4 *Case 3 as an infant with bilateral upper limb phocomelia.*

On the left, the radius was absent, but a hypoplastic thumb was present (Figure 7.6). In both wrists, each row of carpal bones was fused in parallel, transversely, to form two blocks of bone. The bases of two metacarpals in each hand were also fused in parallel. No abnormalities were present in the lower limbs.

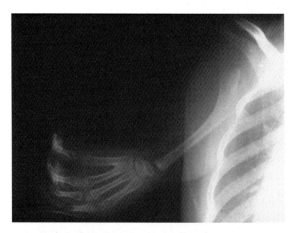

Figure 7.5 *Right arm of Case 3: humero-ulnar fusion with absent radius and thumb at age 9 years. There are fused carpal bones and fused bases of two metacarpals.*

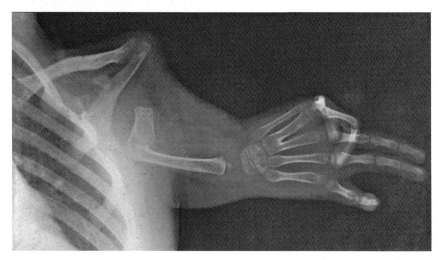

Figure 7.6 *Left arm of Case 3, with absent radius and hypoplastic thumb.*

Case 4

Case 4 was born in 1961 with tetraphocomelia. A photograph in infancy shows the extent of his reduction deformities (Figure 7.7). The similarity between this case and the baby on the cover of the book (a sketch by Goya) is very striking, and it illustrates the ability of thalidomide to mimic sporadic deformities.

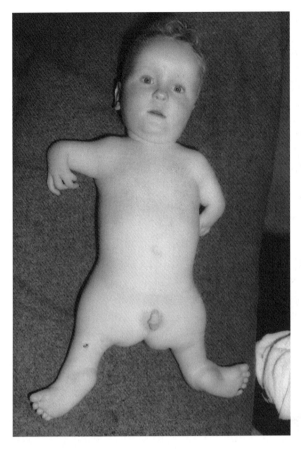

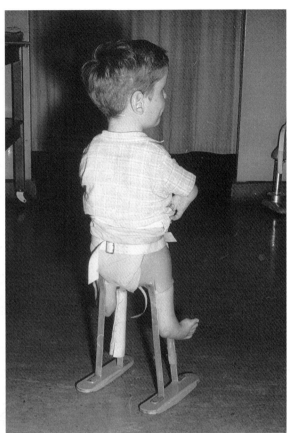

Figure 7.7 *Case 4 as an infant with tetraphocomelia.*　　　**Figure 7.8** *Case 4 learning to walk.*

This child learned to walk suspended by a sling attached to a rocking device which can be manoeuvred forward by swaying the trunk from side to side (Figure 7.8). The several reasons for inability to bear weight upon his feet are depicted in radiographs at the age of 10 years:

- The *foot is dislocated at the ankle* with inversion, causing the dorsal surface of the foot to present to the ground, while the plantar surface is uppermost (Figure 7.9). Within each lower leg is a single slender bone, which is difficult to identify, having mixed features of tibia and fibula. Orthopaedic surgeons christened such bones 'tibulae', in recognition of their conglomerate characteristics.

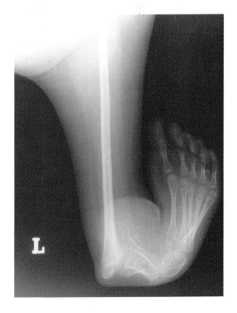

Figure 7.9 *Left leg of Case 4 at age 10 years: absent tibia and dislocated ankle. These features were bilateral.*

Figure 7.10 *Case 4 at age 10 years: absent acetabula, hips, proximal femora, and pubes. Absence of both tibiae.*

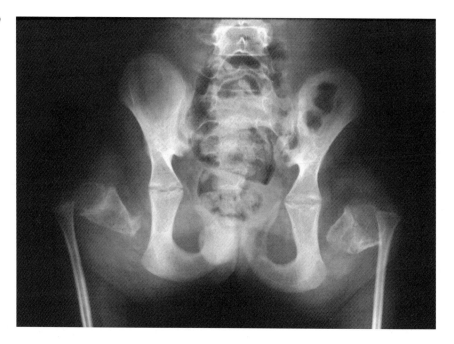

- *Absence of hip joints.* The most striking features of the pelvis are total absence of the hip joints and absence of the proximal three-quarters of both femoral shafts (Figure 7.10). Each femur is represented by a conical distal fragment bearing the distal epiphysis at its base. Articulation of the knee joint appears to be inadequate, with poor modelling of the femoral condyles and absence of the tibial joint surface. There is no evidence of formation of either femoral head or of either acetabular cavity. The lateral walls of the pelvis appear to be vertical, with a tendency to convexity at the site of the missing acetabular concavity. The horizontal rami of the pubes are incompletely formed, so that each obturator foramen is incomplete superiorly.

Absence of the hip joint, knee joint and much of the tibia and eversion of the ankle means that normal weightbearing would be impossible. When left to his own devices, this child shuffles about on his buttocks, swivelling from side to side on his ischial tuberosities. This unusual weightbearing activity may explain their apparent hypertrophy.

Upper limb radiographs are almost symmetrical (Figure 7.11). Both show hypoplasia of the scapula, with some reduction of its glenoid process. The humeral head is small and does not

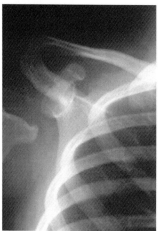

Figure 7.11 *Right arm of Case 4 at age 10 years: absence of radius and upper humerus; dislocated shoulder joint.*

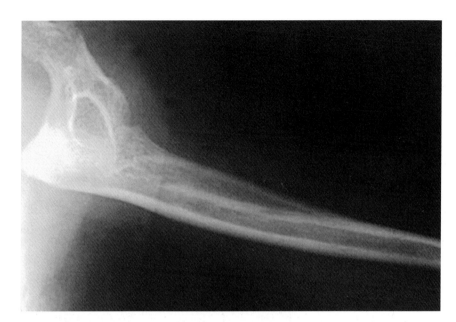

Figure 7.12 *Left arm of Case 4 at age 10 years: aplasia of proximal humerus; hypoplastic elbow; three radial cortices where radius and ulna are synostosed.*

approximate to the glenoid, with consequent dislocation. The humerus comprises a triangular block of bone, based at the elbow, where the bone modelling is consistent with incomplete formation of the distal end.

The right elbow joint is present, but it lacks the normal depth of concavity of the trochlear notch. On the left, there is partial fusion across the joint space. In both arms, the ulnae are relatively slender and the radii are absent distally. A modified radial head is visible, but this is incorporated, by fusion, within the proximal ulnar shaft. Further evidence of this fusion is the observation of three cortical surfaces converging into two in the midshaft. Thus the single forearm bone is a complex of radius and ulna (Figure 7.12).

Both hands are set at right-angles to the forearm in the clinical 'club-hand' position. Only four discrete carpal bones can be discerned in the right wrist, associated with three metacarpals and four digits, one of which is hypoplastic. Five carpal bones are present in the left wrist, plus four metacarpals and four digits. Both thumbs are absent.

Case 5

Case 5 was a boy aged 9 years, with amelia or total absence of the left arm (Figure 7.13). The left scapula and the lateral end of the clavicle were hypoplastic. The right arm was normal proximal to and including the metacarpals and thumb.

There was soft tissue fusion of the bases of the second and third digits (Figure 7.14). There was tapering of the distal ends of the

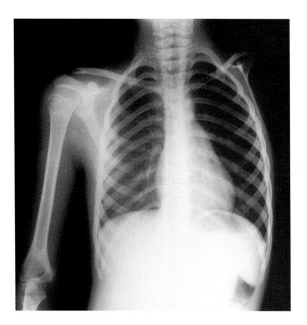

Figure 7.13 *Case 5: boy aged 10 years with left upper amelia.*

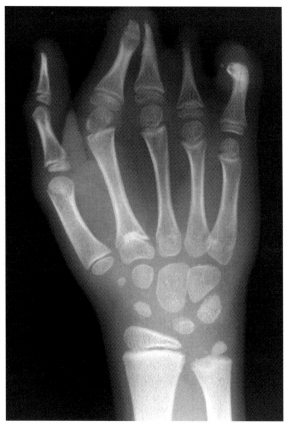

Figure 7.14 *Fused tapered fingers of right hand of Case 5.*

proximal phalanges, most marked in the third and fourth digits, which lacked both middle and distal phalanges. Short remnants of middle phalanges were present on the index and fifth fingers, which lacked terminal phalanges.

This child's mother mentioned that he had a soft lump over the lumbo-sacral spine. On examination, this had the clinical characteristics of a lipoma. An anteroposterior view of the lumbar spine showed spina bifida occulta at S1 and S2, deep to the lipoma (Figure 7.15). Above this, the arches of L5 and L4 were intact, but a second spina bifida occulta was evident at L3.

The right lower limb was normal. The left leg was normal as far as the forefoot. Distal to the metatarsals, the three medial toes were united by soft tissue fusion, and lacked distal phalanges. The proximal phalanges were tapered distally, similar to the appearance in the right hand.

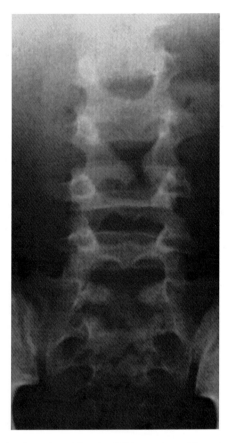

Figure 7.15 *Case 5: lumbar spine with spina bifida occulta at L3, and at S1, 2, with an overlying lipoma here.*

Method of analysis of the disease pattern

The radiographic features of each bone and each joint in the limbs of these five deformed children were summarized in tabular form (Tables 7.1 and 7.2). The abnormalities noted in each bone and joint could then be collated on the horizontal axis across the tables, to achieve a single statement concerning that bone or that joint.

These rather cumbersome data could be compacted again in a summary column in order to extract a general statement that would describe what the disease could do to any bone or any joint. This was done by listing all observations about all bones and all joints. Many observations were common to several bones or joints. All observations were included within the final two statements of what this disease did to bones and joints.

Table 7.1 Malformations in the upper limbs of five children (Cases 1–5)

	Case 4		Case 3		Case 5		Case 1		Case 2	
	Right	Left	Right	Left	Right	Left	Right	Left	Right	Left
Shoulder girdle	Hypoplastic		Hypoplastic	Hypoplastic	Normal	Hypoplastic	Normal	Normal	Normal	Normal
Shoulder joint	Hypoplastic Small glenoid, vestigial head, no humero-glenoid approximation		Hypoplastic No glenoid Tiny head		Normal	Absent	Normal	Normal	Normal	Normal
Humerus	Vestigial triangular block		Vestigial, fused to ulna in a hockey-stick-shaped combination		Normal	—	Normal		Normal	
Elbow joint	Shallow joint space	? Fused	Fused, no joint space		Normal	—	?Normal		?Normal	
Ulna	Hypoplastic		Hypoplastic		Normal	—	Short		Short	
Radius	Either absent or partly present and fused to ulna		Absent		Normal	—	Absent		Absent	
Wrist joint	'Club-hands' perpendicular to the forearm		Normal alignment of hand to forearm, but hypoplastic or fused bone components		Normal	—	'Club hands' perpendicular to the forearm		'Club hands' perpendicular to the forearm	
Carpal bones	3	5	2 Each row fused in parallel: 2 blocks	2	Normal	—	Not ossified		Not ossified	
Metacarpals	3	4	4 2 fused each side	5	Normal	—	4	5	5 1 hypoplastic	5
Digits	4	4	4	5	Phalanges: absent distal, fused or absent middle, tapered proximal	—	4	5	6	5½
Thumb	(1 hypoplastic) Absent thumbs		Thumb absent	Thumb hypoplastic			Thumb absent	Thumb hypoplastic	Thumbs hypoplastic	

Table 7.2 Malformations in the lower limbs of five children (Cases 1–5)

	Case 4 Right	Case 4 Left	Case 3 Right	Case 3 Left	Case 5 Right	Case 5 Left	Case 1 Right	Case 1 Left	Case 2 Right	Case 2 Left
Pelvis	Abnormal pelvis, abnormal horizontal ramus of pubis		Normal	Normal	Normal		Normal		Normal	Normal
Hip joint	Absent acetabula, no femoral head, no approximation of femur to pelvis		Normal	Normal	Normal		Normal		Normal	
Femur	Vestigial triangular block, apex proximal, and formed lower femoral epiphysis appears normal intrinsically		Normal	Normal	Normal		Normal	Short	Normal	
Knee joint	Poorly apposed		Normal	Normal	Normal		Normal		Normal	
Tibia	Absent		Normal	Normal	Normal		Normal		Normal	
Fibula	Slender, hypoplastic		Normal	Normal	Normal		Normal		Normal	
Ankle joint	Foot medially inverted in hook-shaped deformity, toes and plantar surface point superomedially		Normal	Normal	Normal		Normal		Normal	
Tarsal bones	Twisted relations as above		Normal	Normal	Normal		Normal		Normal	
Metatarsals	Normal		Normal	Normal	Normal		Normal		Normal	
Digits	Normal		Normal	Normal	Normal	3 fused toes, absent distal phalanges, tapered proximal phalanges	Normal		2 fused toes	Normal
Other anomalies	0		0		S1/2 spina bifida lipoma	L3 spina bifida occulta	Duodenal atresia		Probable ano-rectal agenesis	

Results

A summary of the effect of thalidomide upon the skeleton derived from radiographs is as follows.

Bones

The bones may be present and *normal*, or *absent* altogether. Between these two extremes, the bones may be *short* in length, *narrow* in width and *deformed* in shape. They are frequently *united* to their neighbour in parallel. They are sometimes *tapered*, and occasionally they are *duplicated* or *supernumerary*. The bones are not abnormal in texture or density. Both periosteal and epiphyseal bone growth appear to be intrinsically normal.

Joints

The involved joints are either *absent* altogether, or *underdeveloped* in size and shape, with poor articulation, *subluxation* or *dislocation*. *Absence* of the joint occurs if one or other component is missing, or when there is *fusion* of the two components. In either case, there is a basic *failure of formation* of the joint.

Analysis of this disease pattern

These two statements comprise a broad but accurate definition of the pattern or radiological spectrum of the disease process as observed in the limbs of five proven thalidomide cases. From the tables, information emerges concerning the distribution of this disease within the skeleton.

Upper versus lower limbs

For instance, in this small series, deformities predominated in the upper limbs. All five cases had upper limb defects, while four had lower limb abnormalities. Thus the ratio of upper to lower limb defects was 5:4.

Symmetry and asymmetry

The series displayed a tendency to left-sided defects in a ratio of 3:1 in those cases where there was asymmetry. Symmetry, or at least relative symmetry, was a striking feature of the condition. Absolute symmetry between left and right sides is unusual in nature. The concept of relative symmetry allows for a small range of differences between the two sides. This flexible approach to interpretation of symmetry was adopted in order to avoid the pitfalls of rigid definition, which have hampered attempts at classification. The process being sought was probably a confluent, continuous whole, rather than a series of subdivisions. One therefore attempted to remain sensitive to the merging and overlapping of the natural morphological variants through which the process was expressed. In these terms, it could be said that four of the five cases had relatively symmetrical defects in the upper limbs. The fifth case was asymmetrical, with absence of one arm and minor defects in the fingers of the other hand.

As far as the lower limb defects were concerned, the only case with gross reduction deformities of the legs was symmetrical. Two cases with abnormalities of the toes were asymmetrical. One case with slight shortening of the left femur was also asymmetrical. The overall tendency to symmetry was therefore 5:4. It cannot be said that this disease is always bilateral and/or always symmetrical. The presence of one case in five with gross difference between the two sides of the body indicates that asymmetry must be included as part of the spectrum of this disorder.

Predominant lesion

The most striking and frequent single radiological observation was *absence of the radius*, wholly or in part, associated with absence or hypoplasia of the thumb. Nine out of ten radii were missing in these five children, and nine out of ten thumbs were either absent or hypoplastic. Aplasia or hypoplasia of radius and thumb was the most common feature within the spectrum of the condition as defined.

Extent of the disease in the skeleton

These observations provided a concept of the boundaries of the *disease pattern* within the skeleton.

The visceral disorders were put aside at this stage, until some sense could be made of the skeletal disorders.

Discussion

Analysis of the predominant lesion was my first approach.

A 90% incidence of *aplasia or hypoplasia of the radius and thumb* was singularly impressive, even in a small series of five cases. This was too focal and too frequent to be an accidental phenomenon, and it implied an organization underlying the distribution of the disease.

What sort of disease might produce this distribution of bony deficiency? Was this an intrinsic disease of bone itself?

A radiologist presented with the pattern of an unknown pathology will at this stage seek to match it with that of a known disease. Pattern matching is employed by a radiologist throughout the working day, every time the images of a patient with an unknown disease are put up on the viewbox for analysis.

Basic patterns of bone diseases

Within the spectrum of bone diseases, certain typical *patterns of distribution* are recognizable radiologically:

Generalized

Bone disease may be *generalized*, affecting *all* bones (e.g. osteoporosis and other metabolic disorders). There was no abnormality of texture or density in bones adjacent to those that were hypoplastic or absent. The residual bones in the vicinity showed normal ossification, in spite of complete or partial obliteration of their neighbour.

- Thalidomide embryopathy did *not* present a generalized distribution.

Focal

Another recognized pattern of distribution of bone disease is that of abnormality in *particular zones* of the bone, such as the *epiphysis, metaphysis* and *diaphysis*. Many diseases, such as bone dysplasias, have these typical locations throughout the skeleton.

- Thalidomide embryopathy did *not* follow such an intrinsic, focal pattern of distribution.

Random

A third classical alternative is a *random* distribution of disease, where one bone (*monostotic*) or multiple scattered bones (*polyostotic*) are affected by disease. Metastases, Paget's disease and fibrous dysplasia exemplify this distribution. Within any collection of these cases with random distribution of disease, there is no repetition of involvement of particular bones, such as radius and thumb, as observed in thalidomide embryopathy.

- The distribution in thalidomide embryopathy was non-random.

Thalidomide embryopathy did not fit any of these three major patterns of bone pathology. This raised the possibility that it was not primarily a bone disease.

A primary mesodermal disease?

Non-appearance of a longitudinal row of bones was particularly curious. It was difficult to envisage a disease that repeatedly eliminated a longitudinal row of bones. If the pathology were of bony origin, an arrest of embryonic bone development would be unlikely to seek out the same sequence of bones repeatedly, unless there were some reason for this selection.

Subdivisions within bones. In Case 4, there was evidence that the head of the radius was still present and fused to the adjacent ulna. In four limbs in the series, the thumb was present, at least in part, but slender and hypoplastic. In other words, the pathological process was capable of eliminating either whole bones, or parts of bones, the parts being longitudinal strips of the original skeleton. It would be quite uncharacteristic of a primary disease of bone itself to eliminate longitudinal strips *within one* bone or *within a series* of bones such as radius, metacarpals and phalanges. This seemed even less likely when it can be observed from the radiographs that the section of bone that remains has normal trabecular structure, normal mineral density, and no evidence of previous disease within it.

No bone disease in the repertoire of radiology causes repeated elimination of a particular bone or a row of bones from the blueprint of the limb.

Perhaps this was not a bone disease at all. Perhaps the drug did not act upon the mesoderm of the embryo.

For these reasons, I began to doubt the assumption that thalidomide embryopathy was a mesodermal disease. I started to consider alternatives. I looked at anatomical systems in the limb that had a longitudinal layout.

A vascular disease?

Could a *vascular* disease in the embryo account for these findings? The embryonic blood supply to the limb buds is rich in anastomoses as the buds develop. Anastomoses are vessels that link up the main ones. They convert the early blood vessels into a net-like reticulation, with multiple links and bypasses. Anastomoses would mediate against infarction (death caused by blocked blood supply) of a distal part. Although the arterial supply to a limb is somewhat segmental in distribution, it is not absolutely segmental, because anastomoses, such as the arterial arcades that persist in the hand and foot, prevent the development of an end-organ relationship. Repeated elimination of radius and thumb, bilaterally, seemed unlikely to be explained on a vascular basis.

An abnormality of the nerves?

On the other hand, *peripheral sensory nerves* to the skin of the limbs are classically segmental in distribution. The pattern of neural segments related to the vertebrae and spinal cord is very ancient in evolutionary terms, and each primitive segment has the segmental nerve in its core. Blood vessels are usually intersegmental, i.e. placed between rather than within the neural segments. Furthermore, nerves classically maintain an end-organ relationship with their peripheral fields of supply and remain loyal to those areas of supply. The absent bones or bony parts seemed to fall into segments that might relate to the dermatome map of the arm.

An ectodermal disease?

Could the drug act on ectoderm rather than mesoderm?

In the absence of maps of the segmental sensory nerve supply of the skeleton, the maps of the skin segments or dermatomes could be consulted.

Dermatome subtraction?

Let us suppose that the 6th cervical dermatome and its underlying bone and muscle are subtracted from the arm (Figure 7.16). Then the remaining parts of the bones could be theoretically amalgamated into

Figure 7.16 *Theoretical subtraction of structures beneath the 6th cervical dermatome creates radial aplasia and absent thumb.*

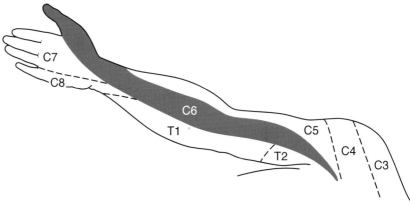

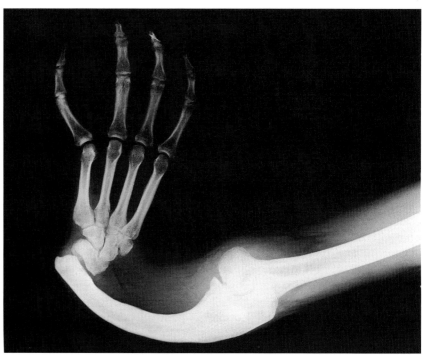

a residual arm that would have the morphology of radial aplasia. Thus the distribution of bone defects suggested the possibility of pathology in the cervical sensory nerves of the embryo as the explanation of radial aplasia. Nerves are of ectodermal, not mesodermal, origin.

That thalidomide acted upon the ectoderm, rather than on the mesoderm, needed to be considered.

Conclusion

Based on radiological evidence from an initial study of five cases, the following hypothesis was suggested:

1. The assumption that thalidomide acts upon the mesoderm is possibly incorrect.
2. Thalidomide-induced radial aplasia with absence of the thumb could be due to action of thalidomide upon the 6th cervical sensory nerve in the embryo.

CHAPTER 8

Verification of the disease pattern: Second radiological analysis (London)

Introduction

The thalidomide epidemic in Australia was limited to fewer than 40 children, now scattered across our large country. The five confirmed cases whose radiographs I had examined in Sydney had provided some insights into the nature of the disease. However, examination of a larger group was necessary, lest those five cases were for some reason atypical. During study leave in UK in 1972 and 1973, I was able to study radiographs of over 100 British thalidomide children at Chailey Heritage, Sussex, and at Queen Mary's Hospital, Roehampton.

Chailey Heritage, once a Victorian workhouse, provided residential, hospital and educational facilities for children whose disabilities were such that adaptation to normal home life was extremely difficult or impossible.

Attached to the general hospital, Queen Mary's Hospital at Roehampton, was the Department of Health Limb Fitting Centre, where limb prostheses could be reviewed and refitted as the children grew. The radiologists and clinicians at these two centres were most generous in their advice and cooperation with my study. Many of the British cases had complete sets of radiographs from birth to 11 years of age, and these were extremely valuable for tracing the effect of the disease upon development of bones, joints and epiphyses during childhood. I was allowed access to a meticulously maintained library of X-ray films of their thalidomide patients.

Materials

Fifty British cases were selected for the second analysis. All had been accepted for compensation, which required prima facie evidence of prescription, tablets, doctors' records, or that a panel of medical

Chapter Summary
- Introduction
- Materials
- Method of case selection
- Method of analysis
- Results
- Conclusion

reviewers had deemed the deformities to be consistent with thalido-mide embryopathy. There are considerable difficulties associated with the latter decisions in the absence of documentation, as described by Lenz,[1] the UK Ministry of Health[2] and Smithells.[3] It is outside the scope of this book, and of my own expertise, to discuss these decisions. For the purpose of radiological analysis, cases were included only if they had been accepted for compensation. This information, if not recorded in the notes, was provided by the clinicians in charge. I am particularly grateful to Drs Claus Newman and Ian Fletcher at Roehampton and Drs Algy Pearson and Philip Quibell at Chailey Heritage.

It has to be remembered that the total range of thalidomide embryopathy varied from minor defects of the digits to lethal complexes of multiple malformations. The present series has been drawn from a population of survivors whose defects were sufficiently severe to require continuous prosthetic care, or episodic hospital-ization, or even an institutional life. The sample is not typical of the entire population within the spectrum of the syndrome, because both extremes have been excluded, i.e. perinatal deaths, and survivors with trivial digital defects. However, the final collection of 50 is typical of the characteristics of the total cases inspected within that band of the disease.

Method of case selection

The only criterion for selection was that the radiographic exami-nation should include as much of the skeleton as possible. The object of this study was to review the whole skeleton in each case – not just those bones with obvious deformities. Some children with minor defects of the hands, for instance, lacked radiographs of the major long bones. These children were excluded in favour of others with more complete radiographic examinations. However, those with radiographs of all four limbs were frequently children with four-limb deformity – hence the clinical indication for more extensive radio-graphy. The effect of this criterion for selection has been to bias the sample towards major and multiple limb malformations, and to exclude minor or unilateral defects. In the absence of radiographs of other limbs, the clinical notes were scanned for information, and if the other limbs were stated to be normal then the clinical description was accepted and such children were also included.

Method of analysis

The X-ray films were examined, and a description of each bone and joint was tabulated in the same manner as described for the Australian cases.

Cases of amelia were treated as having absent bones and joints distal to the shoulder or pelvic girdle.

The term 'hypoplasia' was used in its most general and descriptive sense, i.e. underdevelopment of the part. The morphology of a hypoplastic bone or joint showed certain variations, which were repeated by other cases within the series. These shapes were described and sketched in tabular form, and will be discussed in detail below.

Tibia and fibula were sometimes difficult to identify with any degree of certainty, when a single long bone in the lower leg possessed some characteristics of both. Some bones could be called tibia or fibula with equally good reasons. In order to avoid double-counting, I made an arbitrary decision to call such solitary lower leg bones, of doubtful or composite identity, hypoplastic fibulae, because radiologically they seemed to have predominantly fibular features. This may have been an incorrect choice. At least 20 bones in this group were almost certainly fused composites of tibia and fibula, and could arguably have been counted as hypoplastic tibiae.

Results

Comparison of the results shown in Table 8.1 with the Australian results shows that the radiological features recorded in the five Australian cases are repeated in the larger British series, but in different proportions. The neuropathic pattern of disease was confirmed in this larger series.

In both series, the *bones* are absent, hypoplastic, frequently fused, sometimes tapered, and occasionally supernumerary. No abnormality

Table 8.1 Summary of results of British study

	Upper	Lower
Total number of limbs	100	100
Normal clinically or radiologically	15	38
Amelia	13	1
Hypoplasia of shoulder girdle or pelvis	70	13
Absent shoulder joint or hip joint	57	27
Elbow joint:		
Hypoplastic	39	
Fused	23	
Knee joint absent or dislocated		35
Radius absent or fused	61	
Tibia, fibula absent or fused		39
'Club-hand' deformity of wrist	48	
'Club-foot'		35
Absent thumb	56	
Triphalangeal or hypoplastic thumb	7	
Carpal bones fused in parallel	22	

of trabecular texture, mineral content or other intrinsic feature of bone is seen.

The involved *joints* are absent, hypoplastic, fused or dislocated.

The *most frequent abnormality* in this collection, as in the Australian one, was total or partial absence of the radius, recorded in 76% of cases. Associated with this was absent, hypoplastic or triphalangeal thumb in 69% of all cases. This complex is very striking in its frequency, and it confirms that the high incidence in the first five cases was not due to chance. Associated with this complex was a high incidence of hypoplasia of the shoulder girdle and humerus.

The *distribution* of abnormalities paralleled that in the Australian cases. There were 26 children with defects of upper and lower limbs, 18 with only upper limb defects and 6 with only lower limb defects. The ratio of upper to lower limb defects = was 44:32 = 1.37:1.

Symmetry was striking. There was no case of arm deformity on one side only, but this would have reflected my selection criteria, and could not be accepted as a characteristic component of thalidomide embryopathy. If the limb on the other side had not been X-rayed, and was not recorded as normal in the notes, the case was excluded. This would bias my series towards bilateral malformations. In some cases, there was considerable variation between the two sides, indicating variable degrees of asymmetry in the upper limbs in this selected case group. Two cases had films of one normal and one defective leg. Other lower limb defects were relatively symmetrical. *Thus, although symmetry was striking, there was evidence of both asymmetry and uni-laterality;* these apparent exceptions probably represented a larger proportion of actual cases in the whole disease because of sampling bias.

Conclusion

The findings in a series of 50 cases of thalidomide embryopathy in the UK supported the observations in the first five cases in Australia. The hypothesis that thalidomide acted upon the ectoderm (nerves) rather than the mesoderm (skeleton) was supported, not refuted, by analysis of a larger series.

CHAPTER 9

Congenital reductions of the radius

S ince defects of radius and thumb were the single most common abnormality in both series, and also in the medical literature on thalidomide embryopathy, it was essential to find out what was known about the underlying pathology of radial aplasia. The following is a review of the literature.

History

The clinical entity of congenital absence of the radius was first recorded in 1733. Thereafter, it received occasional mention in the 19th century medical literature. Numerous reports are to be found in 20th century journals. These have been reviewed and augmented by Kato,[1] Birch-Jensen,[2] O'Rahilly,[3] Riordan[4] and Heikel[5] prior to the thalidomide epidemic, and by Pardini[6] and Kelikian[7] subsequently. Many more cases caused by thalidomide are contained within series of cases of thalidomide embryopathy, in which, as we have just seen, radial defects were the most common presentation. Such cases are not separated from other thalidomide-induced birth defects in those series.

The advent of diagnostic radiology at the turn of the 19th/20th century provided anatomists and orthopaedic surgeons with anatomical information that was not previously available except by surgery or autopsy. Case reports, series and reviews thereafter included radiographic illustrations.

Definition and classification

Synonyms for congenital radial aplasia include radial ray defect, congenital absence of the radius, radial hemimelia, radial club-hand, radial meromelia, congenital defects of the radius, hypoplasia of the radius, radial hypoplasia, and reduction of the radius or radial reduction.

Chapter Summary
- History
- Definition and classification
- Aetiology
- Incidence
- Clinical features
- Associations
- Anatomy
- Bones and joints
- Muscles
- Arteries
- Nerves
- Pathogenesis
- Review of past theories
- Another theory: Is radial aplasia due to segmental sensory neuropathy of the 6th cervical nerve?
- References

Nuances of definition and individual preference for particular terms are irrelevant and distract from the fact that all belong to the same basic group of congenital malformations. The difficulty in achieving a universally satisfactory definition results from the inconstancy and variability of all features of the complex. Classification systems are beset by similar difficulties.[3,5] For the present purpose, the term 'radial reduction' will be used to include the possibilities of total absence, partial absence and hypoplasia of the radius. The radial defect is usually associated with absence or hypoplasia of the thumb and first metacarpal, and deviation of the remaining hand to the radial side at an angle with the ulna (radial club-hand). It may be associated with other anomalies of skeletal and other tissues listed later. The scaphoid and trapezium are typically absent, and the lunate and trapezoid are occasionally missing.[3] The second metacarpal and index finger are also occasionally absent or hypoplastic.

Aetiology

The cause of radial aplasia is unknown in most cases, apart from the thalidomide babies born in 1958–62. Genetic and environmental factors, if suspected, are seldom identified. Genetic factors account for less than 10% according to most authors. Pardini,[6] for instance, found only 5 of his 39 cases with any form of congenital malformation in the family, and he stated firmly that hereditary cases were uncommon, in spite of the popularity of genetic theory at that time. He drew attention to the complicated terms such as variable expressivity, variable penetrance and low penetrance, which are sometimes invoked to imply a genetic basis when genetic laws do not fit. He infers that such terms are:

> 'merely pegs on which to hang our hat of ignorance as to certain aspects of the mechanisms of human heredity'.

The cases of radial reduction in children whose mothers took thalidomide certainly illustrated a non-genetic, toxic, environmental aetiology. It has to be emphasized that the thalidomide victims started their intrauterine life with normal genes and chromosomes, and that the embryos were attacked by the drug between 21 and 42 days' gestation.

Other proven environmental factors include maternal riboflavin deficiency,[8] unstable diabetes and X-irradiation.[9]

Incidence

Before thalidomide, the incidence of congenital radial defects in the normal Danish population was estimated to be of the order of 1 in 55 000.[2] Since thalidomide, the general incidence worldwide has become more frequent. In 1972, Lamb[10] noted that this condition, which was previously a rarity in British orthopaedic practice, in the aftermath of thalidomide had become a not-uncommon surgical problem.

Clinical features

These depend on the degree of deformity of structures within the arm. The affected upper limb is shorter than normal – a constant feature of longitudinal reduction deformities of the limbs. The shoulder and upper arm may be normal or, less commonly, may be underdeveloped, with some restriction of movement. The elbow joint may be normal or limited in its range of flexion. The forearm is shortened, sometimes curved, and the wrist joint may show limitation of movement. In mild cases, there may be little or no deviation of the hand. In severe cases, the axis of the hand lies at right-angles to the axis of the forearm, or even at an acute angle so that the radial border of the hand touches the forearm, making a loop or hook at the wrist. Generally, the radius and thumb are affected together, but variants include cases where the radius is present but the thumb is absent, or the converse, where the radius is absent but the thumb is present. The affected thumb may be totally or partially absent, or present but hypoplastic or triphalangeal.

Associations

The following abnormalities have been reported in association with congenital radial aplasia: congenital heart disease, scoliosis, eye and ear defects, cleft lip and palate, polydactyly, ulnar defects, renal disease, aplastic anaemia, mental deficiency, tracheo-oesophageal fistula, oesophageal or laryngeal atresia, and agenesis of the lung.[11]

Anatomy

The anatomy of radial aplasia has been described by many investigators.[1,3–5,12–16] These reports and reviews present consistent findings in the arm, with a limited range of variation from case to case. Particularly valuable data, based on dissection, have been published by O'Rahilly,[3,15] Heikel,[5] and Skerik and Flatt,[16] and details may be found in their articles. Their observations are summarized here in order to derive an underlying pattern from the abnormal anatomy. Major rather than minor defects are included in the summary, using the paper of Skerik and Flatt[16] as the baseline.

Bones and joints

The capitate, hamate, triquetrum, and the four ulnar metacarpals and their phalanges are free from defects in almost all cases. The trapezoid, lunate and pisiform are normal in 90% of cases; when abnormal, they show fusion, underdevelopment and delay in ossification.

The remaining bones of the arm show some degree of abnormality in many cases. The *humerus* is typically shorter than normal, which is obvious in unilateral cases, where the normal limb can be used for comparison. In bilateral cases, the humeri may be equal in length, but still shorter than normal. If one side is more severely involved than the other, the humerus on the worse side tends to be shorter. The distal end of the humerus tends to be poorly formed, with absence or underdevelopment of the capitulum, coronoid fossa, intertubercular sulcus or medial condyle. The trochlea or olecranon fossa is usually shallow and poorly formed. The distal humeral epiphysis may show delayed or reduced development in relation to the severity of the radial lesion. The capsular ligaments of the elbow may be lax, but are more often tight, with limitation of flexion.

The *ulna* is commonly shorter and wider than normal. It is often curved, concave towards the midline of the body when the hand is pronated. The trochlear notch is shallow, and is sometimes dislocated posteriorly on the humerus. The olecranon process tends to be defective, and the coronoid process is frequently missing.

The *radius*, if not completely absent, may be partially absent. The residual proximal part varies in size and shape, either lying free or fused to the ulna. Sometimes, the proximal rather than the distal radius is absent. Some reports describe a fibrous band in place of the radius, not visible on radiographs, which provides attachment for some of the muscles that normally arise or insert on the radius.

The *scaphoid* is absent in the majority of cases. If present, it is said to be normal rather than fused to other carpals. The *trapezium* is frequently absent, and, if present, tends to be rudimentary. The *thumb and its metacarpal* are absent in 60–80% of cases. Less frequently, the thumb is rudimentary, with absence of the thenar eminence. Hypoplastic and triphalangeal thumbs are not unusual. The *wrist joint* is absent or underdeveloped, with no true joint cavity or articular cartilage, and the bones are bound together with tough fibrous tissue. Movement at the wrist joint is half the normal range. The interphalangeal joints also show limitation of movement.

The above anatomical description of the bones and joints correlates almost exactly with my own radiological analysis of the thalidomide victims' radial defects. Thus there is little or no difference in the pattern of radial defects whether due to thalidomide or to some other as-yet unknown cause.

The general pattern may be summarized as absence, hypoplasia or fusion of bones and joints, with partial absence or underdevelopment of parts of bones and joints and occasional dislocation.

Muscles

Dissections of post-mortem specimens show relatively constant anomalies of certain muscles. At the shoulder, the pectoralis major and the deltoid may be hypoplastic, be fused together or have abnormal insertions. The deltoid may be fused to the triceps. Hypoplasia of the deltoid allows the head of the humerus to sublux from the glenoid, and in such cases the acromioclavicular joint is prominent and angular. The biceps is frequently anomalous, being totally or partly absent or rudimentary, especially the long head. Its origin may be abnormal, and if it is present in radial aplasia, it inserts into the lacertus fibrosis. Muscles arising from the radial epicondyle of the humerus, the radius and the interosseous membrane are frequently absent, or confluent, or abnormally inserted, sometimes into the fibrous band lying in the line of the radius. Muscles that are commonly absent include the following: brachioradialis, extensor carpi radialis longus and brevis, extensor digitorum communis, extensor indicis, supinator, pronator teres, pronator quadratus, flexor and extensor carpi radialis, the thenar muscles, flexor and extensor pollicis longus, and abductor pollicis longus. When the thumb is missing, the muscles acting on it are also missing. Extrinsic tendons to the index finger may also be inserted abnormally. Muscles that are normally present are flexor carpi ulnaris, flexors digitorum sublimis and profundus, the hypothenar and interosseous muscles, and the lumbricals. Changes in these muscles are uncommon and are of minor degree.

Arteries

The radial artery is frequently absent, and, if present, it is small. The ulnar artery is usually present and normal in the forearm. The interosseous arteries are usually well developed, and sometimes replace the radial and ulnar arteries. The residual hand has an adequate blood supply.

Nerves

In 1963, Diezel,[17] a pathologist from Heidelberg University, examined the spinal cords and peripheral nerves of two deceased infants with radial defects due to thalidomide. There was no reduction in the anterior horn (motor neurons). Peripheral nerves tapered towards the periphery, with increasing distal loss of the myelin sheath and ribbon-like distensions of axoplasm. The changes were particularly marked in the radial nerves. Diezel added that this nerve damage might possibly be significant in the formation of radial defects, and may support the concept of a significant formative relationship between peripheral nerve fibres and the extremities.

Disturbances of the normal pattern of nerve supply may be profound, and extend proximally to the *root of the brachial plexus*, according to Skerik and Flatt.[16] They note that some of the main branches of the brachial plexus contain fibres from a higher cervical segment than normal. Plexus atrophy was described by Kato.[1] Schaeffer and Nachamofsky[13] described unusually large nerve trunks in their case.

The *axillary and ulnar* nerves are described as normal. The ulnar nerve may supply the entire flexor digitorum profundus, and may have a sensory distribution beyond its normal limits.

The *median* nerve is always present, but its termination is much more extensive than usual. It supplies the muscles of the anterior compartment of the arm that are normally supplied by the musculo-cutaneous nerve. The median nerve also provides both sensory and motor innervation to the structures normally supplied by the terminal branches of the radial nerve.

The *musculo-cutaneous* nerve is frequently missing, and, if present, it is anomalous and connected with the median nerve.

The *radial* nerve usually ends at the elbow after supplying the triceps.[1,4–6,14] *Its end fields (if present) are supplied by the ulnar and median nerves.*

Pathogenesis

The pathogenesis of congenital radial aplasia is not known. There are a number of theories in the literature.

Review of past theories

Before the advent of thalidomide, three main theories were extant, as summarized by Kelikian:[7]

- external compression or amniotic adhesions
- atavism
- focal deficiency or necrosis

External compression or amniotic adhesions

The first theory suggests that the embryo is deformed by external pressure or amniotic adhesions, both of which provide mechanical compression on the embryo or fetus and are postulated to prevent a certain part from forming. Forbes[14] regarded this theory as unlikely, because successive cases of radial aplasia have relatively uniform features, and are frequently bilateral. Apart from the difficulty in producing repeatedly similar and bilateral defects, 'it is almost impossible to conceive of extraneous pressure that could affect such a localised area' in a tiny embryo of 5 weeks' gestation (10 mm).[14]

Kelikian[7] noted that radial aplasia:

'pursues a distinct morphological pattern which cannot be expected to have been reproduced time after time by haphazard mechanical influences. Not uncommonly, radial ray deficiency is accompanied by a defective interventricular septum, which is well protected from external pressure.'

In short, the first theory does not explain the uniformity, bilaterality, or the associated defects, and it is therefore unsatisfactory as an explanation.

Atavism

The second theory of reversion to ancestral form, or atavism, had support from comparative anatomy. Gegenbaur[18] (quoted by Kelikian[7]) proposed the archipterigial theory, namely that the skeleton of vertebrate limbs evolved from the fin rays of dipnoan fish, the upper limb being based on the stem and four secondary rays of the pectoral fin. This theory fell out of fashion[14] in favour of more complex biological theories. Nevertheless, there may still be a fundamental truth in Gegenbaur's hypothesis. For instance, in the evolution of the primate hand, opposition of the thumb with the fingers is regarded as a late modification relating to tree dwelling and manual dexterity. Both Hughlings Jackson[19] in the English literature and Bretscher and Tschumi[20] in the German have suggested that recent evolutionary modifications are more susceptible to damage than the more ancient paw. Goodrich[21] stressed the constant relationship between the rays of the fishes' fins and the nerves supplying those rays. The second theory can explain to some extent the pattern, recurrence and bilaterality of the defect, but it cannot account for the associated defects, nor does it propose a mechanism by which the regression is achieved.

Focal deficiency or necrosis

The third theory is based upon Streeter's theory of focal necrosis.[22] Then Huxley and De Beer[23] proposed that the limb is polarized along the anteroposterior axis. Their postulate was based on the fact that the anterior portion of the limb disc always gave rise to the radius and thumb structures, even though it was grafted in abnormal orientation. They did not investigate the mechanism of this orientation.

O'Rahilly[15] combined Streeter's concept of focal necrosis with Huxley and De Beer's concept[23] of polarization to evolve a system of classification of congenital limb defects. He used radial hemimelia as an example:[15]

'Such defects are usually attributed to a site of focal deficiency, that is, an area where a congenital or hereditary malconstitution of the germ-plasm results in imperfect histogenesis. When this aberration of development affects the polarised limb-field before regional differentiation has occurred, a greater or lesser defect of a limb ray may result. The parts of the ray above and below the affected area may develop normally in some instances and an intercalary form of defect may be produced.'

O'Rahilly[15] established a system of classification that was in use until the 1970s, when it was replaced by a new classification based upon the analysis of thalidomide defects by Henkel and Willert.[24] Henkel and Willert showed that the intercalary defects were a spurious interpretation of anatomy. The concept of 'intercalary defects' was deleted from their classification. O'Rahilly did not explain either the nature of the polarization or the nature of focal deficiency. In another paper, he states:[3]

> 'Successive longitudinal development of the limb means that a compact area of "focal deficiency" (whatever that signifies and however it arises) at an early stage may thus be expected to result in a longitudinal type of defect, such as occurs in paraxial hemimelia under natural or experimental conditions.'

In his own words, O'Rahilly lays bare one part of the essential puzzle: What is focal deficiency and how does it arise? He does not answer this question, or the second one: What is the nature of the polarization of the limb? Both notions are constructs based on observations, but without any explanatory mechanisms.

The third theory, therefore, can be put aside for want of a mechanism. Furthermore, the theory of focal necrosis suffers from the same deficiencies as the theory of external compression. It cannot explain bilaterality. Why should two separated areas of the embryo undergo focal necrosis at the same time? It does not explain the few familial cases. Why should successive embryos be afflicted with similar focal deficiencies? Some genetic factor must be introduced to answer this, which adds a third variable to the other two. Again, focal necrosis fails to explain the association of radial aplasia with malformations of the heart, spine and other organs. It is possible to envisage multiple areas of focal necrosis in scattered parts of the embryo, but it is difficult to understand how the radial ray of the upper limb and the septum of the heart are affected together and so frequently. Of the British thalidomide cases with congenital heart disease, 90% had significant defects in the upper limbs.[25] Such a strong coincidence of random defects is a statistical improbability of the highest order. It is more probable that the linkage is a result of an orderly but still unrecognized underlying mechanism.

Another theory: Is radial aplasia due to segmental sensory neuropathy of the 6th cervical nerve?

The radial aplasia complex as described in the literature was reproduced, repeatedly, in thalidomide embryopathy. It was the most common limb defect in all large collections of thalidomide embryopathy on record, as well as in my own two initial studies. Therefore the unknown pathogenesis of radial aplasia was an open question and central to my investigation.

The simple idea that the absent structures lay beneath the 6th cervical dermatome was obviously a novel approach, which pointed to involvement of the sensory nervous system in embryogenesis. The idea certainly warranted further exploration.

References

1. Kato K. Congenital absence of the radius. *J Bone Joint Surg* 1924; **22**: 589–626.

2. Birch-Jensen A. *Congenital Deformities of the Upper Extremities.* Copenhagen: Munksgaard, 1949.

3. O'Rahilly R. Morphological patterns in limb deficiencies and duplications. *Am J Anat* 1951; **89**: 135–94.

4. Riordan DC. Congenital absence of the radius. *J Bone Joint Surg* 1955; **37A**: 1129–40.

5. Heikel HVA. Aplasia and hypoplasia of the radius: studies on 64 cases and on epiphyseal transplantation in rabbits with imitated defect. *Acta Orthop Scand Suppl* 1959; **39**: 1–155.

6. Pardini AG. Radial dysplasia. *Clin Orthop* 1968; **57**: 153–77.

7. Kelikian H. *Congenital Deformities of the Hand and Forearm.* Philadelphia: WB Saunders, 1974.

8. Warkany J, Nelson RC. Skeletal abnormalities in the offspring of rats reared on deficient diets. *Anat Rec* 1941; **79**: 83.

9. Warkany J, Schraffenberger E. Congenital malformations induced in rats by roentgen rays. *AJR Am J Roentgenol* 1947; **57**: 455.

10. Lamb DW. The treatment of radial club hand. *Hand* 1972; **4**: 22–30.

11. Warkany J. *Congenital Malformations: Notes and Comments.* Chicago: Yearbook Medical Publishers, 1971.

12. Stoffel A, Stumpel E. Anatomische studien uber Klumphand. *Z Orthop Chir* 1909; **23**: 1–57.

13. Schaeffer J, Parsons J, Nachamofsky LH. Some observations on the anatomy of the upper extremities of an infant with complete bilateral absence of the radius. *Anat Rec* 1914; **8**: 1–14.

14. Forbes G. A case of congenital clubhand with a review of the aetiology of the condition. *Anat Rec* 1938; **71**: 181–99.

15. O'Rahilly R. Radial hemimelia and the functional anatomy of the carpus. *J Anat* 1946; **80**: 179–83.

16. Skerik SK, Flatt AE. The anatomy of congenital radial dysplasia: its surgical and functional implications. *Clin Orthop* 1969; **66**: 125–43.

17. Diezel PB. Morphological changes in experimental thalidomide neuropathy and thalidomide-induced deformities of the extremities. *MMW Kongresse und Vereine* 1963; **45**: 2265.

18. Gegenbaur C. Zur morphologie der gliedmassen der Wirbelthiere. *Morph J* 1876; **2**: 396–420.

19. Jackson J Hughlings. Evolution and Dissolution of the Nervous System. The Croonian Lectures, delivered at the Royal College of Physicians, London, 1884.

20. Bretscher A, Tschumi P. Gestufte Reduktion von chemisch behandelten *Xenopus*-Beinen. *Rev Suisse Zool* 1951; **58**: 11.

21. Goodrich ES. *Studies on the Structure and Development of Vertebrates.* New York: Dover, 1958.

22. Streeter GL. Focal deficiencies in fetal tissues and their relation to intrauterine ablation. *Carnegie Inst (Wash)* 1930; **414**(22): 1–44.

23. Huxley JS, De Beer GR. *Elements of Experimental Embryology.* Cambridge: Cambridge University Press 1934; 223–4.

24. Henkel H-L, Willert H-G. Dysmelia: a classification and a pattern of malformation in a group of congenital defects of the limbs. *J Bone Joint Surg* 1969; **51B**: 399–414.

25. Ministry of Health Reports on Public Health and Medical Subjects No. 112. *Deformities Caused by Thalidomide.* London: HMSO, 1964.

CHAPTER 10

Congenital dislocation

The radiographs of each child in this study included serial X-ray examinations over a decade. The observations presented in this chapter and the next were made from the chronological series of examinations, with particular attention being paid to the process of joint formation over time.

In general, the radiological features of the joints ranged from normal through various degrees of hypoplasia to complete absence of joint formation. Absence of a joint took two forms: either dislocation or fusion (synostosis). Dislocation is examined in this chapter and synostosis in the next.

Aim

1. To summarize the radiological features of congenital dislocation of joints, and thus to define the pattern.
2. To compare these features with those of dislocated joints in adults who have suffered longstanding sensory peripheral neuropathy such as Charcot's or neuropathic joints.[1] This is an exercise in pattern matching.

Materials

The radiographs of Australian and British children with thalidomide embryopathy were used to define the pattern of joint dislocation. Radiographs of adults with neuropathic osteopathy were available in the Film Library of the Department of Radiology, Royal Prince Alfred Hospital, Sydney, Australia. The illustrations are composed of these library films, compared with radiographs of appropriate joints from the series of five Australian children. Mr Brian Magee and the Department of Clinical Photography, Royal Prince Alfred Hospital are thanked for assistance with photography and preparation of illustrations, which are reproduced here with permission from *The Lancet.*

Chapter Summary
- Aim
- Materials
- Method
- Results
- Analysis of underlying pathological process
- Conclusion
- References

I also wish to acknowledge the assistance in 1972 of the late Professor Sir Howard Middlemiss, Professor of Radiology at Bristol, UK, then President of the Royal College of Radiologists. He and I used his collection of radiographs of neuropathic bones and joints in African lepers for a second pattern-matching exercise in 1972, comparing them with my films of thalidomide-affected joints in Australian children. Our first discussion of embryonic neuropathy as the underlying mechanism of the embryopathy in general and of the dislocated joints in particular convinced him that my interpretation was correct. He commented that this was the first time radiology had shown the site of pathology of a disease before the pathology was established.

Definition

Congenital dislocation of a joint was defined, for the present study, as absence of any evidence of a parallel alignment of articular bone surfaces, both bones being present and separate. This was observed to be due to total or partial absence of the ends of the bones that would normally form that joint. Some thalidomide children had synostosis or congenital fusion of joints instead of, or as well as, congenital dislocation.

Aetiology and pathogenesis

Thalidomide exposure in utero is the aetiology in these children. The pathogenetic mechanism is unknown.

Pathology

The pathology underlying congenital joint dislocations and fusions is unknown.

Incidence

The incidence of joint abnormalities in the limbs of 50 thalidomide victims from Chailey Heritage, Sussex, and Queen Mary's Hospital, Roehampton, analysed in 1972, was as shown in Table 10.1.

Method

1. Analyse the radiology to deduce the disease pattern.
2. Compare this pattern with adult neuropathic joints.

Radiology of congenital dislocations

Observations were made about aspects of skeletal growth: the epiphyses, periosteal growth, bone density and mineralization, trabecular

Table 10.1 Incidence of joint abnormalities in thalidomide victims from Chailey Heritage and Queen Mary's Hospital

	Percentage
Upper limb	
Hypoplastic shoulder girdle	70
Absent or dislocated shoulder joint	57
Hypoplastic elbow joint	39
Fused elbow joint	23
Fused carpal joints	22
Club-hand deformity of wrist joint	48
Lower limb	
Hypoplastic pelvis	13
Absent or dislocated hip joint	27
Absent or dislocated knee joint	35
Hypoplastic or dislocated ankle	35

structure, and final size and shape of individual bones involved in the dislocated joints.

Epiphyses (growth plates)

Abnormalities of epiphyseal ossification and growth were closely involved with the final morphology of the joint. Observations of epiphyseal development were as follows.

Absence of epiphyses. Where, by the age of 10–12 years, a joint was completely absent (either fused or dislocated), it was noted that epiphyses had never appeared in serial films. This was commonly the case in the elbow joint and the hip, the former resulting in fusion and the latter in dislocation. The end-result could be predicted from the radiographs of the hips in infancy. For instance, a flat lateral pelvic wall with total absence of any acetabular notch in the infant meant that no femoral head would appear, and no hip joint would form. In such cases, absence of the femur and acetabulum ensured dislocation (see Figure 7.10). On the other hand, any sign of a notch or a small acetabular cavity in the infant signalled the presence of an unossified cartilaginous femoral capital epiphysis. This would ultimately ossify and become visible on X-ray, but the process of ossification was delayed in commencement and reduced in volume. A hypoplastic hip joint would result.

Delayed epiphyseal ossification. Delay in appearance of ossified epiphyses was common at an affected joint. Where one limb was more hypoplastic than its fellow, epiphyseal ossification was more delayed and the epiphysis was hypoplastic on the more deformed side.

Epiphyseal growth. In many instances, the epiphyses were abnormal in shape or size, with some degree of asymmetry between the two sides of the body. However, within limitations of this distortion in size and shape, bone growth from the epiphyseal line had taken place normally during the decade.

Radiological observations not related to the epiphyses

Apart from the epiphyses, certain other features of the joints and the bones comprising them require comment.

Periosteal bone growth of the shafts of long bones. This appeared to be normal over the 10-year series, again allowing for initial reduction in the size or shape of the whole bone.

Bone density. This was normal in most instances, indicating that bone mineralization was normal. Occasional cases showed sclerosis of bone ends within dislocated joints.

Trabecular structure within the bones. This was normal in all cases. There was no evidence of disorder of osseous tissue.

Size of component bones. The size of residual bones forming the dislocated joint varied from total absence through different degrees of hypoplasia. All were reduced in length to some degree. Rarely, the appropriate bone appeared to be absent altogether in radiographs of infants before cartilage ossification identified their presence. Later films usually disclosed epiphyseal ossification, which allowed an appropriate long-bone fragment to be identified. Reduced bone growth from the metaphyseal side of such small epiphyses resulted in correspondingly hypoplastic long bones that failed to form a normal articulation (see the femora in Figure 7.10).

Shape of component bones. The shapes of residual bones comprising a dislocated joint were also variable. Reduction in size was always associated with some abnormality of shape. Some short residual long bones seemed completely irregular (e.g. the humerus in Figure 7.12). Others were tapered to a point. Tapering of bone ends was a recurrent feature. Phalanges and metacarpals or metatarsals showed distal tapering (see Figures 7.14). The tibia was repeatedly tapered distally away from the knee, pointing towards the ankle. In contrast, the femur and humerus were characteristically tapered proximally, away from the knee or elbow and pointing towards the hip or shoulder (see e.g. Figures 7.2 and 7.10–7.12).

The most common femoral defect was the malformation known as proximal femoral focal dysplasia, where the proximal end had failed to form, and the residual distal shaft segment formed a triangle based at the knee (see Figure 7.10).

On the other hand, the long bone sometimes terminated suddenly with a transverse or oblique cut-off, short of the joint articulation (see Figure 7.6). A strong similarity to surgical amputation was evident in such cases. Occasionally, when there were two fragments of the bone shaft, there was a false joint or pseudarthrosis between the bone ends.

Pattern of malformations in thalidomide embryopathy

The radiological changes found in thalidomide embryopathy are summarized in Table 10.2.

Table 10.2 Summary of radiological changes in thalidomide embryopathy

Bones
- Absent altogether
- Short
- Sometimes tapered
- Fused in parallel

Joints
- Absent altogether
- Hypoplastic
- Dislocated
- Fused in series or parallel

Skin
- Surface area reduced over short limb
- 'Dermatome' loss?

Summary of disease pattern

In summary, affected joints in thalidomide embryopathy may be *absent, hypoplastic, fused* or *dislocated.*

Involved bone ends may be *absent, hypoplastic, deformed, tapered* or terminated *transversely.*

Bone density and trabecular pattern are *normal* in the majority, with *sclerosis* in some cases. *Pseudoarthrosis* is a rare feature.

This is the pattern of the disease process in thalidomide embryopathy. Does this match any known disease in adults?

A similar pattern exists in Charcot's joints, otherwise known as neuropathic arthropathy (where the joints are disorganized because of diseased nerves).

Radiology of adult neuropathic arthropathy (Charcot's joints)

The following review is to introduce the non-medical reader to the clinical entity of neuropathic arthropathy.

Definition

The term 'Charcot joint' or 'Charcot's joint' was originally coined to designate the destructive joint changes found in the presence of and related to the neuropathy of tabes dorsalis. The condition is now called 'neuropathic arthropathy'.

It was first described in 1868 by the French neurologist Charcot,[1] who recognized the association of painless dislocation of joints with syphilitic patients in the Hôpital Salpetrière in Paris (Figure 10.1). Charcot's conclusions were the more remarkable because they preceded the advent of X-rays, and his clinical observations were confirmed by post-mortem dissections (Figure 10.2).

Other synonyms for the condition include neurotrophic arthropathy, neuropathic joint and neuroarthropathy. The term 'Charcot's joint' has been adopted for similar changes found in other disease entities with sensory neurological abnormalities, such as diabetes, syringomyelia, leprosy, vitamin B deficiency, spina bifida, cauda equina lesions, surgical cordotomy, cervical ribs and congenital indifference to pain.[2] The relative incidence of these causes varies with the particular population surveyed. A number of reviews and case reports have been published.[2–13]

Clinical features

Clinical presentation of joint disease is generally but not always late in the course of the sensory neuropathy – for example 10 years or

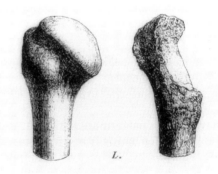

Figure 10.1 *Neuropathic bone – humerus, from Charcot's* Lectures on Diseases of the Nervous System *(1881).[1] The head of the affected humerus on the right has disintegrated. Normal humeral head on left for comparison.*

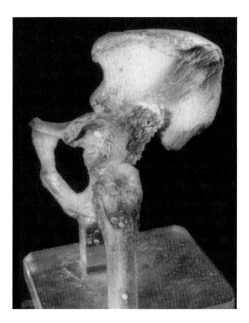

Figure 10.2 *Neuropathic hip joint: both sides have been destroyed. Acetabulum and femoral head have disintegrated. The hip joint no longer articulates.*

more after the initial sensory symptoms. Painless swelling of the joint, with recurrent effusion, is the classical symptom. However, pain, swelling and instability of the joint are also common presentations.[2] Ulceration of the skin is a less frequent finding. The joints of the lower limb are more frequently affected than those of the upper limb, although this distribution varies with the aetiology. Similar joint changes occur in the spine.

Charcot's joints respond poorly to surgery. Attempts to fuse these disorganized unstable joints generally fail.[14,15] Eichenholtz[2] quotes a review of 43 operated cases in the literature, in which only 33% of attempted arthrodeses succeeded. His own 15 attempts at fusion procedures had all failed. He advocated rigid internal fixation, together with prolonged external support and avoidance of weight-bearing until after firm radiological fusion, but even these measures could not ensure success.

Pathology

The skeletal pathology in neuropathies is mainly secondary to damaged sensory nerve supply. Trauma or infection may also be present, and will generate additional features.

The histopathology in bone reflects degeneration of all elements about the joint.[2] In addition to joint effusion, the ligaments, capsule and synovium are infiltrated by oedema, round cells and fibroblastic proliferation. Elastic fibres are scarce or non-existent. The thickened synovium contains areas of haemorrhage and islands of dead bone and dead or living cartilage, as evidence of degeneration of the articular cartilage. Subchondral bone is usually grossly necrotic, fragmented and avascular.

Radiology

Radiological signs of neurotrophic arthropathy are subtle and easily missed in the early stages, although late signs are pathognomonic. Eichenholtz[2] described the evolution of a Charcot joint as 'a logical and usually predictable sequence of changes' when followed by serial radiographs. He described three stages based on X-ray observations of 68 patients.

The *first* stage, of *development*, is characterized by early *breakdown of joint surfaces*. Radiologically, *debris* is seen to be forming, usually beginning at the articular margins. Synovial biopsy at this stage will demonstrate microscopic evidence of bone and cartilage *debris embedded in synovium, which is pathognomonic of the disease*. This proceeds to *fragmentation* of subchondral bone and its articular cartilage, with *effusion*, capsular distention and resultant *subluxation and dislocation*.

The *second* stage, of *coalescence*, is characterized by *absorption* of much of the fine debris, and union of the larger fragments, which then *fuse to adjacent bones*. As a result of disrupted vascularity from the previous disorganization, the ends of the bones tend to become dense and white, termed 'sclerotic'. Bone sclerosis is a classical sign of ischaemia, or reduced blood supply to bone.

The *final* stage, that of *reconstruction*, is marked by revascularization of the bone ends, and *reversal* of the previous *sclerosis*. The bone ends become more rounded, with some attempt at *reformation* of the joint architecture.

In established cases, *disorganization of the joint* is the most characteristic description. Murray and Jacobson[14] stress that whatever the pathological sequence of events, the common denominator is the presence of a *fracture* or fractures (usually *subarticular*), and these become *more numerous, progressing to joint disorganization*. Murray and Jacobson[14] state that a striking feature is the almost complete absence of juxta-articular bone atrophy, i.e. the bone density tends to be *normal* rather than osteoporotic. (This rules out the presence of infection in the bone, because the hyperaemia or increased vascularity caused by active inflammation always induces juxta-articular osteoporosis in the affected joint.)

Occasionally, a *fracture of the shaft of a long bone* occurs. These *fail to unite*, leaving a *pseudarthrosis*.

Extensive absorption of bone causes gross *deformities* in the residual bones, with *tapering* of bone ends[8,16] and abrupt *transverse cut-off* in some cases. Bone absorption may be so extreme that certain bones whittle away, with *disappearance* of the associated joints. This is most obvious in leprosy, where whole digits may absorb, disappear, and give an appearance similar to amputation.

Summary

In summary, neuropathic bones and joints in adults manifest the following signs: destruction of articular cortex, fragmentation, partial or total absorption of subarticular bone, destruction, and disorganization of the joints. Bone fragments may absorb or fuse to one another and to neighbouring bones. Effusion, capsular distention, subluxation and dislocation are typical. Adjacent bone density is either normal or sclerotic. Destruction and absorption leave deformed bone ends that fail to remodel, and are often tapered, shortened and even transversely 'amputated'. Pseudoarthrosis may follow fractures, and failure of surgical fusion is characteristic.

Comparison of congenital dislocation with Charcot's joints

The radiological signs of thalidomide embryopathy and those of adult neuropathic bones and joints were compared. The analogy is illustrated in Figures 10.3–10.8.

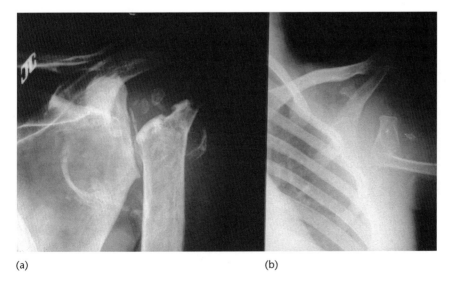

(a)   (b)

Figure 10.3 *(a) A woman with syringomyelia has a neuropathic (Charcot's) shoulder joint. (b) Thalidomide child's shoulder joint. Both show dislocation, with shearing-off of the joint surfaces. The only difference is the bony debris in the adult, resulting from destruction of a formed joint. The infantile joint has failed to form.*

Figure 10.4 *Charcot's hips. (a) An adult with neuropathic destruction and dislocation of hip due to tabes dorsalis. (b) A thalidomide infant with failure of formation of hips and dislocation of both hips and both knees.*

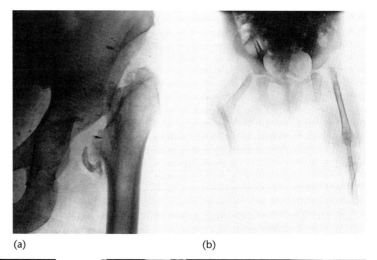

(a)   (b)

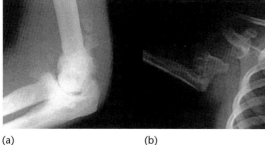

(a)   (b)

Figure 10.5 *(a) Shallow eroded neuropathic elbow joint in syringomyelia. (b) Thalidomide arm with shallow hypoplastic trochlear notch. The adult has bony debris; the child does not.*

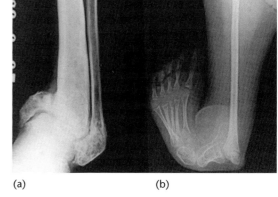

(a)   (b)

Figure 10.6 *(a) Neuropathic ankle in tabes dorsalis: recurrent fractures and malformation of ankle mortise with subluxation and inversion. (b) Thalidomide: absent tibia, ankle subluxation and inversion.*

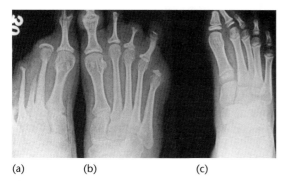

(a)   (b)   (c)

Figure 10.7 *(a, b) Feet of aboriginal leper. (c) Thalidomide child's foot. Tapering and absence of the phalanges are common to both.*

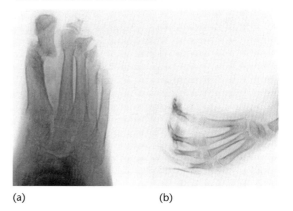

(a)   (b)

Figure 10.8 *(a) Diabetic foot with bony fusion of 1st metacarpophalangeal joint. (b) Thalidomide hand with fusion of each row of carpals and bases of 2nd and 3rd metacarpals.*

Results

Table 10.3 summarizes the extraordinary similarities in the two diseases.

Table 10.3 Comparison of radiological features in adult sensory peripheral neuropathy and thalidomide embryopathy

	Adult sensory peripheral neuropathy	**Thalidomide embryopathy**
Bones	Spontaneus amputation	Absent altogether
	Shortened	Short
	Deformed	Deformed
	Often tapered	Sometimes tapered
		Fused in parallel
Joints	Bone destruction	Absent altogether
	Dislocation	Hypoplastic
	Ankylosis (leprosy)	Fused in series or in parallel
Skin	Loss of sensation	Surface area reduced over short limb
	Trophic ulceration	
Process	Destruction of formed adult bones, joints and skin	Failure of formation of embryonic bones, joints and skin
Cause	Sensory peripheral neuropathy	?

Analysis of underlying pathological process

In adult neuropathy, the essential process can be expressed as *destruction of previously formed tissues*, i.e. of formed bones, joints, skin and soft tissues. In the embryo, the process could be expressed as *failure of formation* of embryonic bones, joints, skin and soft tissues. Both processes can be interpreted as *failure of organized growth* – either failure of organized repair (maintenance growth) in the adult or failure of organized primary growth in the embryo. This concept of failure of organized growth provides a denominator of pathogenesis that is common to the two conditions.

On this basis, a new possibility for a common pathology and pathogenesis arises. The adult condition is known to be caused by sensory peripheral neuropathy. The cause of the embryopathy is unknown, except that the mother took a sensory neurotoxic drug (thalidomide) in early pregnancy. If the two conditions are analogous, as the radiological comparison indicates, then 'embryonic sensory peripheral neuropathy' should be the cause of these congenital dislocations. The site of pathology in the embryo should be sought in the embryonic equivalent of the sensory neuron, namely the neural crest.

Failure of organized repair, or maintenance growth, is the neurotrophic component of adult Charcot's joints. Failure of organized primary growth at a precursor stage of embryonic bones and joints is proposed as the defect of neurotrophism underlying congenital Charcot's joints. Thus both adult and embryonic dislocations are expressions of failure of the normal neurotrophic, growth-provoking stimulus.

Conclusion

Thalidomide induces congenital neuropathic joints in the newborn, consistent with a neuropathic process in the early embryo.

References

1. Charcot JM. *Lectures on Diseases of the Nervous System* (Translated and edited by G Sigerson). London: The New Sydenham Society, 1881 (Republished New York: Hafner, 1962).
2. Eichenholtz SN. *Charcot Joints*. Springfield, IL: CC Thomas, 1966.
3. Hodgson JR, Pugh DG, Young HH. Roengenologic aspects of certain lesions of bone: neurotrophic or infectious? *Radiology* 1948; **50**: 65–71.
4. Martin MM. Diabetic neuropathy: a clinical study of 150 cases. *Brain* 1953; **76**: 594–624.
5. Paterson DE. Radiological bone changes and angiographic findings in leprosy with special reference to pathogenesis of atrophic conditions of digits. *J Fac Radiol* 1955; **7**: 35.
6. Paterson DE. Bone changes in leprosy, their incidence, progress, revention and arrest. *Int J Leprosy* 1961; **29**: 393.
7. Harris JR, Brand PW. Patterns of disintegration of the tarsus in the anaesthetic foot. *J Bone Joint Surg* 1966; **48B**: 4–16.
8. Gondos B. Roentgen observations in diabetic osteopathy. *Radiology* 1968; **91**: 6–13.
9. Norman A, Robbins H, Milgram JE. The acute neuropathic arthropathy – a rapid severely disorganising form of arthritis. *Radiology* 1968; **90**: 1159–64.
10. Schwartz G, Berenyi M, Siegel MW. Atrophic arthropathy and diabetic neuritis. *AJR Am J Roentgenol* 1969; **106**: 523–9
11. Sinha S, Munichoodappa CS, Kosak GP. Neuroarthropathy (Charcot joints) in diabetes mellitus (clinical study of 101 patients). *Medicine* 1972; **51**: 191–210.
12. Campbell WL, Feldman F. Bone and soft tissue abnormalities of the upper extremity in diabetes mellitus. *AJR Am J Roentgenol* 1975; **124**: 7–16.
13. Kraft E, Spyropoulos E, Finby N. Neurogenic disorders of the foot in diabetes mellitus. *AJR Am J Roentgenol* 1975; **124**: 17–24.

14. Murray RO, Jacobson HG. *The Radiology of Skeletal Disorders*. Edinburgh: Churchill Livingstone, 1971.

15. Murray RO. Congenital indifference to pain with special reference to skeletal changes. *Br J Radiol* 1957; **30**: 2–6.

16. Spillane JD, Wells CEC. *Acrodystrophic Neuropathy: A Critical Review of the Syndrome of Trophic Ulcers, Sensory Neuropathy and Bony Erosion, Together with an Account of 16 Cases in South Wales*. Oxford: Oxford University Press, 1969.

CHAPTER 11

Congenital synostosis

Another characteristic of the thalidomide syndrome was con-genital fusion or synostosis of bones and joints. This demanded explanation.

How do two bones come to be joined to one another? How is it that major joints, such as the elbow, fail to form, leaving a compound block of bone at the site of the joint? How do joints form in the embryo, and how could a drug stop the process? The answers to many of these questions could reasonably be sought in the literature on embryology. Embryological facts should be applicable to congenital synostosis as observed in the radiographs. The object of the next exercise was to correlate the radiology of synostosis of joints with the known embryology of the limbs, and to search for processes that might become deranged during the course of joint development.

Chapter Summary
- Radiology
- Embryology
- Discussion: the timing of the injury
- Conclusion
- References

Radiology[1]

Definition

Congenital fusion or synostosis is defined as an embryological fault whereby two or more structures that are normally separate are united at birth. This applies to soft tissues (e.g. horseshoe kidney) and to the skeleton (e.g. syndactyly, fusion of ribs or vertebrae, and other synostoses). Although union of bones and joints was a common finding in thalidomide embryopathy, it generally took place between structures that were also reduced in size and altered in shape. When part of a bone had failed to form, the remainder was frequently united to an adjacent bone. Fused joints united deformed bones, and were part of the structural abnormality.

Incidence and types

In the English series of thalidomide children, the most frequent sites of fusion in the skeleton were as shown in Table 11.1. Congenital

Table 11.1 Sites of fusion in the English thalidomide children, 1972

Elbow joint	22%
Radius and ulna	26%
Carpal bones	25%
Tibia and fibula	20%

fusion was more common in the upper than in the lower limbs. Fusion was never observed in the shoulder joint, hip joint or ankle. These joints, when abnormal, showed dislocation rather than fusion.

Borrowing a classification from physics, two types of congenital fusion were seen: in series and in parallel.

Fusion in series was the union of bones lying in a linear series within a limb (e.g. humero-ulnar fusion).

This always entailed absence or hypoplasia of a major joint. Figure 11.1 is an example where humerus and ulna are united into a bone shaped like a hockey stick or a hunting boomerang, with absence of any joint space for the elbow. This was the most common morphology of elbow fusion in the second thalidomide series.

Fusion in parallel occurred when two or more parallel bones were united en bloc instead of lying separately. It is therefore seen below the elbow and below the knee, where bones are in pairs or multiples. Fusion in parallel did not always involve obliteration of a joint.

Figure 11.2 shows union of proximal radius and ulna, with three cortical surfaces tapering into two in the mid forearm.

Figure 11.3 shows fusion in parallel of carpals, of metacarpals and of phalanges. The 2nd and 3rd metacarpals are fused at their bases without involving a joint space, while the four carpal bones in each row are united into single blocks, with elimination of intervening

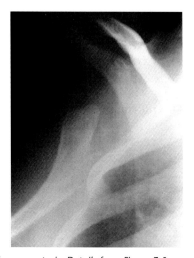

Figure 11.1 *Humero-ulnar synostosis. Details from Figure 7.5.*

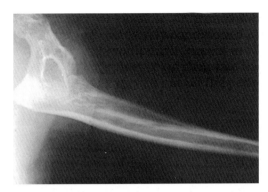

Figure 11.2 *Radio-ulnar synostosis, with three cortical surfaces. The head of the radius is present, but fused to the ulna.*

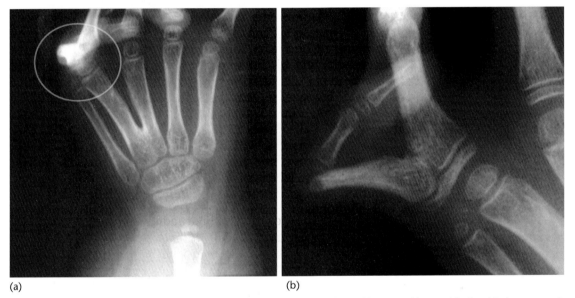

(a)   (b)

Figure 11.3 *Multiple Synostoses. Detail from Figure 7.6. (a) Each row of carpal bones and bases of 2nd and 3rd metacarpals. (b) Fusesd epiphyses of proximal phalanges of index findger and triphalangeal thumb.*

joint surfaces. There is fusion of the epiphyses of the 1st and 2nd proximal phalanges and partial fusion of the adjacent metaphyses. Associated with this, the soft tissues are fused between the proximal parts of the first two digits (index finger and triphalangeal thumb).

Fusion in parallel was most common between radius and ulna (Figure 11.4). It could involve the proximal and/or distal ends of radius and ulna, or their entire lengths. This deformity was at times ambiguous, for it could equally well be interpreted as absence of radius or ulna. However, it was significant that the residual single bone of the forearm was generally shorter and *wider* than either normal radius or normal ulna should have been, which indicated an addition of bone mass to the normal shaft. In shape, such a bone might bear some resemblance to both radius and ulna, with morphological landmarks especially at its ends. It could be interpreted as a morphological complex of elements of both bones. Sometimes,

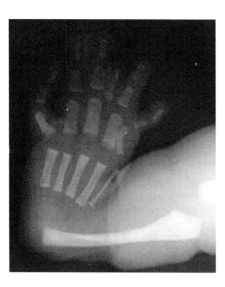

Figure 11.4 *Radio-ulnar fusion with triphalangeal thumb and polydactyly of the 3rd and 4th fingers, which are fused by soft tissues (syndactyly).*

evidence of three cortical surfaces supported the impression of fusion of the two forearm bones, as already illustrated. Both the olecranon and the radial head are discernible, but are united (Figure 11.2).

In the lower leg, fusion in parallel of the tibia and fibula was a frequent observation. The proximal epiphysis was frequently tibial in character, but the shaft was fibular in position and too slender to be tibia. The distal end bore the mortice of the tibial side of the ankle joint, as well as a lateral (fibular) malleolus, giving the same bone a compound identity. Orphopaedic surgeons dealing with these children had christened this complex bone the 'tibula' (Figure 11.5).

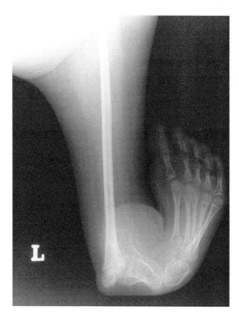

Figure 11.5 *'Tibula' with dislocated ankle joint. The foot is intact.*

Embryology

Any acceptable interpretation of the radiographs of congenital limb malformations should correlate with the known embryology of the limbs. The timetable of chondrogenesis and osteogenesis has a profound bearing on the radiology of congenital synostosis. The embryology of the upper limb is reviewed briefly here. The lower limb undergoes similar development, but lags behind the upper limb in time.

In the human embryo,[2,3] the forelimb buds first appear at *gestational day 28*, the end of the 4th week of life, as lateral bulges of undifferentiated mesenchyme arising from the trunk lateral to the somites. Figures 11.6 and 11.7 are views of the 28-day human embryo provided by Professor H Nishimura of Kyoto from his collection of thousands of dated human abortuses. The spinal nerves are seen penetrating into the limb buds as soon as they are formed.[3,4] This observation will be discussed in detail in Chapter 15. Figure 11.8[3] is a diagram of the cranial and spinal ganglia from a 28-day embryo, with sensory nerves developing in advance of the limb bud itself.

Figure 11.6
Normal 28-day embryo: posterior view. The upper limb buds are emerging from the trunk. (Courtesy of Professor H Nishimura.)

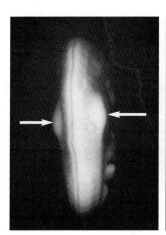
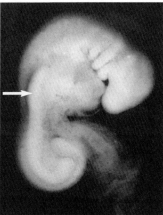

Figure 11.7 *Normal 28-day embryo: lateral view. (Courtesy of Professor H Nishimura.)*

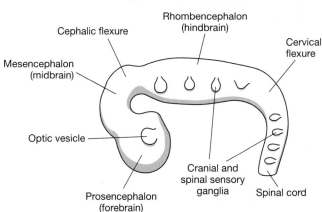

Figure 11.8 *Cranial and spinal ganglia in a 28-day embryo. (After Langman J. Medical Embryology. Baltimore: Williams and Wilkins, 1969.[3])*

At *37 days' gestation*, the human embryo measures *10 mm* and the upper limb now has three visible divisions, as shown in Figure 11.9. Dissection of the sensory nerves of a 10 mm human embryo late in the 5th week of gestation (Figure 11.10) illustrates that the structure of the peripheral nervous system is already well advanced, while the upper limb bud is still a primitive paddle in its external appearance.

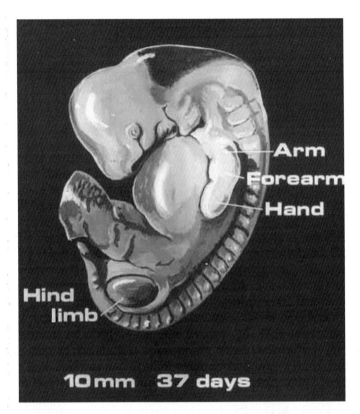

Figure 11.9 *Upper limb in a 37-day human embryo. (From Hamilton WJ, Mossman HW.* Human Embryology. *Cambridge: Heffers/Baltimore: Williams and Wilkins, 1972.[2])*

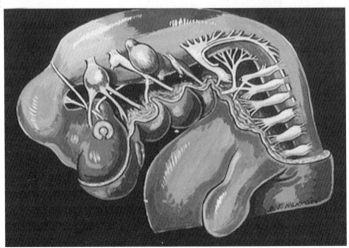

Figure 11.10 *Dissection of a 10 mm human embryo to show advanced development of peripheral nerves while the limb bud is a primitive paddle. (From Hamilton WJ, Mossman HW.* Human Embryology. *Cambridge: Heffers/Baltimore: Williams and Wilkins, 1972.[2])*

Within the limb bud early in the 5th week, mesenchymal condensations become evident at the sites for the future shafts of the major long bones. The limb buds elongate in a caudal direction, and by the end of 5 weeks the buds have become paddle-shaped appendages, as shown in Figure 11.9.

At 5 weeks, the first differentiation of cartilage takes place in the core of the mesenchymal condensations, marking the sites of the central shafts of the long bones. Thus, as early as the end of the 5th week, the humerus, radius and ulna may be separately identified by their individual cartilage centres.

It should be noted that, despite the primitive structure of the limb buds, the peripheral nervous system is comparatively sophisticated in its development relative to the limb bud at this stage. In addition to the above microdissection, a transverse section of human embryo at 5 weeks shows well-developed spinal ganglia with peripheral nerves extending into the mesenchyme of the limb bud.[2] Figures 11.10 and 11.11 show a human embryo at 10 mm, or 37 days. The joints form soon after chondrogenesis begins. The zone of undifferentiated mesenchyme between the primary cartilage centres is flexible, and breaks down into a thin cleft for the joint space.

During the 6th and 7th weeks, the cartilage centres of the long bones enlarge and elongate, until they become recognizable hyaline cartilage models of the future bones. The cartilage model of each bone is clad in a layer of dense *neurovascular* mesenchyme or *perichondrium*.

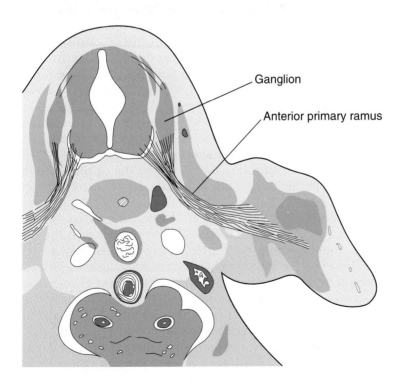

Ganglion

Anterior primary ramus

Figure 11.11 *Transverse section showing nerves in the limb bud mesenchyme in a 10 mm embryo. (Adapted from Hamilton WJ, Mossman HW.* Human Embryology. *Cambridge: Heffers/Baltimore: Williams and Wilkins, 1972.[2])*

The perichondrium of the midshaft develops osteogenic properties (i.e. becomes *periosteum*), and osteoblasts arising from its inner layer start to produce a delicate cylinder of compact bone encircling the midshaft. At about the same time, a vascular bud arises from the inner layer of the periosteum and erupts into the centre of the shaft, carrying with it cells destined to become chondroclasts and osteoblasts. The former break down the primary cartilage, while the latter manufacture layers of bone on the residual cartilage strands. Thus bone is formed at the site and in the shape of the cartilage model originally laid down.

Discussion: the timing of the injury

Let us consider the problem of fusion of the elbow joint. Figures 11.1–11.4 represent suitable examples for discussion, the first two showing the most common elbow morphology in the thalidomide series, and the final two showing some detail of the trabecular structure.

What do these radiographs tell us of the timing of the embryonic error underlying the deformity? We can work backwards from ossification at 8 weeks in search of the origin of synostosis.

In the first place, primary pathology of bone can be dismissed as a cause. The bone density and internal trabeculation are perfect. There are no radiological stigmata of primary bone dysplasia, or of intercurrent bone disease. Ossification appears to have progressed normally, but within an already-abnormal shape. In normal embryological development, the shape of the bone to come is already dictated by the shape of the cartilage model. The conclusion is that the cartilage precursor was already abnormal in shape before ossification commenced, and before the invasion by the vascular bud. This places the embryological error earlier than 8 weeks, and is consistent with the thalidomide-sensitive period (21–42 days' gestation). As well as the timing, the normal bone density also makes a vascular lesion unlikely. Vascular interruption causes ischaemia, and ischaemic bone is always dense. Except at some bone ends as already mentioned, increased bone density was rare in thalidomide embryopathy.

So the insult predated ossification and damaged the cartilage model or its precursor. What had caused the abnormal shape of the cartilage model?

Several possibilities need consideration. Perhaps a cartilage disease such as a destructive arthritis could have intervened between the 5th and 8th weeks. Some types of septic arthritis in adults can repair with joint fusion. However, the radiographic evidence was against this, for there was no scar of any pathological destruction of joint elements, or of repair processes. In the absence of evidence, it seemed unlikely that fusion was a sequel to embryonic arthritis. The radiographs showed no evidence of any joint space within which an arthritic process might have occurred. On the contrary, the bony cortex was smooth and continuous across the site of the joint, with no sign of a diseased articular cortex or articular cleft. Uninterrupted continuity of normal trabeculae in the medullary bone at the anticipated site of the joint also indicated that no embryonic cleft had ever formed. This placed the embryonic error at least in the 5th week, prior to normal cleft formation. A further probability arose as a natural extension of this. Perhaps no zone of intermediate flexible mesenchyme had ever existed. This meant that a single cartilage precursor for all three long bones had arisen from a single centre of mesenchymal condensation where three separate centres are normally found. This possibility would place the embryonic error very early in the 5th week, prior to the earliest condensation of mesenchyme, long before cartilage appears.

Experimental evidence in rats supports the last suggestion. Warkany and Schraffenberger[5] examined the histology of elbow joints in early rat embryos with radiation-induced congenital fusion. They described absence of the intermediate zone of mesenchyme, and continuity of cartilage across the joint site.

Since the essential abnormality appears to be an error in organization of the centres for mesenchymal condensation, an organizer tissue would be the most likely target for the drug.

What organizer tissue is present in the limb bud early in the 5th week? At that stage, the forelimb bud consists of a mass of undifferentiated mesenchyme covered by ectoderm. The latter is thickened at the tip of the bud, into an apical ectodermal ridge (AER), and many scientists believe that the AER has an organizing function. However, this cannot be assumed to be the site of action of thalidomide until all other tissues within the undifferentiated limb bud have been considered, including small blood vessels and nerves. Of the tissues present in the limb bud at that time, the peripheral nerves are the most highly differentiated, far in advance of skeletal structures. Nerves are well recognized as organizers of other tissues.[6]

Clinical evidence from Nowack's study[7] of the 'sensitive period' in thalidomide embryopathy agrees with my deduction of the approximate timing of the error, but pinpoints the time of the injury as closely as was possible from mothers of over 80 confirmed thalidomide babies. Nowack established that malformations of the arms followed maternal ingestion of the drug from day 24 to day 33 of embryonic life (in the 4th and 5th weeks). The timing of the thalidomide injury was 4 days before the appearance of the upper limb bud at day 28, even earlier than I had been able to deduce from the radiological evidence. Not only does the embryonic injury precede mesenchymal condensation in the limb bud, but Nowack's study establishes the fact that congenital fusion is caused by damage inflicted before the limb bud itself exists.

Conclusion

A radiological analysis of congenital fusion of joints corresponds to the timetable of their embryonic development, and shows that fusion is certainly determined before chondrogenesis, when the mesenchymal cells of the limb bud are still undifferentiated and not yet condensed into centres for each bone. The error is timed to be before or during the appearance of centres of mesenchymal condensation, i.e. earlier than the 5th week of gestation. According to embryology textbooks, the peripheral neurons are present and more advanced in development than other cells in the limb buds prior to 35 days' gestation (5th week). This is circumstantial evidence that nerves are present at the time of the injury and could be implicated in the pathogenesis of congenital fusion.

Deductions from the radiographs[1] (to ascertain the advent of congenital joint fusion) coincide with the 'thalidomide-sensitive period'. Nowack's clinical evidence[7] goes further, and pinpoints the time of thalidomide intake by the mother as even earlier than can be deduced from the X-ray films; congenital joint fusion was determined by thalidomide injury incurred before the limb bud was present.

References

1. McCredie J. Congenital fusion of bones: radiology, embryology and pathogenesis. *Clin Radiol* 1975; **26**: 47–51.

2. Hamilton WJ, Mossman HW. *Human Embryology*. Cambridge: Heffers/ Baltimore: Williams and Wilkins, 1972.

3. Langman J. *Medical Embryology*. Baltimore: Williams and Wilkins, 1969.

4. Dyck PJ, Thomas PK, Lambert EH. *Peripheral Neuropathy*. Philadelphia: WB Saunders, 1975.

5. Warkany J, Schraffenberger E. Congenital malformations induced in rats by Roentgen rays. *AJR Am J Roentgenol* 1947; **57**: 445–63.

6. Drachman DM, ed. Trophic Functions of the Neuron. *Ann NY Acad Sci* 1974; **228**.

7. Nowack E. The sensitive phase for thalidomide embryopathy. *Humangenetik* 1965; **1**: 516–36.

CHAPTER 12

The hypothesis of neural crest injury

'He who desires to philosophise must first of all doubt all things . . . and must proceed according to the persuasion of an organic doctrine which adheres to real things, and to a truth that can be understood by the light of reason.'

Giordano Bruno (1548–1600)

The next two chapters introduce the neural crest – the embryonic precursor of sensory and autonomic nerves. Its anatomy and biology are reviewed in the light of its potential to be the target organ for thalidomide and thus the anatomical structure and mechanism, injury to which underlies many birth defects.

On 9 February 1974, the *Medical Journal of Australia* published as its leading article my paper outlining the hypothesis of neural crest injury as the pathogenesis of congenital malformations.[1] It shows the extent to which I had developed the concept of neural crest injury by September 1973, when the paper was written.

Editorial

The paper was accompanied by an editorial entitled 'The pathogenesis of congenital malformations'.[2] Concerning thalidomide in 1961, the editorial says:

'In his original letter McBride indicated that the abnormalities to which he referred were present in the structures developed from mesenchyme.

'After a further lapse of 12 years Janet McCredie, a radiologist, using X-ray findings from some of McBride's cases, published a most interesting radiological review of 5 cases of thalidomide embryopathy and supported the findings with a summary of 50 similar children in Britain. The hypothesis was put forward that the site of teratogenic action is on the neural crest and its derivatives and that the resulting reduction deformities of the limbs represent embryonic peripheral neuropathy. Quite striking radiological evidence was adduced to indicate that the changes seen in the babies were very similar to the trophic complications of sensory peripheral neuropathy revealed in adults suffering

Chapter Summary
- Editorial
- Summary
- Introduction
- Limb growth and the sensory neuron
- The neural crest and its migration
- Embryonic neuropathy – a hypothesis of neural crest injury
- A new concept of reduction deformities
- Supporting evidence
- Conclusion
- References

from diabetes, tabes dorsalis, leprosy and acrodystrophic neuropathy. The idea was proposed that in an embryo of about three weeks if any injury to its primary nervous system developed, the trophic action of the neuron would be destroyed. The unformed nerve of the embryo would fail to develop, and there would be consequent failure of development of bone, joint and skin supplied by that nerve. The focus of attention was shifted away from the mesodermal cells to the central neurons of ectodermal origin, specifically those in the neural crest and its derivatives. It was thought that the mesodermal effects which occurred as part of the development of the deformities were secondary to the neural crest damage.

'On page 159 of this issue, Janet McCredie has taken this hypothesis much further. She puts forward the view that injury or defect of the neural crest and its derivatives is in fact the basic primary lesion sustained by the fetus and that this may consti-tute the underlying mechanism of congenital deformities in general. It is postulated that the destruction of the "trophic" action of the developing neuron will produce all sorts of reduction deformities and that these may not be confined to the limbs but could involve any of the paired structures which normally meet in the midline. The palate, the spinous processes, the septa of the heart and even the circular growth of the components of the hollow viscera could be affected in this way.

'This is an arresting hypothesis . . .'

This chapter is a minor modification of the original paper,[1] but with no literature updates that might alter its context.

Summary

Radiological analysis of the limb deformities of thalidomide children reveals evidence of a sensory neuropathic process. Based on this, a hypothesis of neural crest injury is suggested as the underlying patho-genetic mechanism of many congenital malformations. Using a simple concept of four different modes of growth in the embryo, the hypothesis can explain both skeletal and visceral deformities. Experimental and pathological evidence is presented in its support, and a rational approach to congenital defect syndromes is suggested.

Introduction

The typical manifestations of thalidomide embryopathy were described by Lenz[3] in 1962 as:

'defects of the arms, amelia, atypical phocomelia with absence of thumbs and other fingers as well, aplasia of the radius, defects of the long bones of the legs, especially femora and tibia, absence of the auricles, haemangiomata of the nose and upper lip (wine spot variety), atresia of the oesophagus, the duodenum or the anus, cardiac anomalies and aplasia of the gall bladder and of the appendix.'

Subsequent reports[4] of other associations include anophthalmia and microphthalmia, microtia, abnormalities of the ossicular chain, aplasia and hypoplasia of the otic vesicle, cranial nerve palsies, micrognathia, cleft palate, choanal atresia, spina bifida, meningo-myelocoele, bilobed right lung, genitourinary anomalies, and mal-rotation of the intestine.

During the assessment of thalidomide children for compensation in 1971–72, I was asked to review their radiographs, because some cases were thought to be atypical in age or in clinical features. I was asked whether it was possible to distinguish radiologically between thalidomide and non-thalidomide deformities. There was very little literature on the radiological appearance of these cases, and this question proved impossible to answer. However, I became fascinated by the recurrence of certain deformities within the series. In particular, radial aplasia in four out of five children seemed too frequent to be accidental, and too focal to be acceptable on radiological evidence as a generalized bone disease. It suggested to me the possibility of absence of a dermatome and its underlying bone and soft tissue, and therefore an ectodermal rather than a mesodermal lesion. Based on this observation, I undertook a radiological survey of some of the British children with thalidomide-induced defects during my study leave in the UK in 1972. I reached the conclusion that the radiological signs in their bones were analogous with the trophic skeletal changes in adult sensory peripheral neuropathy and that the deformities could be interpreted as sensory peripheral neuropathy occurring in the embryo.[5,6] Based on this new interpretation of the radiology,[5,6] I proposed the hypothesis that the mechanism of action of thalidomide, hitherto unknown, is on the neural crest and its derivatives, which would link the wide range of abnormalities encountered in the syndrome. I have reviewed some of the literature dealing with aetiology, pathogenesis and the unknown pathology of each mal-formation – not only thalidomide-induced, but of other and unknown cause. This search has revealed sufficient evidence for the proposal of a more general hypothesis to apply to many congenital malformations whose aetiology is not understood. A presentation of the hypothesis, enlarged beyond thalidomide embryopathy, and an outline of some of the supporting evidence, is given in this chapter.

Limb growth and the sensory neuron

The role of the nervous system in the growth of limbs was studied by Singer[7] in 1943, when he investigated the well-known ability of certain amphibians and reptiles to grow a new tail or limb after amputation. Singer established that the limb would regenerate only if the peripheral sensory nerve was intact. If the sensory ganglion was destroyed, the limb failed to regenerate. He concluded that the sensory neuron possessed a 'trophic', or growth-stimulating, quality, essential for limb regeneration.[7,8]

The neural crest and its migration

The sensory ganglia are derivatives of the neural crest of the embryo. This important tissue lies in two strips, one on each side of the neural groove. With the formation of the neural tube, the neural crest migrates to its dorsolateral aspect, and segmentation in this position creates the sensory ganglia of the spinal and some of the cranial nerves.[9–12] In addition to forming the sensory ganglia, neural crest cells also differentiate into sympathetic neuroblasts, Schwann cells, pigment cells and meninges, and take part in the cartilage formation of the face and spinal canal.[10,12] Figures 12.1 and 12.2 trace the

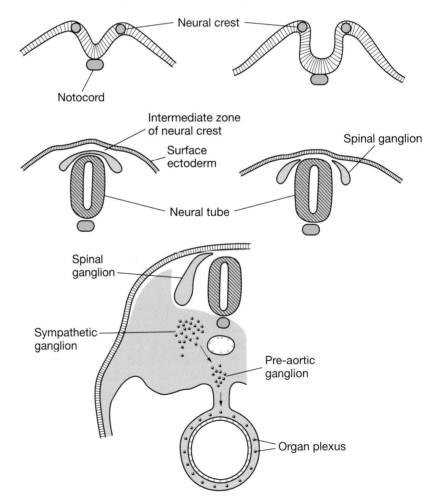

Figure 12.1 *Neural crest development. (After Langman J. Medical Embryology. Baltimore: Williams and Wilkins, 1972.[11])*

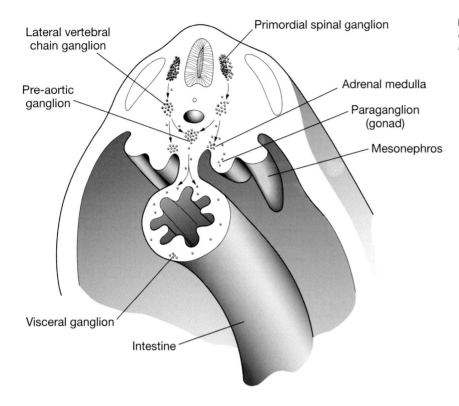

Lateral vertebral chain ganglion

Primordial spinal ganglion

Pre-aortic ganglion

Adrenal medulla

Paraganglion (gonad)

Mesonephros

Visceral ganglion

Intestine

Figure 12.2 *Three-dimensional representation of neural crest development.*

development and migration of the spinal neural crest in forming both the sensory peripheral nervous system and the autonomic nervous system. They show how neural crest cells ultimately migrate to form autonomic ganglia both centrally and distally within the walls of the organs that they supply.

Embryonic neuropathy – a hypothesis of neural crest injury

It is proposed that:

1. An embryo may suffer an injury to its neural crest by a chemical or physical neurotoxic agent.
2. The injury stops the normal migration or axon sprouting of neural crest cells and/or destroys their trophic action.
3. The result is failure of growth of the tissues subtended by that segment of the neural crest.
4. The organ or limb involved is therefore small, or reduced in size at birth.

This hypothesis can be applied to limbs or appendages, to structures that meet in the midline, to cylindrical organs, and to solid organs of the body, as summarized by the following concept.

A new concept of reduction deformities

Limbs

The term 'reduction deformities' is used to describe congenitally short limbs, i.e. limbs that have failed to grow to their destined length. In terms of the limbs, it is a simple concept, for limbs are outward appendages of the trunk, and when short they are obvious to all in their deficiency.

Figure 12.3(a) shows the normal development of the limb, subject to the trophic influence (arrow) of the embryonic sensory neuron. In Figure 12.3(b), embryonic neuropathy has damaged the normal migration, axon growth and/or trophic action of the neural crest (loss of arrow), and the normal limb has failed to form.

What of other body structures, which do not project as obvious appendages, but are nevertheless subject to similar trophic influence and are destined to reach certain points in the anatomic scheme?

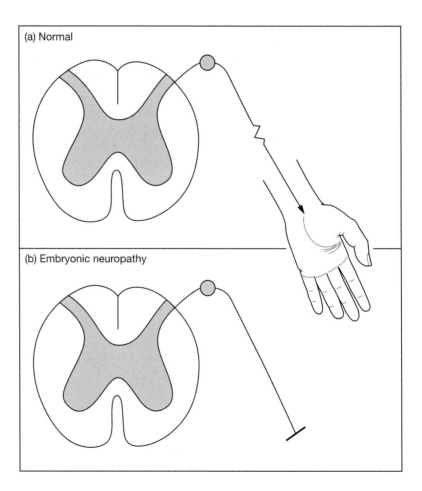

(a) Normal

(b) Embryonic neuropathy

Figure 12.3 *(a) Role of neural crest in normal limb formation. (b) Neural crest injury stops limb growth.*

Midline structures

A number of paired structures are intended to meet one another and fuse in the midline. The palate, for instance, is intended to form by union of two processes, and when this normal growth is halted, a cleft remains. This can be conceived as a reduction deformity, a reduction in length of the palatal process towards the midline. Another midline reduction deformity is spina bifida. Normally, the laminae and spinous processes are supposed to meet and fuse in the midline posteriorly. Impeded growth results in foreshortening of each process, failure to meet in the midline and failure to fuse. Such short unfused processes can also be considered as reduction deformities in terms of their normal growth.

Figure 12.4 illustrates structures that meet in the midline. Subject to normal trophic activity of the neural crest (arrows in Figure 12.4a), the anterior and posterior midline structures meet and fuse normally in the midline. Posteriorly, the spinous processes of the vertebral arches unite. Anteriorly, the palate, the septum between trachea and oesophagus, the septum between rectum and bladder or vagina, and the anterior wall of the trunk attain normal length, and fuse normally. In Figure 12.4(b), damage to the embryonic neural crest has interfered with the migration, axon sprouting or trophic action of the crest (loss of arrows), so that structures are reduced in length, and fail to reach the midline. Posteriorly, this results in spina bifida. Anteriorly, reduction deformities resulting from this are cleft palate, tracheo-oesophageal fistula, gastroschisis, midline hernias, recto-vesical fistula and ectopic bladder.

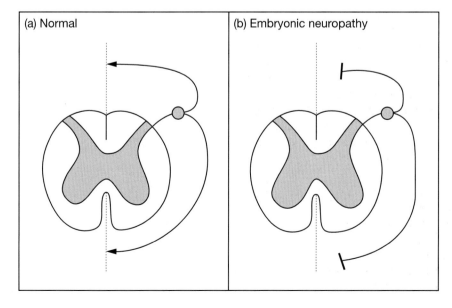

Figure 12.4 *Influence of neural crest on structures that meet in the midline. (a) Normal. (b) Neural crest injury stops growth from reaching the midline.*

Septal defects of the heart can also be regarded as reduction deformities if considered from the point of view of failure of the septum to grow to its normal length. In remaining reduced in length, the septum is left open.

Tubular structures and solid organs

Organs such as blood vessels or the gastrointestinal tract are basically cylinders. A cylinder enlarges by increasing the diameter of its lumen through cell division around the circumference. That is, length and diameter enlarge by growth of the circle.

Reduction in circular growth within a segment would leave a stenosis or atresia in the normal cylinder. Hence the gastrointestinal atresias and stenoses, coarctation of the aorta, and other congenital vascular stenoses can be classed as reduction deformities.

Most solid organs can be considered as spheres, expanding outwards in their normal spherical mode of growth. The eye is an example, and a reduction deformity of the eye would be incomplete expansion (e.g. microphthalmos or anophthalmos).

Coloboma, or failure of closure of the fetal fissure of the eye, is another reduction deformity. The circular growth of the uveal tract is incomplete, with a persisting fissure in the iris and other uveal structures. Agenesis and hypoplasia of kidneys, liver or spleen are different degrees of reduction deformity when looked at from this point of view.

Figure 12.5 illustrates cylindrical growth and spherical growth. The migration of neural crest cells around the normal organs is depicted by the black spots. Absence of neural crest cells in a segment is demonstrated on the right. The tubular organ fails to enlarge within that segment, with resulting stenosis. The best-known example of this is Hirschprung's disease, where the pathological defect is demonstrable absence of autonomic ganglia in the stenotic segment. I believe that this pathological lesion would be found also in many oesophageal, duodenal and other intestinal stenoses, although (as far as I know) it has not been recorded. Coarctation of the aorta is possibly of similar pathology.

Spherical growth is subject to neural crest influence. This is depicted in the lower section of Figure 12.5. Lack of migration or failure of trophic action of neural crest causes cessation of development. Anophthalmos, micropthalmos, agenesis and hypoplasia of solid organs are the result. The best example is the eye.

Supporting evidence

This section presents some of the evidence in support of these concepts of growth and their relation to congenital deformities, exemplified by one or two deformities from each group.

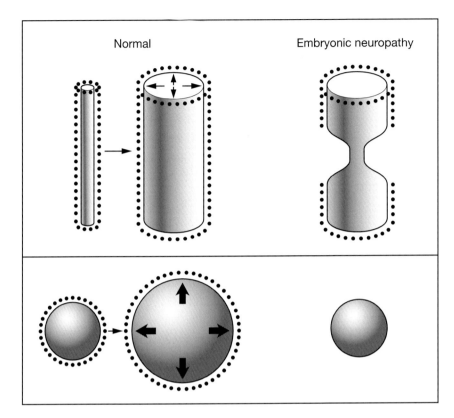

Figure 12.5 *Neural crest injury stops growth of a cylindrical or solid organ anlage. Stenosis or atresia of tubes and aplasia or hypoplasia of solid organs is the result, comparable with longitudinal reduction defects.*

The limbs

Radial aplasia

Absent or hypoplastic radius was the most common skeletal defect encountered in the thalidomide cases reviewed in 1972.[5,6] The possibility that a segmental nerve disease might subtract the 6th cervical dermatome and its underlying structures from the plan for the embryonic arm demanded further research.[13]

Several series of cases of radial dysplasia are available in the literature, and describe fairly constant soft tissue deformities in the affected arm. The muscles of the upper and lower arm may be absent, rudimentary, fused or abnormally inserted. The radial artery is frequently absent or of very small calibre, while the brachial and ulnar arteries are normal. The most striking and constant feature is that the radial nerve ends at the elbow.[14,15] The median and ulnar nerves are present in the forearm, and innervate the residual muscles and skin normally supplied by the radial nerve.

The aetiology of radial aplasia is not known. In 1968, Pardini[14] reviewed the prevailing theories (genetic, intrauterine compression, inflammation, maternal nutritional deficiency, X-rays and drugs). He declared that 'no single theory is strong enough to resist criticism'. He pointed out that only 5 of his own series of 39 cases had any family history of congenital malformations, so that a hereditary factor is the exception rather than the rule.

Based on the radiological findings,[13] I have suggested neural crest injury at the level of C6 as the pathological condition underlying these cases. Injury to the embryonic sensory peripheral nerve with destruction of its trophic action[7,8] would result in aplasia of bones, muscles and skin supplied by the affected nerve.[13] An injury centred on C6 would explain the radiological and surgical anatomy of these cases. Absence of the radial nerve below the elbow may be interpreted as evidence in support of the hypothesis.

The question why C6 should be such a common reduction defect in the arm is difficult to answer. It seems to indicate that there may be gradations of vulnerability between the different segmental levels of the neural crest. Perhaps there are more crest cells in a vulnerable state over a longer period of time at this level. Another idea – philosophical rather than scientific – could be offered in terms of evolution. Opposition of thumb and fingers is a relatively late addition in the evolution of the vertebrate hand, and is a sophisticated action distinguishing humans and certain higher primates from their more primitive brethren. It is possible that this new and complex addition to the blueprint of the forearm within the neural crest is more vulnerable to injury, while the primitive structure of the four-digit paw is more stable. In this context, one might also speculate that fusion between parallel bones, as found in thalidomide embryopathy, is also regression to a more primitive form.

Other reduction deformities of the limbs can be explained on a similar segmental basis. Non-limb deformities such as microtia, anotia, anomalies of ossicles and otic capsule, micrognathia, and other congenital defects of the head may be of similar origin, applying the hypothesis of embryonic neuropathy to the cranial neural crest.

Structures that meet in the midline

The palate

Experimental extirpation of a segment of neural crest has been shown to result in cleft palate in amphibian and chick embryos.[16,17] By labelling neural crest cells with tritiated thymidine, [^{3}H]thymidine, the migration of cranial neural crest cells has been studied in the chick and mammalian embryos.[18] Ventral migration of large numbers of proliferating neural crest cells into the upper facial region is shown to give rise to the embryonic facial processes, 90% of whose mesenchyme is composed of cells of neural crest origin. The maxillary process and the median and lateral nasal processes are thus dependent upon neural crest migration.

In a review of the development of cleft palate, Burston[19] postulates that gross interference with the migration and development of the original maxillary processes could result in reduced size of either or both definitive palatal processes and thus failure to reach the midline. I agree with this part of his interpretation, and also suggest that the failure of growth of the palatal processes is due to impaired migration of the neural crest following an injury such as the surgical experimental extirpation mentioned above. Drug-induced cleft palate is recorded in mice[20] and rabbits,[21] where the time of administration of the drug co-incides with the period of neural crest migration into the face. Similar experience has been noted in humans.[22] Cleft palate was one of the less frequent defects, with or without cleft lip, in the thalidomide syndromes.[4] In previous papers on the radiology of thalidomide deformities,[5,6] the neural crest has been proposed to be the target of the drug. Cleft palate of sporadic incidence and non-specific aetiology could therefore be due to chance neurotoxins entering the embryonic environment at the appropriate moment. Where the incidence is familial, it is difficult to know whether the defect is purely a gene expression, whether the genotype of the neural crest in that family is more fragile than normal and more vulnerable to minimal trauma, or whether two generations have been exposed to the same environmental factors.

The spine and other midline organs

The concept of the trophic quality of the neural crest upon structures formed by union in the midline is summarized in Figure 12.4. Taking any spinal sensory ganglion as an example, the sensory neuron in the diagram represents neural crest derivatives. Neural crest injury, with impaired migration, axon sprouting or trophic influence, would inhibit growth and reduce the final size of the part, Therefore it would fall short of midline union. Theoretically, such a concept could account for anterior midline reduction deformities such as cleft palate, tracheo-oesophageal fistula, gastroschisis and other midline hernias, and ectopic bladder. Posteriorly, the classical example is spina bifida. Evidence in favour of this is the fairly constant histological finding of sensory ganglion cells within the fibrous bands tethering the posterior spinal cord to the site of the bone defect in the spinous processes of cases explored surgically for spinal dysraphism.[23] This seems strong evidence that these bands are in fact damaged sensory nerves, whose injury has prevented complete fusion of the neural arch, resulting in spina bifida. Thus the bone defect in spina bifida may be considered a neural crest defect, or a midline reduction deformity. The neural tube abnormalities such as meningocoele and meningomyelocoele may even be secondary to neural crest damage.

Cylindrical organs

The alimentary tract

A number of theories of pathogenesis of atresias and stenoses of the alimentary tract have been proposed since 1900, when Tandler suggested failure of canalization of the lumen. Other authors have considered mechanical factors to be more likely,[24] such as intrauterine perforation,[25] intussusception,[26] or other injury.[27] Louw and Barnard[28] supported their theory of vascular obstruction with experimental proof in dogs. However, Louw[29] acknowledged that in cases where there are associated malformations in other systems, general rather than local factors are probably responsible, possibly on a basis of multiple vascular insufficiencies. Renal, skeletal, cardiac and other gastrointestinal anomalies are commonly associated with alimentary atresias and stenoses of unknown cause,[30] and were found in embryopathy due to thalidomide.[3,4] Any theory of pathogenesis must explain the whole spectrum as well as the local abnormality.

While the application of previous theories is certainly not denied, the hypothesis of embryonic neuropathy offers a comprehensive explanation of all malformations. According to this hypothesis, failure of migration of cells from the neural crest into the wall of the bowel (Figure 12.1) would result in absence of autonomic plexuses in that segment, and failure of growth (Figure 12.5). Absence of Auerbach's and Meissner's plexuses in the stenotic segment of colon is the recognized histopathology of Hirschprung's disease. This may be interpreted as failure of migration of neural crest cells, or autonomic embryonic neuropathy, manifest by stenosis of the bowel. This principle would apply equally well to many congenital obstructions of the oesophagus, duodenum, bile ducts, small bowel, colon and anus. Very few data are available concerning the neuropathology of these congenital stenoses and atresias. However, autonomic neuropathy is a recognized pathology in the gastrointestinal tract of adults with diabetes or on certain drugs.[31] Neonatal stenosis or atresia is proposed to be the embryonic equivalent.

Solid organs

The eye

In his autoradiographic study of the migration of cranial neural crest cells labelled with [³H]thymidine, Johnston[18] made the interesting observation that 'crest cells almost completely surround the eye cup, except for a small region occupied by mesodermal cells which lie ventromedial and caudal to the eye cup and are continuous with the mesoderm underlying the brain'. Applying the hypothesis of embryonic neuropathy, it is proposed that the neural crest cells normally induce growth of the optic vesicle. Figure 12.5 shows the sphere of the eye expanding like a balloon under the uniform trophic stimulus of its mantle of neural crest cells. Neural crest injury in the very early embryo is postulated to prevent migration of the crest cells around the optic vesicle (anophthalmos). Injury in the later embryo, when migration has already occurred, results in loss of growth stimulus, so that the eye is present but abnormally small (microphthalmos).

Coloboma is explained on the same basis as failure of the trophic action in closure of the fetal fissure of the uveal tract.

These congenital eye defects were part of the thalidomide syndrome,[2] but also occur without known cause, either alone or in conjunction with deformities in other systems of the body.[30,32] Neural crest injury is suggested as a comprehensive theory of pathogenesis of both ocular and associated defects in many of these cases.

Other organs

Aplasia and hypoplasia of other solid organs, such as the kidney, liver and spleen, may be due to injury of the autonomic nerves in the embryo, but evidence to support this suggestion has not yet been found in the literature.

Conclusion

Since the thalidomide epidemic, there has been increasing documentation of congenital defect syndromes. In practice, application of the syndromes as defined is frequently unsatisfactory in particular cases and has thus required a proliferation of subgroups, variants and provisions for atypical features. The custom of subdividing congenital deformities ad infinitum should be re-examined. The alternative is to approach the subject of congenital defects as a whole.

The hypothesis of neural crest injury offers a logical approach to interpretation of many syndromes, and provides a unifying concept to explain many apparently unrelated anomalies.

References

1. McCredie J. Embryonic neuropathy. A hypothesis of neural crest injury as the pathogenesis of congenital malformations. *Med J Aust* 1974; **1**: 159–63.

2. Editorial. The pathogenesis of congenital malformations. *Med J Aust* 1974, **1**:

3. Lenz W. Thalidomide and congenital abnormalities. *Lancet* 1962; **i**: 45.

4. Ministry of Health Reports on Public Health and Medical Subjects No. 112. *Deformities Caused by Thalidomide*. London: HMSO, 1964.

5. McCredie J. Thalidomide and congenital Charcot's joints. *Lancet* 1973; **ii**: 1058–61.

6. McCredie J, McBride WG. Some congenital abnormalities: possibly due to embryonic peripheral neuropathy. *Clin Radiol* 1973; **24**: 204–11.

7. Singer M. The nervous system and regeneration of the forelimb of adult *Triturus. J Exp Zool* 1943; **92**: 297–312.

8. Singer M. The influence of the nerve in regeneration of the amphibian extremity. *Q Rev Biol* 1952; **27**: 169–200.

9. Hamilton WJ, Mossman HW. *Human Embryology*. Cambridge: Heffer/ Baltimore: Williams and Wilkins, 1972.

10. Horstadius S. *The Neural Crest*. Oxford: Oxford University Press, 1950.

11. Langman J. *Medical Embryology*. Baltimore: Williams and Wilkins, 1969.

12. Weston, JA. The migration and differentiation of neural crest cells. *Adv Morphogen* 1970; **8**: 41–114.

13. McCredie J. Segmental embryonic peripheral neuropathy. *Pediatr Radiol* 1975; **3**: 162–8.

14. Pardini A. Radial dysplasia. *Clin Orthop* 1968; **57**: 153–77.

15. Riordan DC, Congenital absence of the radius. *J Bone Joint Surg* 1955; **37A**: 1129–40.

16. Hammond WS, Yntema CL. Deficiencies in the visceral skeleton of the chick after removal of the cranial neural crest. *Anat Rec* 1953; **115**: 393.

17. Hammond WS, Yntema CL. Depletions of the pharyngeal arch cartilages following extirpation of cranial neural crest in chick embryos. *Acta Anat* 1964; **56**: 21.

18. Johnston MC. A radioautographic study of the migration and fate of cranial neural crest cells in chick embryo. *Anat Rec* 1966; **156**: 143.

19. Burston WR. The development of cleft lip and palate. *Ann R Coll Surg Engl* 1959; **25**: 225.

20. Clarke Fraser F, Fainstat TD. Production of congenital defects in the off-spring of pregnant mice treated with cortisone. *Pediatrics* 1951; **8**: 527.

21. Fainstat TD. Cortisone-induced cleft palate in rabbits. *Endocrinology* 1954; **55**: 502.

22. Harris JWS, Ross IP. Cortisone therapy in early pregnancy: relation to cleft palate. *Lancet* 1956; **i**: 1045.

23. James CCM, Lassman LP. *Spinal Dysraphism*. London: Butterworths, 1972.

24. Evans CH. Atresias of the gastrointestinal tract. *Int Abstr Surg* 1951; **92**: 1.

25. Bernstein J, Vauter G Harris G et al. The occurrence of intestinal atresia in newborns with meconium ileus. *Am J Dis Child* 1960; **99**: 804–18.

26. Parkkulainen K. Intrauterine intussusception as a cause of intestinal atresias. *Surgery* 1958; **44**: 1106.

27. Santulli TV, Blanc WA. Congenital atresia of the intestine: pathogenesis and treatment. *Ann Surg* 1961; **154**: 939.

28. Louw JH, Barnard CN. Congenital intestinal atresia: observations on its origin. *Lancet* 1955; **ii**: 1065.

29. Louw JH. Congenital intestinal atresia and stenosis in the newborn: Observations on its pathogenesis and treatment. *Ann R Coll Surg Engl* 1959; **25**: 209.

30. Rubin A. *Handbook of Congenital Malformations*. Philadelphia: WB Saunders, 1967.

31. Smith B. *The Neuropathology of the Alimentary Tract*. London: Edward Arnold, 1972.

32. Norman AP. *Congenital Abnormalities in Infancy*. Oxford: Blackwells, 1971.

CHAPTER 13

The neural crest

Introduction

The sensory peripheral nervous system develops from the neural crest, a primordial and recognizable tissue in the very early vertebrate embryo. In spite of the fact that the neural crest is well recognized as the progenitor of the sensory and autonomic nerves, as an organ it is complex, migratory, elusive and difficult to study. Most research in embryology has used the chick embryo model because of easy access in the egg to the embryo for observation and experimental manipulation. Neural crest cells are shown to migrate and intermingle with other cells, disguised by histological anonymity, indistinguishable from the cells of the part they are invading. More important, their invading axons and dendrites are difficult to find on light microscopy because their diameter is less than 5 nm and beyond the power of resolution of the light microscope.

Horstadius[1] in 1950 described the neural crest as an important but neglected tissue. His classical monograph *The Neural Crest* summarized and evaluated experiments on neural crest from the late 19th century. Now out of print, that book was rescued from obscurity and republished by BK Hall in 1988.[2]

This chapter presents no more than a brief review of some of the known facts and problems of neural crest biology that relate to thalidomide's pathogenesis. For more detailed information, readers are recommended to consult *The Neural Crest* by le Douarin,[3] the book of the same title by Horstadius and Hall,[2] and the publications of Weston[4] and Johnston.[5] Much of the research quoted in this chapter was published after 1974, and was not available when I formulated and first published the neural crest hypothesis.

The aims of this chapter are:

1. To outline the early development of the neural crest and difficulties in defining its limits.

Chapter Summary
- **Introduction**
- **Early neural crest development**
- **Problems with labelling and tracing neural crest migration**
- **Subsequent neural crest development**
- **Neural crest and the thalidomide-sensitive period**
- **Conclusion**
- **References**

2. To examine the chronological relationship between early neural crest development and the thalidomide-sensitive period.

Early neural crest development

The neural crest is a primordial structure. It becomes visible in the human embryo at day 18, as a thickening of the ectoderm around the rim of the neural plate. The thickened edges of the plate become the apices of the neural folds as these rise upwards to reshape the plate into the neural groove. The crests curl towards one another, meet in the midline and convert the neural groove into the neural tube, which will become the central nervous system (brain and spinal cord). This process of 'neurulation' (formation of the neural tube) progresses chronologically from the head end to the tail end of the embryo (craniocaudal sequence), in a movement similar to downward closure of a zipper. The neural tube and the fused neural crest sink beneath the surface ectoderm. The fused crest detaches from the tube, and redivides into two columns that slide apart, one on each side of the back of the neural tube. Thus the rudiments of the peripheral nervous system are moving into place. Motor nuclei lie within the neural tube. Sensory and autonomic nuclei are based within the neural crest at this stage.

Next, the paired sensory ganglia are formed by sequential craniocaudal segmentation of these columns of neural crest, which come to look like two strings of beads, each lying lateral and posterior to the neural tube. All the spinal dorsal root ganglia are of neural crest origin. As far as the cranial nerves are concerned, the ganglia of at least the 5th, 7th, 9th and 10th sensory nerves are derived from the neural crest.[3,5] The origin of the remaining cranial sensory ganglia is debatable.

The neural crest is a unique tissue in that it has only a transient life as a discrete organ. Unlike other organs, it is not confined by a basement membrane. Therefore it is free to merge with and infiltrate other tissues. By means of active cell division and extensive migration, great numbers of neural crest cells leave the original columns and ganglia and disperse widely, yet with precision, throughout the early embryo. Neural crest cells are histologically indistinguishable from mesenchymal cells at this stage.

Neural crest cells play an active role in the formation of a wide range of tissues and organs (Figure 13.1). One population of trunk crest cells (not shown in Figure 13.1) migrates laterally beneath the ectoderm, and will give rise to melanoblasts in the skin. Another large group migrates ventrally as shown. Some of these cells aggregate into the sympathetic and parasympathetic ganglia,[6] while others migrate further to surround the primordia of future internal organs, forming the intrinsic autonomic plexuses such as those of Auerbach and Meissner in the gut, known as enteric nerves.

The number of enteric neurons in vertebrates can exceed the total number of neurons in the spinal cord.[7] The less visible autonomic

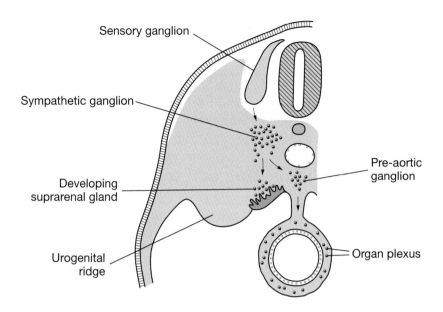

Sensory ganglion

Sympathetic ganglion

Developing
suprarenal gland

Urogenital
ridge

Pre-aortic
ganglion

Organ plexus

Figure 13.1 *Migration of neural crest cells. The ventral migration of neural crest cells gives rise to the sympathetic and parasympathetic ganglia and to the organ plexuses such as those in the gut (enteric plexuses). (From Langman J. Medical Embryology. Baltimore: Williams and Wilkins, 1969.)*

nervous system has a much greater cell population than the well-recognized peripheral motor nervous system.[7]

In addition to the sensory peripheral and autonomic nervous systems, neural crest cells in the trunk give rise to pigment cells, Schwann cells and satellite cells, some of the spinal meninges, and a proportion of the spinal cartilages.[1–6]

As opposed to the trunk crest, the cranial neural crest gives rise to relatively few pigment cells. But, by infiltration and multiplication, it contributes 90% of the mesenchyme that will form the visceral skeleton of the head and face.[5,8–10] By 1975, Le Lievre and Le Douarin[9] had concluded from studies on the quail–chick chimera that the visceral skeleton of the head is entirely derived from neural crest mesenchyme. They inferred that the pattern of cranial neural crest migration is similar in mammalian embryos and that 'a number of spontaneous malformations of the face and brain in the human can be explained by defective neural crest migration and differentiation'.[9]

The various levels of the neural axis from which actual cartilages and bones of the head region originate had been established[9,10] by 1979. These include the mandible, odontoblasts, carotid bodies, and cranial autonomic and sensory neuroblasts in association with ectodermal placodes. Cranial neural crest cells migrate caudally into the thoracic cavity, and form all but the endothelial lining of the aorta and the great vessels arising from it,[5,9] including the septum of the heart.[11]

'Chondromucoid and calcium hydroxyapatite are synthesized by neural crest and placodes, and deposited onto an existing collagenous network. The neural crest also produces calcitonin and thus facilitates the deposition of calcium in bone.'[7]

This function of neural crest cells raises the possibility that it contributes directly to osteogenesis. It begs further investigation, for it has far-reaching implications in medicine.

The mesenchyme derived from neural crest ectoderm has wide developmental capabilities, including differentiation into connective tissues, adipose, dermis, smooth and striated muscles, bone, cartilage, odontoblasts, and vascular structures (excluding vascular endothelium).

Problems with labelling and tracing neural crest migration

The ill-defined margins of the crest at the neural fold stage,[3] the lack of a basement membrane to contain the crest,[12] its non-specific histological appearance and its characteristic wide migration among mesodermal cells of similar histological appearance all present problems that have challenged scientists for over a century. The essential task was to break the histological anonymity by labelling crest cells with a marker that would allow them to be identified during their subsequent travels.

Labelling techniques have varied with the advent of new technologies. The historical development of crest markers and their limitations on mapping the diaspora of neural crest cells is as follows.

Pigment markers[1]

The earliest studies of neural crest by transplantation had to rely on its known control of feather pigmentation as the marker of the neural crest implant. By transplanting crest cells of chick embryos – black donor into white host and vice versa – the destination of particular levels of crest was shown by the colour of skin or feathers in the hatched chicks.

Vital dyes[1]

An alternative method was to stain one embryo with a vital dye, then to transplant stained crest segments into unstained hosts. Neural crest migration could be traced microscopically to an extent limited by progressive dilution of dye intensity because of cell division and diffusion.

In spite of experimental evidence that neural crest ectoderm gave rise to the dentine of teeth and to cartilage of the visceral arches,[13] the concept of an ectodermal contribution to mesodermal structures was slow to find acceptance. One reason was that the 'germ layer theory' of von Baer had dominated embryological thinking since 1828, particularly in the German school that dominated embryology in the 19th and early 20th centuries.[14] This theory maintained that the organs of the body arose specifically from the three separate layers of the embryo: ectoderm, mesoderm and endoderm. The germ layer theory conflicts with the suggestion that an ectodermal derivative such as the neural crest could infiltrate and take part in the formation of mesodermal structures.

Progress in science is always retarded by the slow death of old ideas. Horstadius in his 1950 book[1] presented a convincing case for the critical role of neural crest in formation of many non-ectodermal tissues, drawing on facts established using pigments or vital dyes. His book did not receive the attention it deserved, probably because of the entrenched influence of the germ layer theory.

Tritiated thymidine and autoradiography[4,5]

A significant advance in neural crest biology was made at the US National Institutes of Health (NIH) in the 1960s by a Canadian dental researcher, Johnston,[5] and an American biologist, Weston.[4] They labelled chick embryos with tritiated thymidine, [^{3}H]thymidine, transplanted ^{3}H-labelled sections of neural crest into unlabelled embryos, and traced the subsequent migration of ^{3}H-labelled neural crest cells by autoradiography. This technique enabled the fate of non-pigment-related neural crest cells to be studied in the head and neck[5] and in the trunk.[4] Their observations added very considerably to current knowledge of the timing and extent of neural crest migration and its contribution to the formation of different organs. Weston's classic review[4] of the two decades of experimental work since Horstadius' monograph elegantly summarized the advances in neural crest biology to 1970. However, the radionuclide marker was also subject to dilution, because progressive cell divisions diminished the radioactivity per cell until it became imperceptible on autoradiography.

Japanese quail–chick chimera[3,6,9]

Subsequently, a more stable biological marker was employed in Paris by Le Douarin and her colleagues.[6,9] This technique was based upon the fact that the nuclei of cells in the Japanese quail have a characteristic structure and pattern of chromatin distribution that distinguishes quail crest nuclei from those of the chick. Exchange transplantation of sections of neural tube and crest between Japanese quail and chick embryos created a useful 'quail–chick chimera'. Using this model, neural crest cell migration could be studied more extensively than with the previous marker systems, because it overcame the problem of marker dilution: quail cell nuclei remained histologically different from chick cell nuclei throughout their migration and life cycles. The reader is referred to Le Douarin's monograph[3] for a detailed review.

Nuclei versus axons

The quail–chick chimera overcame the problem of marker dilution that had plagued previous research. But it still shared one problem with its predecessors, namely that the marker is within the nucleus, not the cytoplasm. None of the marker systems so far can identify and track the outline of the whole cell and the outreach of its cytoplasm. During early multiplication and migration, neural crest cells sprout axons and rapidly evolve into sensory and autonomic neurons.[15]

Sensory neurons are extraordinary cells. They are the largest cells in the body by virtue of their very long axons and dendrites. A cytoplasmic extension is still an integral part of one nerve cell, even if the nucleus of that cell lies in a lumbar ganglion in the spinal canal and its axon of continuous cytoplasm terminates in the great toe. Because nuclear markers fail to label cytoplasm with its axonal and dendritic extensions, conclusions drawn from studies based upon nuclear markers have to be limited to statements about the location of nuclei, and not the location of the whole cell. This is a technical limitation common to all nuclear markers.

Another serious limitation of any transplantation experiment is the youngest age at which the embryo will survive the operation. The possibility exists that an early wave of cell migration could occur prior to the earliest transplantation experiments,[16] so that mapping of the earliest neural crest migration may be incomplete. Even more complex issues, such as the laws that govern crest cell migration, await elucidation.

Some studies using nuclear marker methods have concluded that neural crest cells do not migrate into the limb buds. This statement is partly correct. The correct conclusion is that the *nuclei* of neural crest cells have not been seen to migrate into limb buds.

What the *axons* are doing, and whether or not they are present in the limb bud, is another question altogether.

Histochemical mapping of cytoplasm with immunofluorescence

Modern developments in histochemistry allow investigators to identify and assay intracellular enzymes, proteins, transmitters, their precursors and other intracellular constituents. Histochemical mapping promises to identify neural pathways that have been occult to date. This method does not require surgical transplantation.

Fluorescent markers bind to chemicals within cytoplasm. Major nerve bundles become visible by fluorescence of their axoplasm. This is an advance on nuclear markers, and reveals major nerve trunks entering and ramifying into limb buds. But immunofluorescence is not without technical limitations.

The tissue is still inspected by serial sections, and the process of cutting sections of tissue needs to be understood.

The ramification of nerves is similar to the branching of a tree. Nerves branch among other cells, as a tree branches into the air. The trunk of a tree, being larger in mass, is more easily seen than its twigs. Under the microscope, we are inspecting slices through the equivalent of a tree and its branches. By virtue of their large size and characteristic alignment, nerve trunks and major branches are relatively easily seen, reinforced by a content of many axons and their collective fluoresence. But axon numbers decrease and the diameters of axon bundles diminish as they branch further and further. Each branch contains fewer axons than its predecessor. Very small twigs are difficult or impossible to see on light microscopy.

As nerves branch and spread, their alignment departs from that of the plane of the section under the microscope. So there is a geometric problem with identification of smaller and smaller bundles of axons that lie oblique to the plane of section, and are physically seen as inconspicuous dots or ovoids, not as linear streams of cytoplasm.

There is also the chemical problem of a diminishing signal. Small branches containing few axons emit very little fluorescence. The power of resolution of the labelling method declines as the size of the fluorescing object decreases – i.e., the smaller the branch, the less the fluorescent signal. How small a bundle of axons can be demonstrated? Can a single axon (as small as 3 nm diameter) be identified? How strong is the fluorescent signal from a single axon? Can such a miniscule signal be recorded? Herein lies another limitation of immunofluorescence: limitation of its power of resolution.

The absence of a signal does not mean that no axons are present!

When a signal is too weak to detect, the problem becomes that of the limitation of the technology, similar to dilution of nuclear markers, despite the technical advance of getting a marker into the cytoplasm.

Electron microscopy: transmission and scanning

The increased power of resolution of optical instruments in recent decades has of course impacted neuroscience.

Axons of nerves are too small to be visualized by light microscopy (maximum magnification 1000×). But high magnifications (e.g. 30 000× or more) provided by the electron microscope can expose previously invisible structures.

Nerve axons contain inherent histological markers: neurotubules (microtubules) and neurofibrils, subcellular structures that no other cells contain. On electron microscopy, their presence in cytoplasm is diagnostic of axoplasm – the cytoplasm of a neuron (Figure 13.2).

Axons less than 3 nm in diameter are extremely delicate. They can be identified with careful tissue processing that must include optimum methods of fixation, staining, sectioning and examination, as used in neuropathology laboratories for examination of unmyelinated axons in patients with peripheral neuropathy and other

Figure 13.2 *Internal structure of an axon. Transverse section magnified by electron microscopy, allowing microtubules to be identified. These subcellular structures are unique to neurons, and their presence defines such fragments of cytoplasm as belonging to a neuron.*

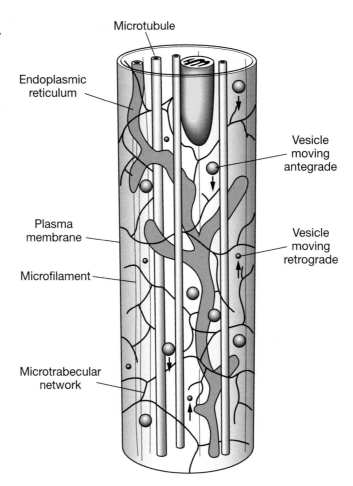

neurological diseases. Transmission electron microscopy (TEM or simply EM) allows bundles of such axons to be identified by their unique inherent microtubular markers. By scanning electron microscopy (SEM), nerves can be traced as they penetrate into other tissues.[17] In our laboratory, Cameron used TEM to search for axons penetrating between the mesenchymal cells of the embryonic limb bud before any mesenchymal condensation (see Chapter 15). He identified axoplasm by the presence of neurotubules.

Tosney[15] studied axonal sprouting from neural crest cells in chick embryo by SEM and showed that:

1. Crest cells appear up to four somite lengths in front of the most recent visible somites.
2. They have processes that traverse intercellular spaces to contact neighbouring cells.
3. At the leading edges of the neural crest, the cells project laterally and extend long filopodia into the cell-free extracellular spaces beyond the crest itself.

4. The extension of a cell process from the lateral edge of the neural crest into a meshwork of fibrils (<7 nm diameter) in the cell free space beyond the crest was traced and photographed on SEM of a stage 12 embryo.
5. All of the above stages of early neurite formation take place *before* the neural crest has subdivided into segments for formation of ganglia, and *prior to any migration of crest cells*.

The axons and dendrites of neural crest cells are much more precocious than has been realized to date.

Using both TEM and SEM, Newgreen et al[19] showed that processes (diameter 3 nm) of neural crest cells rather than the cell bodies penetrate the open surface of the embryonic sclerotome (sclerato-genous zone that will form skeletal parts) in chick and quail. Contrary to von Baer's germ layer theory, this means that ectodermal cell processes invade mesoderm.

By meticulous SEM, Sulik et al[22] have shown the fine processes of neural crest cells in mouse embryo extending far beyond the cell body and its nucleus.

Problems of interpretation of data

Any one of these methods will fail to disclose the complete picture of what is there. Any study will only prove what it is capable of proving to be there. *What has been shown and what is actually there are two different things*.

Conclusions drawn from any experiment need to be carefully and precisely worded, and carefully read. The materials and method, in particular, need to be read critically to avoid misunderstanding. Results and conclusions need to state clearly, for instance, that axons were identified to the point where the limitation of the method was reached (e.g. where the dye, the radioactivity or the fluorescence disappeared). This does not mean that the axons end there, but that the power of resolution of the technique ends there.

'Absence of evidence is not evidence of absence' is a classical scientific axiom that must always be observed. Radiologists are habitually aware of the limitations of the different diagnostic procedures they employ, and the precise language of their reports is part of their quest for accuracy and avoidance of error in diagnoses.

Subsequent neural crest development

Craniocaudal gradient of development

Horstadius,[1,2] Le Douarin[3] and Weston[4] all emphasized the cranio-caudal sequence of neural crest development along the embryonic neuraxis. This is well displayed in serial sections of an embryo at any stage during neurulation. The cranial crest develops in advance of the cervicothoracic crest, which is ahead of the lumbosacral crest. This chronological progression of development, from the head towards the tail, is extremely important, because it establishes a normal gradation of maturity whereby, at any given time, one sensory ganglion is likely to be similar to that on the opposite side, but developmentally different (or in a slightly different phase of development) from those above and below.

The craniocaudal gradient of development thus separates any one segmental level from the others during early embryogenesis. The chronological separation and progressive maturation of neural crest segments can be likened to playing a musical scale, in that only one note in the scale is heard at any particular moment.

> 'One feature of the development of neural crest cells is that they start differentiating only after a phase of migration which brings them to a defined embryonic region. This migration phase appears precisely controlled in all its aspects: timing, pathways, directionality, and sites of arrest. The mechanisms whereby the cells are guided and recognise their way in the three-dimensional network of the developing embryo are among the most fascinating problems of developmental biology.'[3]

Neural crest development has attracted the attention of many scientists, including embryologists, geneticists, neurophysiologists, anatomists, molecular biologists, organic chemists and oncologists. Many questions need to be answered: How does neural crest migrate so specifically? At what stage and how does the crest become programmed to differentiate, or to assist differentiation of very diverse cell types? What environmental factors influence its migration and differentiation? These questions lie outside the scope of this book, and will be solved in due course by neurobiological research. Some aspects related to the subject of this book are briefly summarized here.

Environment and substrate

The substrate over which neural crest cells or axons move has been explored by molecular biologists and chemists, yielding more molecular and chemical data than can currently be integrated with its morphology. Le Douarin[3] emphasized the need to discover more about

> 'the relationships of the migrating cells with the matrix components and with the other cells that they meet on their way, and also about signals that induce the crest cells to stop, settle and begin differentiating.
> 'The question of the relationship between cell commitment and migration is also difficult to answer. It is clear, however, that, once cells have reached their destination, they still can choose between

a number of possible differentiation options, and that these choices are extensively conditioned by extrinsic signals. The fact that the embryonic environment in which the crest cells develop has a major influence on their fate has been very well illustrated by the studies carried out on the peripheral nervous system.'

Environment and axonal outgrowth

Le Douarin included the whole neural crest cell in these statements. The outgrowth of axons and dendrites is included in the environmental interaction depicted. Thus the growth and function of axons and other delicate cytoplasmic extensions can be impacted by chemical intruders into the molecular environment through which unmyelinated and thus unprotected axons are passing.

The relationship between the neural crest and its environment is illustrated by thalidomide embryopathy. Ideally, the relationship could be examined using cultures of crest cells exposed to thalidomide, the effect being compared with unexposed controls. This experiment has not been done, probably because of many difficulties in culturing nerves from pleomorphic crest cells, which tend to dedifferentiate and revert to more primitive progeny in culture.

However, an intriguing experiment was recorded by a marine biologist, Boney.[23] Using cultures of intertidal spores of marine red algae, he tested their filamentous growth against various water pollutants. He included a series tested against thalidomide. Red algae normally develop into four-cell filaments (Figure 13.3a–d). With thalidomide exposure (Figure 13.3e–o), the linear outgrowth was

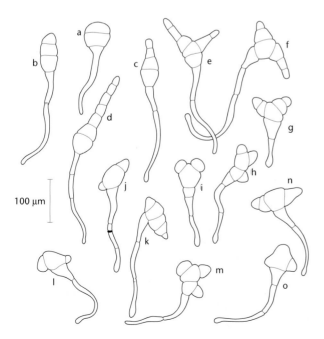

Figure 13.3 *Effect of thalidomide on filamentous growth. (From Boney AD.* Nature *1963; 198: 1069–9.[23])*

deranged in many different ways, with stunting, branching, and other abnormal morphological derangements of the normal anatomy. In the absence of any other data, this experiment tells us something about the impact of thalidomide upon a linear growth pattern, even if the algal model is a multicellular plant. A possible analogy with the outgrowth of axons from neural crest cells invites scientific contemplation!

Neural crest and the thalidomide-sensitive period

Among many facts established by studies of neural crest, four are pertinent to this discussion:

1. The neural crest is a single, primordial, embryonic tissue that is normally implicated in the development of widespread and diverse tissues and organs.
2. The neural crest is the embryonic precursor of sensory and autonomic neurons and their satellite cells.
3. It develops in a craniocaudal sequence from day 18 in the human embryo.
4. Thereafter, segmentation and migration of the neural crest usually take place in a bilateral, symmetrical fashion.

These four facts apply to the potential relationship between neural crest and thalidomide embryopathy.

Multiple organ systems and autonomic nerves

Thalidomide causes defects in widespread and diverse organs. If thalidomide acted specifically upon the neural crest, it would be possible to impair growth in many different organs and tissues, because it is the precursor of the autonomic nervous system (Figure 13.4) as well as the sensory nerves. A single site of action – one target tissue – is a more likely hypothesis than one involving multiple sites and modes of action.

Defects parallel the timing of crest development

Thalidomide malformations occur in a head-to-tail sequence chronologically, in parallel with the evolution of the neural crest:

1. The sensitive period for thalidomide in the human embryo commences at day 21 post conception.
2. The sensitive period for upper limb defects commences at day 24.[24,25]
3. The upper limb bud is first visible at day 28 post conception (Nishimura H, personal communication, 1972; and see any embryology textbook).

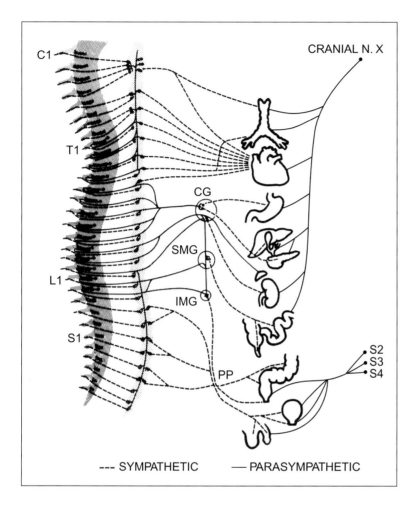

C1

T1

CRANIAL N. X

CG

SMG

L1

IMG

S1

PP

S2
S3
S4

--- SYMPATHETIC   — PARASYMPATHETIC

Figure 13.4 *Segmental arrangement of the autonomic nervous system. (From Netter FH.* The Ciba Collection of Medical Illustrations. Volume 1: Nervous System. *New York: Case-Hoyt, 1975).*

4. Therefore the thalidomide-sensitive period coincides with neural crest development, but not with limb development.

The timing of drug ingestion predates the formation of limb buds and other damaged organs. The upper limb bud is not present until day 28, yet malformations of the upper limb follow thalidomide ingestion after day 24[24,25] of gestation (Figure 13.5). This discordance is emphasized by the short half-life of the teratogen (Chapters 2 and 3). The teratogen acts before the limb bud is formed, but during development of the neural crest and its axons.

Therefore any hypothesis proposing that thalidomide acts upon the limb bud or parts thereof (e.g. the apical ectodermal ridge, the mesenchyme, etc.) is *not* supported by the chronological data.

Figure 13.5 *Chronology of thalidomide embryopathy in relation to neural crest development. The arrow at day 24 is the first thalidomide exposure that induces an upper limb defect. But the upper limb bud is not visible until day 28. The half-life of the drug is 3 hours, so it is no longer there when the limb bud appears. However, the neural crest is present from day 18, and is active throughout the thalidomide-sensitive period. This is circumstantial evidence that thalidomide does not act upon the limb bud, but on some earlier target tissue such as the neural crest.*

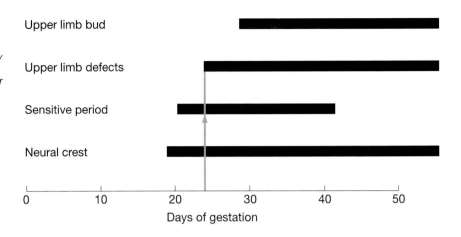

The human sensitive period enables one to state categorically that *thalidomide does not act on the limb bud*. The proposition that it acts on limb buds is simply untenable, irrespective of the elaborate constructs of (invisible and unprovable) 'presumptive limb bud tissues' that have been invented to bolster weak hypotheses.

This does not mean that the effect of thalidomide is not seen in the limbs. The effect most certainly is seen there, and elsewhere. Cause and effect are chronologically separated, but neurologically connected.

Although the upper limb bud is not present in the first 4 days of the thalidomide-sensitive period for upper limb defects, the neural crest has been present since day 18 of gestation and has developed as far as the separation of cervical ganglia by day 28. This is circumstantial evidence that at the earliest appropriate time, *the crest was present, but the upper limb bud was not*. Thalidomide caused upper limb deformities by action before the limb bud existed, but during active neural crest development.

Craniocaudal sequence of thalidomide defects

Chapter 2 describes Lenz's analysis of the sensitive period for thalidomide, and its subsequent refinement into sensitive days for specific malformations by Nowack.[24] Their studies showed that a direct relationship existed between the age of the embryo at the time of drug exposure, and the anatomical malformation that resulted.

Cephalic defects followed the earliest intake (from 20 days' gestational age).

Arm deformities were maximum after ingestion of thalidomide between 26 and 30 days' gestational age, but were reported to commence from day 24 of gestation.

Leg defects were maximum from drug ingestion at days 28–33 of gestation, but congenital dislocation of the hip could occur from day 24 of gestation.

Craniocaudal sequence of development of the neural crest

The normal craniocaudal sequence of development of the neural crest means that no spinal segment is precisely the same as another spinal segment at any given moment. The segments or zones of the whole are therefore separable from one another on the basis of incremental time differences in development within the embryonic timetable.

Thalidomide could block a particular process that was only happening in a short zone or segment of the crest at that moment. The short half-life of thalidomide fits this concept (Chapter 2). Its teratogenic action is delivered as a short pulse, maximum about 1 hour after the mother's ingestion of the drug. The pulse is so short and sharp that it would be capable of a precise focal insult, perhaps as precise as one segment of neural crest that was sensitive at that time. Given the highly organized complexity of neural crest migration and axon outgrowth, and the high mitotic rate of neural crest cells, there would be considerable scope for toxic interference in one particular function, if not all these activities.

Let us look at this from the point of view of structure rather than function. An alternative analogy is that the neural crest can be compared with a roulette wheel in motion. At a precise moment, there is one slot whose position (relative to the ball, directions and speeds) will allow it to capture the ball. So, in the progression of craniocaudal development of the neural crest, there will be one segmental level that is vulnerable to receive (or to be attacked by) thalidomide at a precise moment. The pair (right and left) of neural crest segments at that level will be injured by the neurotoxic intruder at the moment of contact. Because of the normally synchronous maturation of pairs of neural crest segments, the damage will be bilateral and symmetrical in the majority of embryos. The initial injury is bilateral chemical disruption to the sensory peripheral and autonomic arms of the peripheral nervous system, and to any other neural crest derivatives from that spinal segment. The chemical wounds may not be visible, but the scars that they leave are revealed in the newborn baby.

The craniocaudal sequence of thalidomide defects in time reflects the general craniocaudal sequence of embryonic development: head structures are developing in advance of the upper limb and thorax, which develop ahead of the lower limb, etc.

Symmetry, asymmetry, bilaterality and unilaterality in normal human embryos

Finally, the symmetry and bilaterality of thalidomide-induced malformations requires comment. A misconception has arisen that all thalidomide defects are bilateral and symmetrical. The evidence is that *most, but not all*, thalidomide malformations are bilateral and symmetrical. The following authors reported their cases to be 'mostly' or 'usually' symmetrical:

- Pfeiffer and Kosenow[26]   170 cases
- Henkel and Willert[27]   287 cases
- Smithells[28]   154 cases

Henkel and Willert[27] commented that in the asymmetric minority, the difference between the two sides was not great, and the symmetry remained within a narrow range of morphological limits, which is in agreement with my own observations. It should be noted that we are not using the terms 'symmetry' and 'asymmetry' in their strict geometric context, where any lack of symmetry about an axis constitutes asymmetry. We are speaking of biological symmetry, with standard deviations.

Symmetry in higher plants and animals under normal conditions is not exact, either in external appearance or in internal structure.

> 'In external appearance, although the human form is grossly bilaterally symmetric, there are always defects that break the symmetry, e.g. the finger prints of one hand are *not* mirror images of the other hand. The hand or foot on one side is almost always slightly longer than the other side.'[29]

The symmetry of thalidomide deformities in the British Ministry of Health survey[30] can be calculated as follows, but is only approximate because of the limitations of their published data:

- Upper limb: 268 cases   210 symmetrical (78%)
- Lower limb: 142 cases   110 symmetrical (77%)

Willert and Henkel[31] published a series of thalidomide limb defects in which asymmetry was 16%. Asymmetry is at least 16% and up to 23% of a large collection of thalidomide cases.

This high degree of symmetry is because the majority of embryos develop in a symmetrical manner. The neural crest also develops in a symmetrical fashion. Hypothetical injury to some aspect of neural crest development at a precise moment would impede both sides of the segment or zone of neural crest, leading to bilateral defects in the anatomical field/s dependent upon that zone of the crest.

The group of asymmetric deformities, such as the fifth Australian case, represent the minority (approximately 20%) of normal embryos in which one side lags behind the other in its development by up to 2 days (Nishimura H, personal communication, 1972). Professor Nishimura examined tens of thousands of normal human abortuses and established the fact that approximately 20% of normal human embryos exhibit asynchronous development between the two sides of up to 2 days. The left and right sides of these embryos are out of step in growth and development. In such an embryo, an injury at one particular moment would affect different segments of neural crest on the right and left sides, and the result would be asymmetric defects in the child.

Thus the proportion of asymmetrical embryos observed within a large representative sample of normal human embryos is the same as the proportion observed in thalidomide embryopathy.

Conclusion

Studies of normal neural crest migration and development provide evidence of a complex and incompletely understood mechanism, whereby a single ectodermal primordium is normally implicated in the differentiation of widespread and diverse organs.

The biological data concerning the neural crest and its development correspond to the established timetable and distribution of thalidomide malformations. Very early development of axons that penetrate intercellular spaces coincides with the precocious teratogenic activity of the drug before the limb bud exists.

References

1. Horstadius S. *The Neural Crest: Its Properties and Derivatives in the Light of Experimental Research.* Oxford: Oxford University Press, 1950.

2. Horstadius S, Hall BK. *The Neural Crest.* Oxford: Oxford University Press, 1988.

3. Le Douarin N. *The Neural Crest.* Cambridge: Cambridge University Press, 1982.

4. Weston JA. The migration and differentiation of neural crest cells. *Adv Morphog* 1970; **6**: 41–114.

5. Johnston MC. A radioautographic study of the migration and fate of cranial neural crest cells in the chick embryo. *Anat Rec* 1966; **156**: 143–56.

6. Le Douarin NM, Teillet M-AM. Experimental analysis of the migration and differentiation of neuroblasts of the autonomic nervous system and of neurectodermal mesenchymal derivatives, using a biological cell marking technique. *Dev Biol* 1974; **41**: 162–84.

7. Northcutt RG, Gans C. The genesis of neural crest and epidermal placodes: a reinterpretation of vertebrate origins. *Q Rev Biol* 1983; **58**: 1–28.

8. Johnston MC, Sulik KK. Some abnormal patterns of development in the craniofacial region. *Birth Defects* 1979; **15**: 23–42.

9. Le Lièvre CS, Le Douarin NM. Mesenchymal derivatives of the neural crest: analysis of chimaeric quail and chick embryos. *J Embryol Exp Morphol* 1975; **34**: 125–54.

10. Johnston MC. The neural crest in abnormalities of the face and brain. *Birth Defects* 1975; **11**: 1–18.

11. Kirby ML, Gilmore SA. A correlative histofluorescence and light microscopic study of the formation of the sympathetic trunks in chick embryos. *Anat Rec* 1976; **186**: 437–50.

12. Newgreen DF, Ritterman M, Peters EA. Morphology and behaviour of neural crest cells of chick embryo in vitro. *Cell Tissue Res* 1979; **203**: 115–40.

13. Platt JB. Ectodermal origin of the cartilages of the head. *Anat Anz* 1893; **8**: 506–9.

14. Opitz JM. Editorial Comment. The developmental field concept. *Am J Med Genet* 1985; **21**: 1–11.

15. Tosney KW. Early migration of neural crest cells in the trunk region of the avian embryo: an electron microscopic study. *Dev Biol* 1978; **62**: 317–33.

16. Weston JA, Ciment G, Girdlestone J. The role of extracellular matrix in neural crest development: a reevaluation. In: Trelsted RL, ed. *The Role of Extracellular Matrix in Development*. New York: Alan R Liss, 1984: 433–60.

17. Erickson CA, Weston JA. An SEM analysis of neural crest migration in the mouse. *J Embryol Exp Morphol* 1983; **74**: 97–118.

18. Newgreen DF. The rostral level of origin of sympathetic neurons in chick embryo studied in tissue culture. *Am J Anat* 1979; **154**: 557–562.

19. Newgreen DF, Scheel M, Kastner V. Morphogenesis of sclerotome and neural crest in avian embryos: in vivo and in vitro studies on the role of notochordal extracellular material. *Cell Tissue Res* 1986; **244**: 299–313.

20. Newgreen DF, Erickson CA. The migration of neural crest cells. *Int Rev Cytol* 1986; **103**: 89–145.

21. Cameron J, McCredie J. Innervation of undifferentiated limb bud in rabbit embryo. *J Anat* 1982; **134**: 795–808.

22. Sulik KK, Johnston MC, Ambrose LJH et al. Phenytoin (Dilantin)-induced cleft lip and palate in A/J mice: a scanning and transmission electron microscopic study. *Anat Rec* 1979; **195**: 243–55.

23. Boney AD. Abnormal growth of sporelings of a marine red alga induced by thalidomide. *Nature* 1963; **198**: 1069–9.

24. Nowack E. The sensitive phase for thalidomide embryopathy. *Humangenetik* 1965; **1**: 516–36.

25. Knapp K, Lenz W, Nowack E. Multiple congenital abnormalities. *Lancet* 1963; **ii**: 725.

26. Pfeiffer RA, Kosenow W. Thalidomide and congenital abnormalities. *Lancet* 1962; **i**: 45–6.

27. Henkel H-L, Willert H-G. Dysmelia: A classification and pattern of malformations in a group of congenital defects of the limbs. *J Bone Joint Surg* 1969; **51B**: 399–414.

28. Smithells RW. Defects and disabilities of thalidomide children. *BMJ* 1973; **i**: 269–72.

29. Rosen J. *Symmetry Discovered*. Cambridge: Cambridge University Press, 1975.

30. Ministry of Health Reports on Public Health and Medical Subjects No. 112. *Deformities caused by Thalidomide*. London: HMSO, 1964.

31. Willert H-G, Henkel H-L. *Klinik und Pathologie der Dysmelie: Die Fehlbildungen an den oberen Extremitäten bei der Thalidomid-Embryopathie*. Berlin: Springer-Verlag, 1969

CHAPTER 14

Neurotrophism

Introduction

Dinsmore and Mescher comment in their chapter in *Cellular and Molecular Basis of Regeneration: From Invertebrates to Humans*: 'Phylogenetically, the first true nerve cells in the animal kingdom evolved in coelenterates such as the hydroids. The extraordinary regenerative abilities of hydra, discovered by Abraham Trembley in 1740, have subsequently proven to be dependent on factors found in and secreted by its nerve cells.'[1]

This chapter introduces the biology of neurotrophism, a subject not taught in most medical courses. Neurotrophism is a vital component of embryology and dysmorphology. Without it, most birth defects cannot be understood.

Definition

The dependence of growth and repair upon nerves is known as neurotrophism. Nerves are said to have a trophic or growth-stimulating effect upon the tissues they supply.

In a Ciba Foundation Symposium on 'Growth of the Nervous System' in 1968, Singer[2] defined neurotrophism as 'that quality of the neuron, represented possibly in a neural secretion, responsible primarily for the structural maintenance and growth of the axonal processes but also for the morphological and structural integrity of the tissues upon which the axon terminates and of the myelin sheath which enfolds it'.

In 1974, at a New York Academy of Sciences conference on 'Trophic Functions of the Neuron', Drachman[3] defined neurotrophism as 'any long-term relationship in which nerve cells and target cells interact so as to influence the structure or function of either member of the pair'.

Chapter Summary
- Introduction
- Definition
- Neurotrophism in regeneration
- Neurotrophism in amphibia
- Principles of neurotrophism
- Classical experiments
- The neural mechanism of neurotrophism
- Quantitative and threshold factors
- Nerves at the amputation site in regeneration
- Neurotrophism stimulates mitosis
- Phases of regeneration
- The chemical basis of neurotrophism
- Neurotrophism in other species
- The early nerve-dependent phase of limb regeneration
- References

Neurotrophism in regeneration

There have been many papers published on different aspects of neurotrophism, and many conference reports and books discussing the role of nerves in regeneration of body parts. It is beyond the scope of this book to attempt to review that extensive literature, a task that has already been accomplished comprehensively in the book *Cellular and Molecular Basis of Regeneration: From Invertebrates to Humans*, edited by Ferretti and Géraudie.[4] Chapter 4 of that book, 'The role of the nervous system in regeneration', by Dinsmore and Mescher,[1] summarizes the history of experimental studies of regeneration and neurotrophism in various species and tissues, including abundant data on various 'putative trophic factors from nerves' that have come from molecular biology. Dinsmore and Mescher stress the important point that several compounds – strong claimants for roles as neurotrophic factors – 'at least act as potentiators of mitosis'. They note the lack of any 'developmental principle on which to organise these putative trophic factors'.

Neurotrophism in amphibia

The nature of nerve-dependent regeneration became an issue of scientific interest in 1823, when Todd first demonstrated the inhibitory effect of denervation on the regeneration of salamander limbs. The salamander remains the best-studied model of neurotrophism in regenerative growth. Neurotrophism in amphibia is easily demonstrated and is accessible to experimental manipulation. A great deal more was discovered about trophic *effects* than about trophic *mechanisms*.[3,5]

Principles of neurotrophism

The biological principles of neurotrophism have been formulated by Singer and his colleagues since the 1940s from classical studies on salamanders and other amphibia. From 1943, when Singer's PhD thesis was serialized in the *Journal of Experimental Zoology*, a lifetime of experimental work has shown that:

1. Sensory denervation prevents limb regeneration.
2. Motor denervation does not prevent regeneration, although all nerves have a limited trophic ability. This and point 1 established the important principle that *sensory nerves are more important than motor nerves in neurotrophism.*
3. *Neurotrophism is quantitative*, and depends on the *amount* of the nerve supply. Augmentation of supply by nerve deviation experiments can force regeneration of limbs in species that do not normally regenerate. A *threshold principle* operates, in that a certain quantity of nerve supply must be available before regeneration takes place.

4. Regeneration involves *two* sequential phases:
   (a) the first is *nerve-dependent*, and comprises *simple cell division*, i.e. a phase of simple mitotic activity rather than morphogenesis;
   (b) the second is *nerve-independent* and morphogenetic, regulating cell *differentiation* rather than simple cell division.

Classical experiments

In his initial experiment, Singer submitted two groups of the newt *Triturus viridescens* to cervical laminectomy and sectioning of the cervical nerves on one side (Figure 14.1). In one group, the motor roots of the nerves to the forelimbs were severed. In the second group, sensory roots were cut. Both forelimbs of both groups were then amputated, leaving each armless animal with an operated side and a control (unoperated) side. In terms of its cervical nerve supply, each animal had one normal side and the other side denervated. The animals were convalesced in aquaria for several weeks. Limb regeneration was then assessed. In all animals, the forelimbs on the unoperated side regenerated to normal. So had the limbs with motor denervation. However, there was little or no regrowth in the sensory-denervated limbs.

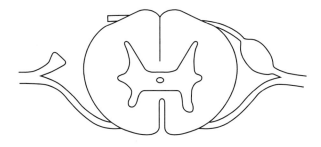

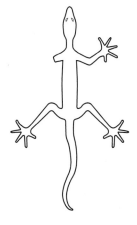

Figure 14.1 *Singer's classical experiment. Sensory denervation at the time of amputation of the limb prevents its regeneration. Any regeneration that occurs is directly proportional to the mass of residual dorsal root ganglion.*

Singer then extended his experiment by a simple, important step that is all too rarely taken. Instead of assuming that he had cut the sensory nerves as intended, he checked the actual damage. He killed the sensory-denervated group and made serial transverse sections of their spinal cords and cervical ganglia in order to measure the surgical injury. Microscopically, he found that where the sensory ganglia had been totally crushed or avulsed at surgery, no limb regeneration took place. Where the ganglia were partly damaged, some regeneration occurred. The *size* of the regenerate was *directly proportional* to the *volume* or *mass* of residual ganglion tissue. He concluded that limb regeneration depends upon the integrity of the sensory neuron, and, conversely, that the sensory neuron has a trophic or growth-stimulating function in relation to limb growth.[6]

The neural mechanism of neurotrophism

It has been shown that all neurons have some trophic effect, but that of the sensory neuron is dominant and the greatest in degree. Neither central connections nor reflex circuitry are required, for the trophic action is independent of the polarization of the neuron, and is always *centrifugal* in direction, emanating from the cell body and flowing thence into the distal neuronal processes.[7] This may sound contradictory in sensory nerves, whose well-known electrical impulses flow in a *centripetal* direction from peripheral sensory receptors to the brain. But the truth is that there is traffic both ways. In another experiment, Singer showed that normal cytoplasmic flow within nerve axons is *in two directions* (Figure 14.2).

Subsequent work by neurological scientists has shown that there are two speeds of centrifugal axoplasmic flow: fast within the neurotubules to convey neurotransmitter substances, and slow within axoplasm for transport of maintenance materials such as nutritional and waste products. Axoplasmic flow of proteins and other substances in a centrifugal direction in nerve fibres is a function completely separate from the centripetal conduction of electric sensory stimuli to the brain and spinal cord.

The neuron provides an existing cell structure and mechanism whereby a neurotrophic influence can be brought to bear upon growth at the cellular level. Neurotrophism needs to be recognized as another physiological function of sensory and autonomic nerves in addition to their function as conductors of sensory and autonomic impulses. Recognition of the principles of neurotrophism has been slower in medicine than in the biological sciences.

Quantitative and threshold factors

A quantitative factor became apparent early in the course of Singer's experiments. He observed that the more damaged the ganglia, the smaller the regenerate. A direct relationship was apparent between the

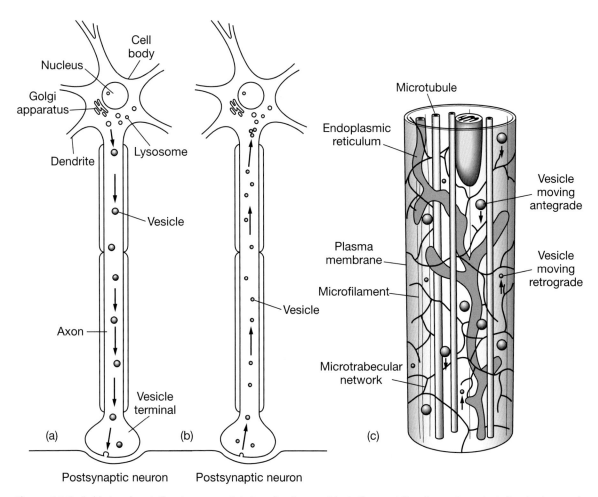

Figure 14.2 *(a,b): Axoplasmic flow in an axon is in two directions: nutrients flow centrifugally; waste products flow back towards the cell body. (c) Enlargement in three dimensions to show neurotubules and other organelles in the axon.*

volume of the regenerate and the amount of its residual nerve supply. At first, it was thought that there must be a threshold number of nerve fibres at the amputation surface for limb regeneration to occur.[8–10] Below this threshold, regeneration does not take place; above it, regrowth always occurs. But the speed and size of regrowth is not related to the number of fibres.[11] Instead, this threshold was shown to relate to the *cross-sectional area of axoplasm presenting at the amputation site*. The effectiveness of the individual neuron as an agent of growth is directly related to the cross-sectional area of its axon.[12]

Singer[13] emphasized the dependence of axonal processes upon their cell bodies for maintenance of their own growth and integrity. He proposed that both extracellular and intracellular growth influences are the same, and that nerve fibres continuously leak trophic substance into the tissues at the periphery. He thought that some degree of trophic ability is shared by all living cells, but that the neuron, *with its extraordinarily large volume of peripheral cytoplasm*, had overtaken smaller cells in the production of trophic substance or substances.

Nerves at the amputation site in regeneration

After amputation of an amphibian limb, cells at the cut surface of the stump rapidly deregulate into more primitive cells that epithelialize and seal off the wound. The following resume of events after amputation is from Dinsmore and Mescher:[1]

> 'The newly formed wound epithelium becomes richly supplied with regenerating axons of sensory nerves,[14] and the underlying dedifferentiating tissues are still more densely supplied with growing axons, which branch repeatedly and penetrate the area around the mesenchymal cells in great numbers.[15]
>
> 'At all stages of limb regeneration, the cells at the distal end of the limb stump are in close proximity to axons growing from the cut nerves.
>
> 'As differentiation proceeds distally, the diffusely arranged growing axons reorganise in the new limb as anatomically distinct nerve bundles with synaptic connections in motor end plates and sensory receptors.
>
> 'Nerves primarily effect the mitotic activity in dedifferentiating cells which give rise to the limb regeneration blastema.[15,16] Denervation at the time of limb amputation does not prevent epithelial closure of the wound, inflammation, or the onset of histolysis, which normally precede blastema formation. However, dedifferentiating cells do not proliferate in the absence of growing axons and no blastema forms.'

Denervation later, after a blastema has formed, reduces the rate of mitotic activity, but does not prevent differentiation of cells and subsequent limb morphogenesis. The resulting regenerate limb is smaller than normal.[15] Stocum and others have subsequently analysed the biosynthetic and gene activity in late-denervation regenerates. They conclude that the general reduction in macromolecular synthesis appears to reflect the decreased mitotic activity in the blastema after removal of growing axons. There is no evidence in this system that denervation alters specific gene activity.[16]

Once the regeneration blastema has formed, its growth enters a 'nerve-independent' phase, when differentiation of its parts is completed, but its size may be smaller than normal because of a reduced mitotic rate.

Singer showed that neurotrophism is quantitative, not qualitative. The amount of axoplasm at the amputation site is what matters, not the type of nerve. Sensory fibres comprise by far the most abundant population of nerves in newt forelimbs, and they can meet the quantitative demands alone. All cells probably possess some trophic ability, but nerves, by virtue of their large size, play the main role in trophic functions. Augmentation of nerve supply has been shown to induce regeneration in various experimental models. Again, it is the quantity of nerve supply that counts.

Neurotrophism stimulates mitosis

The trophic substance has eluded investigators. Possibly there is more than one chemical involved. Singer thought that there was a chemical cascade between the end of the axon and the target cell. This cascade might be complicated in a chemical sense, but its final message is essentially simple: it instructs the target cell to *divide*.[15] In other words, the trophic message is *to stimulate mitosis*. It is now agreed in regeneration biology that nerves primarily affect *mitotic activity* in dedifferentiating cells (at the surface of the amputation), which give rise to the regeneration blastema or growing stump.[16]

Phases of regeneration

The timing of denervation is critical.[1,17]

Denervation first, amputation later

Dedifferentiating cells do not divide and proliferate in the absence of growing axons. No blastema forms in a denervated area.

Simultaneous amputation and denervation

The neurotrophic effect is most obvious when denervation is done at the same time as amputation, as in Singer's original study.

In denervation at or soon after amputation, adequate numbers of cells do not enter the cell cycle, leading to their failure to proliferate and form a blastema; the percentage of cell divisions remains very low.[17] This not only causes regeneration to fail, but also prevents the repair of injured tissues.[1] Continuation of the state of denervation leads to gradual regression in volume as dedifferentiating cells die.[17]

Amputation first, denervation later

If denervation is done some time after amputation, at a stage when there is a well-formed regeneration blastema, the subsequent rate of mitotic activity is still reduced, but cell differentiation and morpho-genesis are not prevented. Such late denervations have been shown to reduce the size of the final regenerated limb, and to reduce the DNA replication (by up to 50%), the synthesis of all classes of RNA, overall protein synthesis, and production of glycosaminoglycans.[16] The general reduction in these macromolecular syntheses reflects the *decreased mitotic activity with the loss of live axons*.

There is no evidence that denervation alters the specific activity of genes or their expression.[16]

Denervation after the formation of a blastema results therefore in small regenerates with documented low mitotic rates, but no interference with tissue differentiation.[18–20] This indicates that the nerve-independent stage of regeneration has been reached, and the effect of subsequent denervation is therefore less.

The chemical basis of neurotrophism

A search for the trophic factor or factors has continued to the molecular level in the wake of Singer's original work, and the problem is not yet resolved (see the review by Dinsmore and Mescher[1]). All evidence points to the nerve axons being responsible for transportation of critical proteins such as transferrin to the early blastema, even substituting for capillaries if the stump has been rendered avascular.[21] There is strong evidence that neurotubules in axons may act as extremely fine conduits for the safe delivery of trophic factors essential for cell division, transmission being via the fast, microtubular component of axonal transport.[22,23]

Neurotrophism in other species

Experiments on regeneration have largely been confined to amphibia, in which the phenomenon of limb regeneration is so obvious. Higher vertebrates have lost the capacity to regenerate adult limbs, yet the facts of evolution may be cited in support of a neurotrophic influence upon the formation of vertebrate limbs in general. The fish and amphibia of 150 million years ago were the forebears of both present-day newts and higher vertebrates, including *Homo sapiens*. Fossils of these ancient amphibia display classic pentadactyl limbs, primitive variants of our own. Darwin himself pondered over the phenomenal similarity of limb anatomy throughout the vertebrate kingdom:[24]

> 'What can be more curious than that the hand of man, formed for grasping, that of a mole for digging, the leg of a horse, the paddle of a porpoise, and the wing of a bat should all be constructed on the same pattern, and should include similar bones in the same relative positions?'

There is no evidence to suggest that the neurotrophic dependence of limb formation (as exhibited in newts of today) has been abandoned or superseded during evolution by an alternative mechanism of limb formation in higher vertebrates, especially as the overall pentadactyl pattern has remained constant over millions of years. The basic morphology of pentadactyl limbs is common to ancient fossils, modern newts and all higher vertebrates. The inescapable likelihood is that the underlying mechanism of limb morphogenesis is, and has always been, common to all vertebrates.

Pisces

The ability to regenerate pectoral fins is believed to be an inherited property from a common ancestor.[25] The same rules of regeneration appear to apply to the regrowth of fins in fish as to limb regeneration in amphibia, although the events are completed more rapidly in some fish.[26–28] As in amphibia, denervation completely inhibits the ability of amputated fins to regenerate. From a study of five genera of teleosts, Géraudie and Singer[26] found a close correlation between nerve supply and regenerative capacity. A battery of genes is reactivated in the injured fin to contribute to its regeneration. These are the same genes as those identified in limb regeneration in higher vertebrates.[29]

Marsupials

Following in the footsteps of Singer's augmentation experiments, Mizell and Isaacs[30] induced regeneration of amputated hind limbs in newborn opossum (*Didelphys virginiana*). This marsupial is born at an embryonic stage (12 days, which is equivalent to 2 months' human gestation) and it slowly matures in the pouch during the next few weeks. Mizell and Isaacs implanted neural tissue (cerebral cortex) close to the base of the newborn limb, then amputated the limb 2–4 days later. In their controlled experiments, 8 of 30 young opossum limbs regenerated. They concluded that mammalian embryonic limbs are capable of regeneration when additional nervous tissue is supplied.

Higher animals

Many zoologists regard the newt as an adult creature that has retained certain embryonic properties such as the ability to form limbs. Adult members of the higher ranks of vertebrates have lost the embryonic property to generate limbs and to repeat embryonic limb morphogenesis later in life. Several theories exist as to how and why this property was lost during evolution, but discussion of these is peripheral to the purpose of this book.

Humans and wound healing

It has been recorded that amputated fingertips in young children will tend to regenerate if the wound is kept open rather than sutured.[31]

There are several well-established examples in medicine of the trophic effect of nerves upon maintenance and growth of other structures. When nerves are cut, muscles waste. Taste buds and other sensory organelles degenerate. Poliomyelitis damages motor nerves and reduces growth in affected limbs. After a stroke (cerebrovascular accident), there is wasting of muscles on the hemiplegic side of the body.

Wound healing in adults is slow and incomplete in sensory neuropathic tissues. One example is the problem of indolent, trophic ulcers on the feet of diabetic patients with sensory peripheral neuropathy. Another is incomplete healing of fractures and dislocations in neuropathic bones.

The relevance of neurotrophism to wound healing and other human diseases where sensory nerves are damaged is reviewed in Chapter 30.

Nerves dominate the character of muscles

The speed of conduction within a nerve fibre is either slow or fast. The contractility of muscle fibres is also intrinsically slow or fast. By crossed innervation experiments between fast and slow muscles and fast and slow nerves, Eccles[32] showed that the nature of the nerves dominates the nature of the muscles. If slow nerves are surgically attached to fast muscles, those muscles will change from fast to slow.

The early nerve-dependent phase of limb regeneration

Figure 14.3 shows the results of experiments by Wallace,[22] in which he counted mitotic figures per thousand cells in the early stages of newt limb regeneration before digit formation. The dashed curve depicts a big surge of mitotic activity immediately after amputation at day 0, causing an undifferentiated blastema to emerge from the amputation site from day 3. The mitotic activity subsides as differentiation takes over and digits become delineated around day 18.

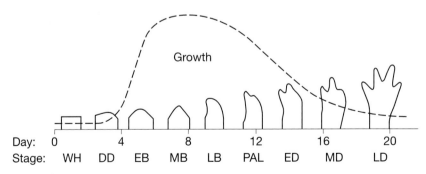

Figure 14.3 *Temporal relationship between cellular proliferation (growth: dashed curve) and the progressive stages of limb regeneration. The dashed curve representing growth is an approximation of relative labelling indices at each stage based on data from Wallace.[22] The stages illustrated are as follows: WH, wound healing; DD, de-differentiation; EB, early bud; MB, medium bud; LB, late bud; PAL, palette; ED, early digits; MD, medium digits; LD, late digits. (From Ferretti P, Géraudie J, eds.* Cellular and Molecular Basis of Regeneration: From Invertebrates to Humans. *Chichester: Wiley, 1998:190.)*

This important study has profound implications for understanding the pathogenesis of birth defects. It defines the nerve-dependent phase of limb regeneration. The question is whether the embryo has a similar early phase of nerve-dependent mitosis before the genes activate differentiation. If so, a neurotoxin administered at or before this phase could theoretically halt mitosis, reduce the final number of cells in the limb bud, and reduce the cell mass of the limb bud within which the genes will subsequently act during differentiation.

But it is said that there are no nerves in embryonic limb buds, and thus no neurotrophic influence can influence limb morphogenesis in the embryo.

That belief is examined in the next chapter.

References

1. Dinsmore CE, Mescher AL. The role of the nervous system in regeneration. In: Ferretti P, Géraudie J, eds. *Cellular and Molecular Basis of Regeneration: From Invertebrates to Humans*. Chichester: Wiley, 1998.

2. Singer M. Penetration of labelled amino acids into the peripheral nerve fibre from surrounding body fluids. In: *Growth of the Nervous System: Ciba Foundation Symposium*. London: Churchill, 1968: 200–219.

3. Drachman DB. Trophic actions of the neuron: an introduction. *Ann NY Acad Sci* 1974; **228**: 3–5.

4. Ferretti P, Géraudie J, eds. *Cellular and Molecular Basis of Regeneration: From Invertebrates to Humans*. Chichester: Wiley, 1998.

5. Guth L. Trophic effects of vertebrate neurons. Overview and discussion: What do we mean by the 'trophic' function of the neuron? *Neurosci Res Prog Bull* 1969; **7**(1): 43–54.

6. Singer M. The nervous system and regeneration of the forelimb of adult *Triturus. J Exp Zool* 1943; **92**: 297.

7. Singer M. Neurotrophic control of limb regeneration in the newt. *Ann NY Acad Sci* 1974; **228**: 308–22.

8. Singer M. The nervous system and the regeneration of the forelimbs of the adult *Triturus*. The influence of the number of nerve fibres. *J Exp Zool* 1946; **101**: 299–337.

9. Singer M. The nervous system and regeneration of the forelimb of adult *Triturus*. IV The stimulating action of a regenerated motor supply. *J Exp Zool* 1946; **101**: 221–40.

10. Singer M. The nervous system and regeneration of the forelimb of adult *Triturus*. VII The relation between number of nerve fibres and surface area of amputation. *J Exp Zool* 1947; **104**: 251–65.

11. Singer M, Induction of regeneration of the forelimb of the post metamorphic frog by augmentation of the nerve supply. *J Exp Zool* 1954; **126**: 419–472.

12. Singer M, Rhezak K, Maier CS. The relation between the calibre of the axon and the trophic activity of nerves in limb regeneration. *J Exp Zool* 1967; **166**: 89–98.

13. Singer M. The trophic quality of the neuron: some theoretical considerations. In: Singer M, Scháde JP, eds. *Mechanisms of Neural Regeneration.* Amsterdam: Elsevier, 1964: 228–32.

14. Singer M. The invasion of the epidermis is of the regenerating forelimb of the urodele *Triturus* by nerve fibers. *J Exp Zool* 1949; **111**: 189–209.

15. Singer M. The influence of the nerve in regeneration of the amphibian extremity. *Q Rev Biol* 1952; **27**: 169–200.

16. Stocum D. *Wound Repair, Regeneration and Artificial Tissues.* Austin, TX: RG Landes, 1995.

17. Tassava RA, McCullough WD. Neural control of cell cycle events in regenerating salamander limbs. *Am Zool* 1978; **18**: 843–54.

18. Singer M, Craven L. The growth and morphogenesis of the regenerating forelimb of adult *Triturus* following denervation at various stages of development. *J Exp Zool* 1948; **108**: 270–308.

19. Maden M. Neurotrophic control of the cell cycle during amphibian limb regeneration *J Embryol Exp Morphol* 1978; **48**: 169–175.

20. Boilly B, Oudkhir M, Lassalle B. Control of the cell cycle by the peripheral nervous system during newt limb regeneration: continuous labelling analysis. *Biol Cell* 1985; **55**: 107–12.

21. Kiffmeyer WR, Tomusk EV, Mescher AL. Axonal transport and release of transferrin in nerves of regenerating amphibian limbs. *Dev Biol* 1991; **147**: 392–402.

22. Wallace H. *Vertebrate Limb Regeneration.* Chichester: Wiley, 1981.

23. Scadding SR. Treatment of brachial nerves with colchicine inhibits limb regeneration in the newt *Notophthalmos viridescens. J Exp Zool* 1998; **247**: 56–61.

24. Darwin C. *Origin of Species by Means of Natural Selection.* 1859.

25. Thouveny Y, Tassava RA. Regeneration through phylogenesis. In: Ferretti P, Géraudie J, eds. *Cellular and Molecular Basis of Regeneration: From Invertebrates to Humans.* Chichester: Wiley, 1998.

26. Géraudie J, Singer M. Relation between nerve fiber number and pectoral fin regeneration in the teleost. *J Exp Zool* 1977; **199**: 1–8.

27. Géraudie J, Singer M. Necessity of an adequate nerve supply for regeneration of the amputated pectoral fin in the teleost *Fundulus. J Exp Zool* 1985; **234**: 367–74.

28. Géraudie J, Singer M. The fish fin regenerate. In: Taban C, Boilly B, eds. *Keys for Regeneration.* Basel: Karger, 1992: 62–72.

29. Géraudie J, Akimenko M-A, Smith MM. The dermal skeleton. In: Ferretti P, Géraudie J, eds. *Cellular and Molecular Basis of Regeneration: From Invertebrates to Humans.* Chichester: Wiley, 1998.

30. Mizell M, Isaacs JJ. Induced regeneration of hind limbs in the newborn opossum. *Am Zool* 1970; **10**: 141–55.

31. Illingworth CM. Trapped fingers and amputated finger tips in children. *J Pediatr Surg* 1974; **9**: 853–8.

32. Eccles JC. The effects of nerve cross-union on muscle contraction. In: Milhorat AT, ed. *Exploratory Concepts in Muscular Dystrophy and Related Disorders.* Amsterdam: Excerpta Medica 1967: 151–63.

CHAPTER 15

Nerve in limb bud

T he experiment described in this chapter was carried out by Dr John Cameron as part of his PhD project in the Department of Medicine, University of Sydney, where the Neurological Laboratory is fully equipped for the investigation of peripheral neuropathies. Professor JG McLeod's encouragement, criticism and guidance in this research were invaluable. Miss Virginia Best provided expert assistance with histological, electron microscopic and photographic preparations. Mrs Diana Shaw typed the manuscript, and the illustrations were made by the Department of Illustration, University of Sydney. The study was financed by a generous grant from the Ramaciotti Foundations of New South Wales. This experiment was published in *The Lancet*[1] and in the *Journal of Anatomy*[2] The first part of this chapter is adapted from the latter journal, with permission. The illustrations are from Dr Cameron's Thesis, with permission.

Chapter Summary
- Introduction
- Materials and methods
- Results
- Discussion
- Summary
- Review of some literature published after the above work
- Conclusion
- References

Introduction

In the wake of the thalidomide disaster of 1958–62, several theories have been proposed concerning the mechanism of teratogenic action of this drug. One theory is that thalidomide deformities were secondary to neural crest injury, and that the neural crest was the target organ for the action of thalidomide in the embryo.[3–5] The most important outcome of this hypothesis is that it provides a mechanism that might explain the majority of sporadic congenital malformations unrelated to thalidomide. Thereby it could unify the understanding of many teratogenic influences through provision of a common mechanism.

The neural crest hypothesis has been criticized by O'Rahilly and Gardner,[6,7] Poswillo,[8] and Wolpert,[9] because certain aspects of the hypothesis appear to contradict present-day concepts of morphogenesis. One fundamental criticism concerns the precise timing of innervation of the limb bud relative to its differentiation. In their comprehensive review of limb bud development, O'Rahilly and Gardner[6] contended that there exists a significant delay in the appearance of nerve fibres within the proximal parts of the human limb bud (stage 14–15) compared with the emergence of the limb bud as a structure at stage 12. Furthermore, they maintained that condensation of mesenchyme to form the nidus of future skeletal components of the hand and foot plates seemed to precede the ingrowth of nerve fibres. O'Rahilly and Gardner based their opinions predominantly upon the detailed studies of limb development carried out by Bardeen and Lewis[10] and Lewis.[11] The latter authors described the earliest condensation of forelimb mesenchyme in the site of the future humerus at the beginning of the 4th week of life. They observed that nerve fibres at that stage extended only as far as the base of the limb bud, implying that condensation of mesenchyme precedes the entry of nerve axons into the limb.

Because the neural crest hypothesis requires nerve fibres to be present at the site of initial condensation and differentiation in the limb bud, the criticism of O'Rahilly and Gardner,[6] based upon Lewis's observations,[10] would appear to be reasonable. However, unmyelinated axons, and embryonic axons prior to myelination, are exquisitely delicate, and are easily destroyed during fixation and embedding, especially when hot paraffin is used. Furthermore, these axons are often difficult to detect and to identify by light microscopy, even with ideal tissue preparation and good microscopic resolution. The histological methods available to Bardeen and Lewis in 1900 would not be considered as adequate for this task by modern standards of tissue preparation and microscopy.[10] On purely technical grounds, therefore, a potential discrepancy can be seen to exist between the observations of Bardeen and Lewis and the true situation. Before the criticism of O'Rahilly and Gardner can be upheld, it is necessary to establish whether embryonic nerve fibres are present or absent at the site of early mesenchymal condensation. The following experiment was designed for that purpose, using modern methods of tissue preparation and inspection, including electron microscopy.

Materials and method

The rabbit embryo was chosen as a model for this study of mammalian limb buds and their innervation, because neural crest development has been studied extensively in this species[12–16] and because the rabbit is susceptible to thalidomide.[17–25] It has been established that the rabbit embryo is sensitive to thalidomide between 8 and 14 days' gestation, and that cartilage is first visible within the forelimb bud on the 13th day (320 hours' gestation). It was decided to study the upper limb buds at 260 and 290 hours' gestation, because at the former time the limb bud consists of undifferentiated mesenchyme, and at the latter time early mesenchymal condensation has begun, but has not yet proceeded to chondrogenesis.

Two laboratory-bred Castle Hill White rabbits were mated naturally, and the time of copulation was recorded as zero-hour. The does were then removed from the breeding cage, placed in separate cages, and allowed free access to water and food pellets. One doe was anaesthetized at 260 hours' and the other at 290 hours' gestation, using oxygen–halothane (1%) inhalation. Through a midline laparotomy incision, the uterine horns were exposed, and the products of conception were removed by careful division of the embryonic membranes. The adult rabbit was killed by an intracardiac injection of thiopentone.

All embryos were fixed by immediate immersion in Karnovsky's solution[26] at room temperature, and allowed to fix for 2 hours. Each specimen was rinsed in buffered sodium cacodylate solution and post-fixed for another 90 minutes in Dalton's solution.[27] After a second rinsing in buffered cacodylate, the specimens were dehydrated slowly through solutions of increasing strengths of ethanol up to 100%, followed by further dehydration in absolute acetone. Each embryo was obliquely transacted to separate the forelimbs prior to impregnation and embedding in Spurr's medium.

Two embryos, one typical of 260 hours' gestation and one typical of 290 hours' gestation, were selected for study of innervation of the limb buds (Figure 15.1).

Serial longitudinal sections, each 1 μm thick, were cut throughout one entire upper limb bud and the adjacent trunk of each embryo in a cephalocaudal direction (Figure 15.2a). Serial sections, also 1 μm thick, were cut from the tip of the opposite limb bud in a disto-proximal direction transverse to the axis of the limb bud (Figure 15.2b). Sections were stained with 0.2% toluidine blue and examined serially by light microscopy for the presence of neural tissue before further sectioning proceeded.

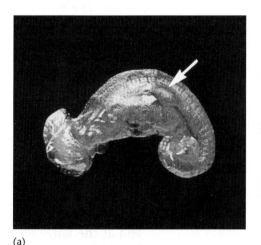

(a)

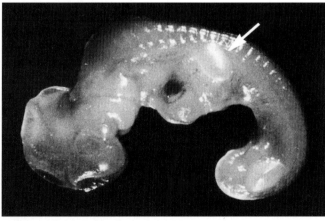

(b)

Figure 15.1 *Rabbit embryos of 260 hours' (a) and 290 hours' (b) gestation. Arrows indicate upper limb buds.*

Figure 15.2 *Planes of
section: (a) in longitudinal axis
of limb bud; (b) transverse to
long axis of the limb bud.*

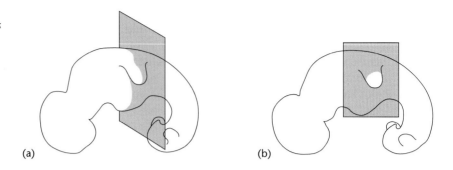

(a)   (b)

Areas of tissue that were thought to show bundles of embryonic
nerve fibres at light microscopy were prepared for electron microscopy.
Sections were cut on an LKB Ultramicrotome at 60–90 nm thickness.
They were placed on copper grids and stained with lead citrate for 5
minutes, then with uranyl acetate for 5 minutes. They were examined
under an electron microscope (Siemens 102 Elmiscope).

Results

Embryo of 260 hours' gestation

The embryo selected for study at 260 hours' gestation had a crown–rump
length of 6 mm. The maximum length of the upper limb bud was found
to be 0.5 mm, by measurement of serial longitudinal sections throughout the limb bud under a light microscope fitted with an eyepiece gratic-
ule. The maximum transverse diameter of the limb bud at its base was

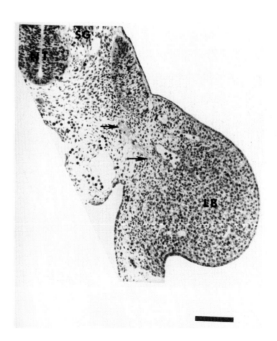

Figure 15.3 *Low power,
longitudinal section of 260-
hour embryonic limb bud;
arrows indicate the nerves
entering it. Scale bar 150 μm.*

measured by the same method, and was found to be 0.6 mm. The mesenchyme within the limb bud was still undifferentiated at this stage, and the limb bud lacked any external differentiation.

From these serial longitudinal sections, the outgrowth of nerve bundles from the early condensing sensory ganglia and from the ventral neural tube was traced to its furthest extent at the most proximal region of the limb bud (arrows in Figure 15.3).

Embryo of 290 hours' gestation

The embryo selected at 290 hours' gestation had a crown–rump length of 8 mm. The maximum length of the forelimb bud was 1.4 mm, with a maximum base diameter of 1.1 mm. Macroscopically, however, condensation and early differentiation of mesenchyme had begun within the proximal part of the bud. The distal part of the limb bud was still composed of loosely packed, undifferentiated mesenchymal cells (Figure 15.4).

The sensory ganglia adjacent to the limb bud had condensed and showed spindle-shaped and transitional globular neuroblasts as described by Tennyson[12] (Figure 15.5). A well-developed outgrowth of

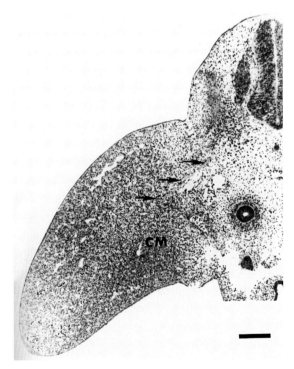

Figure 15.4 *Low power, longitudinal section of 290-hour limb bud; arrows indicate nerve trunk extending into upper third. CM, condensing mesenchyme. Scale bar: 200 μm.*

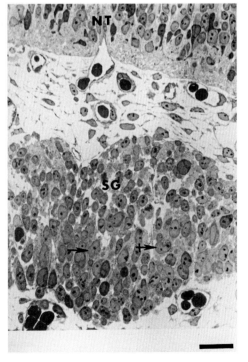

Figure 15.5 *High power of neuroblasts in sensory ganglion (SG). Arrows indicate neuroblasts. NT, neural tube. Scale bar: 25 μm.*

nerve bundles could be traced from both the sensory ganglia and the ventral neural tube to the junction of the proximal and middle thirds of the limb bud (Figures 15.6 and 15.7), at its maximum visible extent by light microscopy. The extent of this innervation was confirmed by serial transverse sections of the opposite forelimb bud of the same embryo (Figures 15.7–15.9). At the most distal extent of this ingrowth, the nerve bundles were observed to arborize into fine protoplasmic processes within the region of mesenchymal condensation (Figure 15.7).

Electron micrographs of transverse sections where the nerve bundles had been seen by light microscopy showed the typical mosaic patterns of developing axons described by Tennyson.[13,14] The axons were of uniform size, and each contained numerous neurotubules and neurofilaments, with occasional mitochondria (Figures 15.10–15.12). Many bundles of axons were surrounded by almost continuous cytoplasm of immature Schwann cells (Figure 15.10).

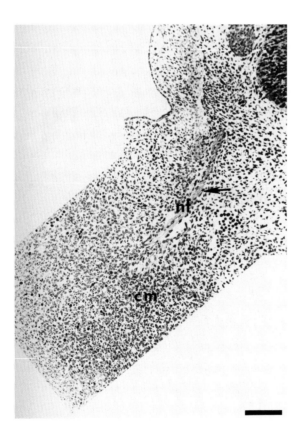

Figure 15.6 *Longitudinal section montage of nerve fibre ingrowth (NF) at 290 hours' gestation. CM, condensing mesenchyme at site of nerve fibre ingrowth. Scale bar: 500 μm.*

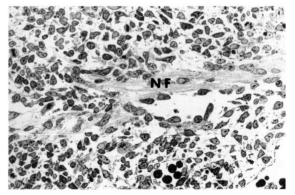

Figure 15.7 *High power of nerve fibres in 290-hour limb bud. Nerve fibres (NF) sprouting to left are infiltrating into condensing mesenchyme.*

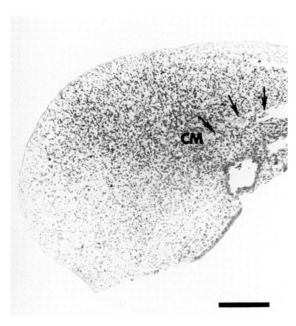

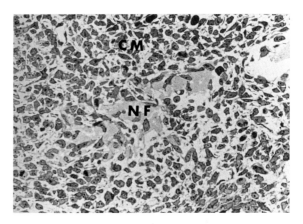

Figure 15.9 *Transverse section, high power, of nerve fibres ingrowth (NF) in the 290-hour limb bud shown in Figure 15.8. CM, condensing mesenchyme. Scale bar: 50 µm.*

Figure 15.8 *Transverse section, low power, of nerves within a 290-hour limb bud. CM, condensing mesenchyme around nerve fibres. Scale bar: 200 µm.*

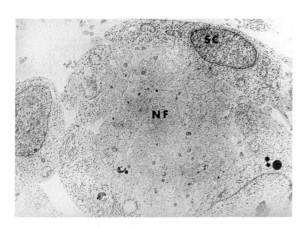

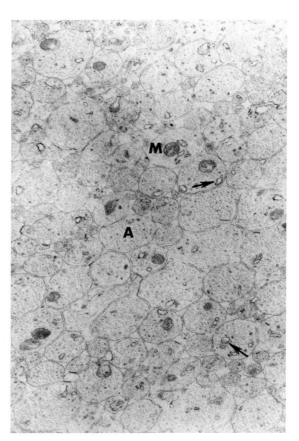

Figure 15.10 *Electron microscopy of transverse section of a bundle of axons in 290-hour limb bud (NF). Axons make a mosaic pattern and contain many neurotubules, microfilaments and a few mitochondria. SC, a Schwann cell starting to wrap around the bundle of axons. Magnification × 13 000.*

Figure 15.11 *Transverse section of axons in 290-hour limb bud, forming a fine mosaic. EM × 13 000 and enlarged photographically. Axon (A), mitochondrion (M), arrows on vesicles. Fine dots are neurotubules.*

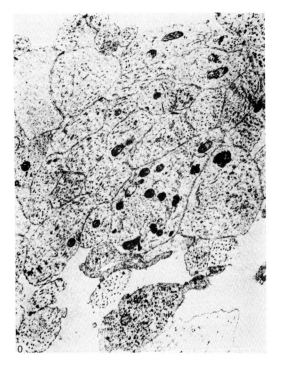

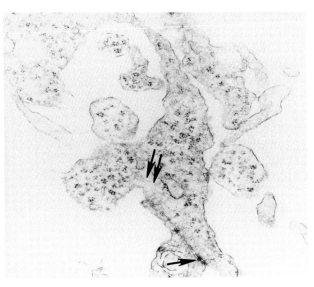

Figure 15.13 *Cytoplasmic processes of a primitive neuroblast at 290 hours' gestation. Single arrow indicates a gap junction. Double arrows indicate neurotubules. EM × 30 000.*

Figure 15.12 *Transverse section of axons: black spots are mitochondria and fine dots in the axoplasm are neurotubules, a diagnostic marker. EM × 60 000.*

Discussion

The innervation of the undifferentiated forelimb bud of the rabbit has been shown by this study to be more extensive than hitherto realized. In a previous study of the development of the ventral horn of the spinal cord in rabbits, Romanes[28] briefly described the early innervation of the forelimb. His observations were made upon rabbit embryos fixed in alcohol–ammonia, impregnated with pyridine–silver, and sectioned at 10 μm thickness. In a 5 mm embryo, he was unable to trace the nerve outgrowth further than the junction of fibres from the sensory ganglia and the ventral horn. However, he noted that more distal mesenchymal cells were orientated along the axis of projected outgrowth, beyond the limit of visible fibres. In an 8 mm embryo, he noted a more developed outgrowth of nerve fibres from both motor and sensory sources. However, the outgrowth appeared to cease abruptly at the base of the limb bud. The inability of Romanes to demonstrate the extent of innervation seen in the present study may have been due to his tissue preparation and the thickness of his sections. The extent of nerve fibre growth that is apparent in silver preparations is not necessarily the real limit of the extent of axonal growth, since the fine protoplasmic processes at the tips of nerve fibres tend not to take up the silver stain, and may also be beyond the limits of resolution of light microscopy.[29–31]

Bardeen and Lewis[10] based their observations upon published drawings, photographs and waxplate reconstructions of human embryos up to 20 mm in length. The initial method of tissue fixation was not specified. The thickness of their sections for microscopy varied from 10 μm to 50 μm. The 3-week-old embryo in which they studied limb development was sectioned at 20 μm intervals. Bardeen and Lewis[10] observed that:

> 'the Wolffian ridge and limb buds, which appear during the third week, consist, therefore, at the end of this period, merely of a mass of mesenchyme which intervenes between the coelom and the ectoderm lateral to the axis of the body. This mesenchyme contains a vascular plexus.'

Spinal ganglia and nerve roots were described in the trunk of this embryo, but the presence of nerve fibres within the limb bud was not documented. Nerves were first recorded entering upper and lower limb buds during the 4th week, although these extended 'for no considerable distance into the limb bud' at a stage when mesenchymal condensation for the future humerus was visible.

The rabbit embryos used in the present experiment are at equivalent stages of development to the human embryos described by Bardeen and Lewis.[10] Immediate fixation, a cold embedding technique and serial 1 μm sections have revealed that nerve bundles are present within the proximal third of the limb bud at the time of mesenchymal condensation and early differentiation in that area. Arborization of axons within the region of mesenchymal condensation indicates an earlier and more intimate relationship between embryonic nerves and mesenchyme than has been recognized in the past.

Our findings are supported by studies in lower vertebrates. Taylor[29] made a detailed study of early innervation of the forelimbs of frog larvae. Tadpoles were fixed in Bouin's or Zenker's fluid, embedded in paraffin, and stained with silver and Mallory's azar triple stains. Taylor's reconstruction of serial sections showed a well-developed nerve supply penetrating into the limb bud before mesenchymal condensation had begun. He reported a reticulum of very fine protoplasmic nerve fibres within the undifferentiated mesenchyme, similar to that observed in the present study of the rabbit embryo. He concluded that differentiation in the limb bud occurs *after* the mesenchyme has been invaded by nerve fibres, and *after* the major branches of the nerve trunks have formed. Our findings indicate that a similar conclusion can be drawn in relation to the mammalian limb bud.

Such a conclusion has important implications for the understanding of the control of embryonic differentiation. It is commonly believed that limb buds are self-differentiating systems[32] and that nerves play no part in their differentiation.[6-9] What governs differentiation has remained a subject for debate. Initial elongation of the undifferentiated limb bud has been shown to be due to rapid proliferation of cells at the distal tip of the bud, known as the apical ectodermal ridge.[33-35] It has been suggested that this basic pattern of development is common to all vertebrates, such that the musculoskeletal system is laid down within the limb buds in a proximodistal sequence.[36,37] The fact that this proximodistal gradient of differentiation is in the opposite direction to the initial distoproximal production of mesenchyme from the tip of the limb bud has stimulated several hypotheses. Saunders[33] believed that the apical ectodermal ridge played an inductive role, in that 'there is no further elaboration of distal structures such as hands or fingers, once the ridge has been removed'. Bell, Kaighn and Fassenden[38] and Bell, Saunders and Zwilling[39] correlated their findings and agreed that limb development may proceed in the absence of an apical ectodermal ridge, but that distal outgrowth may depend upon the presence of a 'refractile' layer beneath the ridge.

Wolpert[9] has sought to explain the proximodistal gradient of differentiation by a hypothesis of positional awareness. He has proposed that mesenchymal cells are able to sense their position in space by reference to a 'three-dimensional grid' based on cell–cell contact. He suggests that differentiation occurs in relation to the spatial orientation of cells. The lack of any anatomical framework for such a complex grid casts doubt upon Wolpert's hypothesis. Another inherent weakness is that this hypothesis bestows upon primitive mesenchymal cells the sophisticated function of consciousness of position in space. (This is a normal property of neurons, known as proprioception. It seems unlikely that simple mesenchymal cells should possess a neural property for a short period in embryogenesis.)

Our serial sections showed nerves branching proximodistally within the condensing mesenchyme prior to differentiation. The direction of nerve growth parallels the gradient of differentiation in time and space. The nerves provide an anatomical framework, linked to the neuraxis, through which neurotrophic influences might be brought to bear upon mesenchyme during condensation and early differentiation. It is also possible that an insult to these axons by a neurotoxin such as thalidomide could result in derangement of mesenchymal differentiation within a zone being innervated at that time. The presence of axons prior to mesenchymal differentiation provides a feasible anatomical basis through which a neurotrophic influence might be exerted.

The question of whether or not there is a role for nerves in differentiation has not been explored in the present study, although, in view of the results, such a possibility exists. In the past, some in vitro studies, using cultured or grafted limb buds, have suggested that the 'non-innervated' limb bud is a self-differentiating system. The state of innervation of limb buds used in such experiments would need to be checked by suitable neurohistological methods as described here, lest early innervation be overlooked and a false conclusion be drawn.

Summary

The concept that there are no nerves in the limb bud of mammalian embryos prior to differentiation has been re-examined and refuted. Rabbit embryos were collected at 260 and 290 hours' gestation, which is prior to cartilage formation in the forelimb at 320 hours. Forelimb buds and adjacent neural tube were excised, fixed and embedded for light and electron microscopy. The limb buds were sectioned in two planes by serial 1 μm sections and inspected by light microscopy. Bundles of nerve fibres were seen within the proximal third of the limb bud, with distal ramification into adjacent zones of condensing mesenchyme. Electron microscopy confirmed the presence of axons and associated immature Schwann cells. These results demonstrate the existence of an anatomical framework through which a neurotrophic influence might be brought to bear upon mesenchyme prior to early differentiation.

Review of some literature published after the above work

Subsequent to publication of the above work in 1978 and 1982, the controversy about innervation of the limb bud continued. Following the 1978 *Lancet* publication of our research, some biologists continued to resuscitate the old theory of nerveless limb buds.

In a paper presented in Berlin in 1980, Lewis,[40] from Wolpert's laboratory, challenged our *Lancet* paper of 1978 on this topic with an experiment on 2-day chick embryos, attempting to eliminate the sensory component of wing innervation by ultraviolet light reflected with mirrors. No evidence was provided that this aim could be or had been achieved. The method as described required that the egg be moved during treatment and microscopy, with no proof that the UV beam remained focused on the target. Lewis nevertheless asserted that he had confirmed 'the old view that the development of the limb skeleton is independent of innervation'. This claim was based on an unproven method of injury, coupled with silver staining/light microscopy, despite the known limitations of both in defining the distal ends of nerve axons. Many older studies relied on silver stains and drew the wrong conclusions. The distal extremes of unmyelinated axons are not revealed by silver stains, and their presence has gone undetected because of limitations in the methodology.

Lewis's method lacks the power of resolution needed to support his conclusion – a classical false negative. His study did not refute what we found by using electron microscopy. Electron microscopy has superseded silver stains in medical neuropathology laboratories because of its reliability and superior power of resolution for imaging distal axons.

In the light of our experiment, we propose that any limb bud, at any stage, contains axons and growth cones until proven otherwise by appropriate neurohistology and electron microscopy, when read by an experienced neuropathologist. Application of this principle to past limb bud experiments enables them to be re-interpreted, and a more rational process of limb development emerges.

On the matter of early innervation of the limb bud, discord exists between what is taught in biology and in neurology. The following statement based on Taylor's work[29] appears in Dyck and Thomas's 1975 textbook on peripheral neuropathy:[41]

> 'Nerve sprouts are found in the limb buds as they form, and when a frog's limb bud is less than 1 mm long, the major limb nerves can be recognised. At this early stage, muscle and bone are represented only by condensing mesenchyme.'

Bancroft and Bellairs[42] showed in chick embryo that neural crest cells tend to overlap one another and that they have filopodia that contact other crest cells. Cameron in our laboratory found similar cytoplasmic processes as part of neural crest cells (Figure 15.13).

Varon and Bunge,[43] leaders in nerve cell culture, stress the precocity of sensory neuritic growth cones advancing ahead of Schwann cells.

Of critical concern is the period just before the limb bud emerges from the trunk. Thalidomide induced arm defects from day 24, but the limb bud only appears on day 28 (stage 12). What is the nerve supply doing in those 4 critical days? What is the chronological relationship between neurite outgrowth from neural crest cells and the emergence of the limb bud from the wall of the trunk?

Tosney[44] showed by scanning electron microscopy that axons arise from crest cells very early, prior to segmentation of the crest into ganglia, and prior to any migration of neural crest cells (Chapter 13). Nerve cells and their fibrillar processes are so shaped that they can invade the intercellular spaces of other tissues and organs with their fine protoplasmic extensions, irrespective of where the nuclei of the nerve cells actually reside. This complements observations by Taylor and ourselves that nerve bundles are already present in the proximal limb bud when it first arises from the trunk. The fibrils seen by Tosney on scanning electron microscopy must lie distal to the nerve trunks that we observed. More powerful tools probe deeper into the truth.

In adults, many nerve fibres are easily seen by virtue of the myelin sheath surrounding them. Their identification in the embryo is more difficult. Myelination of peripheral nerves does not begin until 8 weeks of age in the human embryo. In the earlier embryo, the first peripheral axons are delicate unprotected filaments of protein, potentially vulnerable in vivo to circulating toxins, particularly neurotoxins. In vitro, they are destroyed by harsh fixatives and by hot wax embedding processes. These intercellular filaments are seen in histological section as minute fragments (0.3 µm) that are inevitably overlooked by the untrained eye using the relatively coarse method of light microscopy (with its limitation of resolution 0.5 µm).

Newgreen et al[45] have shown cytoplasmic extensions from neural crest cells penetrating into the embryonic sclerotomes, recorded by scanning electron microscopy. This intrusion of an ectodermal structure into a mesodermal derivative reveals an anatomical pathway whereby nerves can potentially influence other embryonic layers.

Conclusion

In view of the presence of nerves in the limb bud, the following two statements are refuted:

- Limb buds have no nerve supply.
- Limbs develop as self-differentiating systems.

From their inception, limb buds have a nerve supply whereby they are linked to the neuraxis even before their appearance as anatomical entities. It follows that they cannot be autonomous in their development, insofar as they cannot escape the influence of their nerve supply. Whether or not limb morphogenesis is influenced by very early damage to neural tissue, lying medial to the limb bud before the bud exists, is the subject of Chapter 17.

If nerves have not been reported in past experiments where they were not sought, or could not be seen, this does not mean that they do not exist.

References

1. McCredie J, Cameron J, Shoobridge R. Congenital malformations and the neural crest. *Lancet* 1978; **ii**: 761–3.

2. Cameron J, McCredie J. Innervation of the undifferentiated limb bud of rabbit embryo. *J Anat* 1982; **134**: 795–808.

3. McCredie J. Thalidomide and congenital Charcot's joints. *Lancet* 1973; **ii**: 1058–61.

4. McCredie J. Embryonic neuropathy. A hypothesis of neural crest injury as the pathogenesis of congenital malformations. *Med J Aust* 1974; **1**: 159–63.

5. McCredie J. Neural crest defects. A neuroanatomic basis for classification of multiple malformations related to phocomelia. *J Neurol Sci* 1976; **28**: 273–87.

6. O'Rahilly R, Gardner E. The timing and sequence of events in the development of the limbs in the human embryo. *Anat Embryol* 1975; **148**: 1–23.

7. Gardner E, O'Rahilly R. Neural crest, limb development and thalidomide embryopathy. *Lancet* 1976; **i**: 635–6.

8. Poswillo D. Mechanisms and pathogenesis of malformations. *Br Med Bull* 1976; **32**: 59–64.

9. Wolpert L. Mechanisms of limb development and malformation. *Br Med Bull* 1976; **32**: 65–70.

10. Bardeen CR, Lewis WH. The development of limbs, body wall and back in man. *Am J Anat* 1901; **1**: 1–36.

11. Lewis WH. The development of the arm in man. *Am J Anat* 1902; **1**: 145–183.

12. Tennyson VM. Electron microscopic study of the developing neuroblast of the dorsal root ganglion of the rabbit embryo. *J Comp Neurol* 1965; **124**: 267–317.

13. Tennyson VM. The fine structure of the axon and growth cone of the dorsal root neuroblast of the rabbit embryo. *J Cell Biol* 1970; **44**: 62–79.

14. Tennyson VM. The fine structure of the developing nervous system. In: Himwich WA, ed. *Developmental Neurobiology*. Springfield, IL: Charles C Thomas, 1970: 47–116.

15. Tennyson VM. Light and electron microscopy of dorsal root and sympathetic ganglia. In: Dyck PJ, Thomas PK, Lambert EH, eds *Peripheral Neuropathy*, Vol 1. Philadelphia: WB Saunders, 1975: 74–103.

16. Cameron J. A histological study of the effect of thalidomide on the developing nervous system of the rabbit. PhD dissertation, University of Sydney.

17. Somers GF. Thalidomide and congenital abnormalities. *Lancet* 1962; **i**: 912.

18. Spencer KEV. Thalidomide and congenital abnormalities. *Lancet* 1962; **ii**: 100.

19. Seller MJ. Thalidomide and congenital abnormalities. *Lancet* 1962; **ii**: 249.

20. Felisati D, Nodari R. Toxic and teratogenic effects of thalidomide on rabbit foetus. *J Suisse Med* 1963; **93**: 1559–62.

21. Dekker A, Mehrizi A. the use of thalidomide as a teratogenic agent in rabbits. *Bull Johns Hopkins Hosp* 1964; **115**: 223–30.

22. Vickers TH. Dysmelic lesions found in thalidomide embryopathy of rabbits. In: *Proceedings of 5th Annual Meeting of the Congenital Anomalies Research Association of Japan*, 1965: 15.

23. Vickers TH. The thalidomide embryopathy in hybrid rabbits. *Br J Exp Pathol* 1967; **48**: 579–91.

24. Vickers TH. Concerning the morphogenesis of thalidomide dysmelia in rabbits. *Br J Exp Pathol* 1967; **48**: 579–91.

25. Vickers TH, Wrba H. Further observations on the thalidomide embryopathy in rabbits. *Exp Pathol* 1970; **4**: 81–97.

26. Karnovsky MJ. A formaldehyde–glutaraldehyde fixative of high osmolality for use in electron microscopy. *J Cell Biol* 1965; **27**: 137.

27. Dalton AJ. Chrome osmium fixative for electron microscopy. *Anat Rec* 1955; **121**: 281.

28. Romanes GJ. The development and significance of the cell columns in the ventral horn of the cervical and upper thoracic spinal cord of the rabbit. *J Anat* 1941; **76**: 112–30.

29. Taylor AC. Development of the innervation pattern in the limb bud of the frog. *Anat Rec* 1943; **87**: 379–413.

30. Gasser HS. Properties of the dorsal root unmedullated fibres on the two sides of the ganglion. *J Gen Physiol* 1955; **38**: 709–28.

31. Egar M, Yntema CL, Singer M. The nerve fiber content of *Amblystoma* aneurogenic limbs. *J Exp Zool* 1973; **186**: 91–6.

32. Hamilton WJ, Mossman HW. *Human Embryology*. Cambridge: Heffers/ Baltimore: Williams and Wilkins, 1972.

33. Saunders JW. The proximo-distal sequence of origin of the parts of the chick wing and the role of the ectoderm. *J Exp Zool* 1948; **108**: 363–403.

34. Tschumi PA. The growth of the hind limb of *Xenopus laevis* and its dependence upon the epidermis. *J Anat* 1957; **91**: 149–73.

35. Streeter GL. Developmental horizons in human embryos. A review of the histogenesis of cartilage and bone. *Contrib Embryol* 1949; **33**: 149–67.

36. Ede DA. Control of form and pattern in the vertebrate limb. *Symp Soc Exp Biol* 1971; **25**: 235–254.

37. Stocum DL. Outgrowth and pattern formation during limb ontogeny and regeneration. *Differentiation* 1975; **3**: 167–82.

38. Bell E, Kaign ME, Fessenden LM. The role of mesodermal and ectodermal components in the development of the chick limb. *Dev Biol* 1959; **1**: 101–24.

39. Bell E, Saunders JW, Zwilling E. Limb development in the absence of ectodermal ridge. *Nature* 1959; **184**: 1736–7.

40. Lewis J. Defective innervation and defective limbs: causes and effects in the developing chick wing. In: Merker H-J, Nau H, Neubert D, eds. *Teratology of the Limbs*, Berlin: Walter de Gruyter, 1980: 235–42.

41. Dyck PJ, Thomas PK, Lambert E. *Peripheral Neuropathy*. Philadelphia: WB Saunders, 1975.

42. Bancroft M, Bellairs R. The development of the notochord in chick embryo studied by scanning electron microscopy and transmission electron microscopy. *J Embryol Exp Morphol* 1976; **35**: 383–401.

43. Varon SS, Bunge RP. Trophic mechanisms in peripheral nervous system. *Annu Rev Neurosci* 1978; **1**: 327–61.

44. Tosney KW. Early migration of neural crest cells in the trunk region of the avian embryo: an electron microscopic study. *Dev Biol* 1978; **62**: 317–33.

45. Newgreen DF, Erickson CA. The migration of neural crest cells. *Int Rev Cytol* 1986; **103**: 89–145.

CHAPTER 16

Regeneration and embryogenesis

Amphibian amputees and mammalian embryos both commence limb growth by the formation of limb buds containing simple undifferentiated mesenchymal cells.

Regeneration and embryogenesis are both expressions of growth – either regrowth of a previously existing part or primary formation of a part in the embryo. Each process can be considered as a function of growth, mathematically speaking. Both processes have been intensively studied in the limbs, and a large literature exists in each field. Are they two separate processes, or two expressions of the same process?

Similarities and differences

The relationship between limb regeneration and limb embryogenesis has been debated for over a century.

Parallels between the two fields were summarized by Faber[1] in 1971. He noted that investigators have tended to keep these two research areas apart. Scientists in one rarely quoted results from the other. There is a well-founded reluctance in science to extrapolate data, or even principles, from one species to another. Few scientists are as courageous as Darwin, daring to visualize the entire animal kingdom through a wide-angled lens!

Faber[1] recognized that close parallels between regeneration and embryogenesis were constantly emerging in science. In attempting a synthesis, he concluded that the problems confronting investigators in the two fields were the same. The only difference between the two systems was that:

'the regeneration blastema is dependent upon innervation for its development, whereas the embryonic limb bud is not'.

Reviews in 1998 by Gardiner and Bryant[2] and Carlson[3] updated the comparisons between these two fields of research, and included new

---

Chapter Summary
- Similarities and differences
- Evidence against nerve dependence of embryonic limb buds
- Evidence for nerve dependence of embryonic limb buds
- Deficient mesenchymal mass
- Where, when and how does thalidomide act in regeneration?
- Neurotrophism and embryogenesis – a new proposal
- Conclusion
- References

findings from molecular biology. Carlson[3] summarized the extensive biological literature on pattern formation. He concluded that:

'A regenerating limb appears to utilise many of the same fundamental pattern-forming mechanisms as does a developing one.'

He listed these as follows:

The same molecules are present

At the molecular and genetic level, the same trophic substances, such as transferrin and its gene, have been found in the cells of amphibian regenerates and of many organ rudiments in the embryo.[4]
Results from recent studies:

'demonstrate that regardless of how outgrowth is initiated, the molecules involved in the control of growth and pattern formation have equivalent functions in both limb development and regeneration'.[2]

The same genes are involved

The *HoxA* complex of homeobox – containing genes have been investigated in relation to current concepts of 'pattern formation' in developing limbs,[5–7] in which the genes are expressed in discrete spatial domains related to the limb segments (in the sense of upper arm, forearm, hand). During regeneration, *HoxA* genes are expressed in the same unique spatial domains as in embryonic limb development.[8] Gardiner and Bryant[2] headed one section of their paper thus: 'The same genes are involved in limb regeneration as in embryonic limb development'.
While there are some differences in the steps involved in the activation of *HoxA* expression:

'the eventual expression patterns, and the limb parts to which they correspond, are the same in the blastema and in the limb bud'.[2]

There are similar tissues and structures in both systems . . .

Both embryonic limb bud and the regeneration blastema contain undifferentiated cells of mesenchymal type.
There is a specialized epidermis at the apex of the limb bud and at the tip of the regeneration blastema. In the embryonic limb bud, this is called the apical ectodermal ridge (AER). In the amphibian regenerate stump or blastema, it is called the apical epidermal cap (AEC). The importance of this specialized apical area of epidermis is debatable. Its importance has probably been overestimated in embryogenesis, where

developmental biologists have studied the AER very thoroughly indeed in the past decades. Concentration upon the AER as a hypothetically independent entity (believed to be capable of inducing limb structures in its wake) has diverted attention from nerve supply, to the extent that nerves are never mentioned in limb bud embryology. On the other hand, nerves are the prime movers in limb regeneration, and their influence has been thoroughly investigated, as reviewed in the 1998 volume edited by Ferretti and Géraudie.[9]

. . . But there is one difference: innervation

Finally, the review by Gardiner and Bryant[2] states:

> 'A difference between the two processes is that *limb regeneration, but not limb development, is dependent on nerves.*'

Nearly 30 years elapsed between the reviews by Faber[1] and by Gardiner and Bryant.[2] The belief that there are no nerves in embryonic limb buds persists, despite existence of contrary data in the medical literature. This creates an impasse in scientific thought, hopefully to be unblocked by this chapter.

Chapter 14 quoted the principles of limb regeneration and neurotrophism established in amphibian biology. This included the fact that regeneration is biphasic:

- Phase 1 is *nerve-dependent* and comprises simple cell division, i.e. mitosis.
- Phase 2 is *independent of nerves*, and involves differentiation and morphogenesis.

No comparable principles exist for early embryogenesis.

Evidence against nerve dependence of embryonic limb buds

Support for the idea that limb embryogenesis is independent of nerves appears to rest on two concepts:

- that there are no nerves in the limb bud;
- that there are 'aneurigenic limbs' that can regenerate.

The concept that there are no nerves in the limb bud

If there are no nerves present in limb buds, it follows that there can be no nerve dependence of limb bud growth. However, the alleged absence of nerves is based on a combination of misquotation and unsuitable laboratory methods, as discussed in Chapter 15. This misquotation of results of Bardeen and Lewis[11] is deeply embedded in embryology and developmental biology textbooks. That error has not been transmitted into neurology, where the contrary view is held (Chapter 15). Embryology is at odds with medicine and the neurological sciences on this subject.

The actual statement by Bardeen and Lewis[11] – that they *saw* no nerves in limb buds of embryos – would be true for the materials and methods they used in 1900. It is not true when the search is repeated with modern methods of neurohistology, including high magnification provided by electron microscopy as described in Chapter 15. Neuroscientists recognize the superior power of resolution of the electron microscope to identify axons, as discussed in Chapter 15.

The statement that 'there are no nerves in the limb bud' is false and needs to be excised from embryology texts. Those who have believed it without checking it for themselves have been misled. The error has been quoted widely and transmitted into the literature on limb regeneration, where it now impedes progress in a second scientific field.

The concept of 'aneurigenic limbs' that can regenerate

Yntema[13] removed the neural tubes from one group of amphibian embryos, and then grafted them onto the backs of a second group of embryos. He argued that these piggybacked or 'parabiosed' embryos without neural tubes had no nerve supply to their limb buds, and that if and when they developed limb buds, these were 'aneurigenic' (nerveless) limbs that could regenerate after amputation, despite the assumed absence of nerves.

Yntema concluded from this complicated experiment that limbs that have never been innervated during their embryonic development can regenerate in the absence of nerves. His claim supported the old belief that limbs develop without nerves, during both regeneration and early embryogenesis.

His embryo-to-embryo grafts had another problem. The grafts had to be performed when both embryos were mature enough to survive the surgery, at which stage the nervous system was already well developed. Yntema actually stated in his original method that the grafts were carried out *after neural crest migration*, in order to ensure survival of the graft. But, thereafter, the possible presence of axons in the limb buds was neither considered nor sought.

This concept presented a challenge to Singer's group. The basic notion of 'aneurigenic limbs' was questioned by Singer. It contradicted all the observations of his research group – that limb regeneration requires sensory innervation. He invited Yntema to his laboratory in Cleveland to construct 'parabiosed' embryos, in order that their state of innervation could be checked. Egar, Yntema and Singer,[14] using electron microscopy, found that *62% of the so-called 'aneurigenic limbs' contained nerve fibres*, and that others contained ependymal channels, suggesting the previous presence of nerves. Yntema's assumption that his parabiosed embryos had no nerves was refuted.

The concept of 'aneurigenic limbs' was thus shown to be flawed. Truth was established by electron microscopy.

The term 'aneurigenic limb' is a contradiction, and its use should be discontinued. It can never be assumed that axons are not present unless they have been sought by electron microscopy, histochemical mapping or other high-resolution methods. On first principles, the opposite assumption is more logical: that axons are present until otherwise proven. Many past studies based on light microscopy need to be repeated with electron microscopy – or at least critically reassessed to dispel the confusion that has arisen around the subject of limb bud innervation.

The literature has already been shown to contain articles that claim to prove the absence of nerves, using methods such as light microscopy and silver stains that for different reasons lack the power of resolution needed to resolve that problem (Chapters 13 and 15). The truth has been obscured in the past by inadequate methodology.

Concepts must change as new technologies reveal new evidence. Understandable but erroneous conclusions from the past have been superseded by using more powerful tools.

Evidence for nerve dependence of embryonic limb buds

There is evidence that early limb development *is* nerve-dependent. Thalidomide can stop embryonic limb development altogether (amelia) or alter the pattern of limb development (phocomelia). Thalidomide is therefore a unique research tool to use when asking questions about *when*, *where* and *how* limb embryogenesis can be stopped or grossly disrupted.

Thalidomide and embryogenesis

When does thalidomide act in embryogenesis?

We know that thalidomide induces longitudinal reduction deformities of human limbs from exposure during the 'sensitive period' of 21–42 days' gestation. It was shown in 1965 by Nowack[15] that thalidomide ingested by the mother from day 24 caused arm defects, although the upper limb bud does not appear until day 28. From the thalidomide epidemic in humans, the answer to *when* thalidomide starts to act is 4 days *before the limb bud exists.*

Vickers[16] confirmed that the thalidomide-sensitive period in rabbits (7–11 days' gestation) *predated* the appearance of the limb buds at day 12–13. He found that malformations developed in areas where initial mesenchymal proliferation was deficient.

This timing was confirmed in non-human primates. Barrow et al[17] induced phocomelia in rhesus monkeys by administering thalidomide 'either *immediately before or during* the appearance of the limb buds'. Neubert et al[18] used macaque monkeys, and they agree that the timing of thalidomide's action is precocious – certainly three embryonic stages *before* the appearance of the apical ectodermal ridge. That structure therefore plays no part in the induction of phocomelia.

Although they observed that thalidomide acted very early, *before formation of the limb bud*, none of these scientists considered a role for the neural crest or its axons. They defined *when* the drug acted, but not *where*. Neubert et al[18] theorized that it acts deep within the trunk, possibly on mesonephric mesenchyme. Although they did not lead to the target tissue, these contributions are very valuable in defining *a period of embryonic vulnerability prior to limb bud formation*.

Where does thalidomide act in embryogenesis?

The neural crest is present from day 18 in the human, and its cells are dividing, migrating and sprouting axons during the 'thalidomide-sensitive period' of 21–42 days' gestation (Chapter 13), i.e. prior to and during early limb bud formation. This is circumstantial evidence that the neural crest should at least be suspected as the target – it was present at the right time. Additional evidence has been presented in previous chapters and is summarized here in the present context:

- Thalidomide is a proven sensory neurotoxin, i.e. it has an affinity for sensorineural cells (Chapter 4).
- Sensory neurons possess the property of neurotrophism, whereby they stimulate other cells to divide by mitosis (Chapter 14).
- Thalidomide exposure in the pre-limb-bud period stops limb growth (amelia) or induces longitudinal reduction deformities (dysmelia or phocomelia) in the limbs of the vertebrate embryo (Chapters 2 and 5–11).

It follows that *the first phase of limb embryogenesis* (24–36 days' gestation) *is nerve-dependent*. Nowack called this phase the 'thalidomide-sensitive period' (Chapter 2)

This brings limb embryogenesis into line with limb regeneration. Both processes can now be seen as biphasic, the first phase being nerve-dependent, and the second independent of nerves (Chapter 14).

How does thalidomide act in embryogenesis?

Normally, initiation of the embryonic limb bud comprises simple cell division. By repeated mitoses, a mass of mesenchyme is generated from the base to create the incipient limb bud, in preparation for the second phase of differentiation and morphogenesis to follow.

Deficient mesenchymal mass is the earliest sign of a thalidomide-induced limb defect in animals.

Deficient mesenchymal mass

How does thalidomide reduce mesenchymal mass? Does thalidomide stop mitosis in the embryonic mesenchyme by direct or indirect action on dividing cells?

Is the drug acting directly on mitosis?

It is possible that thalidomide stops mitosis *directly*, without mediation through the sensory nervous system. This possibility underlies part of the recent rationale for using thalidomide against cancer.

If the drug has a direct action on dividing cells, it has two distinct actions, the other being its proven sensory neurotoxicity. By Occam's Razor, a single action would be a better scientific proposition. Nevertheless, the possibility of a separate, direct antimitotic action has to be considered.

The relationship between thalidomide and mitosis was explored in an experiment by Salzgeber in Paris (described in Chapter 3).[19] A distinguished chick embryologist, Salzgeber had already investigated the effect of nitrogen mustard on chick embryos. Nitrogen mustard is a spindle poison that disrupted formation of the mitotic spindle. The limb buds of chick embryos exposed to nitrogen mustard showed multiple disorganized and incomplete mitotic figures – a direct effect upon mitosis. At the time of the thalidomide epidemic, Salzgeber wondered if thalidomide had the same mode of action. To her surprise, there were no mitotic figures in the limb buds of thalidomide-exposed chick embryos, and no damaged spindles.

Subsequently, when she and I discussed her findings, we concluded that as thalidomide did not interfere directly with spindle formation in embryonic mitosis, it had to be acting in some other way to reduce or stop cell division. One possibility was that thalidomide prevented the neurotrophic stimulation of mitosis. This could be mediated through a primary insult to neural crest cells and their axons, with absence of mitoses being secondary to damaged axons and/or damaged neurotrophism.

Salzgeber's observations refute the case for direct action of thalidomide on mitotic cells.

Does thalidomide stop mitosis indirectly?

Indirect action via disrupted neurotrophism is only slightly more complex than direct antimitotic action on the mesenchyme, but it makes more sense, because it connects the drug's two actions: teratogenicity and neurotoxicity. It satisfies Occam's Razor by resolving two phenomena into one unified mode of drug action.

There is much evidence to support an indirect action on mitosis mediated through the neural crest. The fact that dysmelic malformations are neuropathic in character, and specifically reveal evidence of an embryonic sensory neuropathy, indicates that thalido-mide damages the neural crest. The steps in the proposed mode of action that follow from recognition of phocomelia as nerve injury (in previous chapters) are listed here:

1. Thalidomide damages neural crest cells (and axons).
2. Axonal function/signal transmission fails.
3. There is reduced or nil trophic signal to mesenchyme.
4. Mesenchymal cell division is reduced or nil.
5. The final mesenchymal mass is deficient.
6. Subsequent differentiation is quantitatively incomplete.
7. Morphogenesis is quantitatively incomplete.
8. Reduction deformities result.

The number of cells in the mass of undifferentiated mesenchyme that comprises the early limb bud is reduced, particularly within the zone supplied by the damaged nerves. In the following phase of differ-entiation and morphogenesis, the reduced cell mass is insufficient for construction of the normal anatomical parts supplied by that nerve. Longitudinal reduction deformities result. Bones and other anatomi-cal structures are absent or reduced in size.

This indicates that thalidomide stops the induction of mitosis by damage to nerves and their trophic function.

Where, when and how does thalidomide act in regeneration?

Thalidomide and amphibian regeneration

If the early 'thalidomide-sensitive period' of limb embryogenesis is nerve-dependent, it follows that this 'sensitive period' should correspond to the early nerve-dependent phase of amphibian limb regeneration. This proposal can be verified or refuted in amphibia, again using thalidomide as the tool. Does thalidomide injure amphibian limb regeneration or not? If not, the proposal is refuted. If it does, then when, where and how does the drug act?

Does thalidomide affect limb regeneration? If so, when?

This question was addressed in an elegant study performed in 1977 on an amphibian model by Bazzoli, Manson, Scott and Wilson (American teratologists).[20] They gave oral thalidomide to limb-amputated newts during and after the nerve-dependent stage of upper limb regenera-tion. They recorded a 75% malformation rate in limb regenerates of phocomelic type when thalidomide was given during the nerve-dependent phase. There were no malformations following thalidomide administration at later stages of development.

A comparable incidence of reduction deformities was observed by

these researchers after similarly-timed dosing with EM12, a teratogenic analogue of thalidomide, but not after treatment with a non-
teratogenic analogue, EM87. The authors did not explore the nerve
supply or inquire whether there was damage to, or quantitative
reduction in, the nerves. No definite conclusion concerning cause and
effect was drawn.

In the present context, this is precious data:

- It proves that amphibian amputees do react to thalidomide if it is
  given in the nerve-dependent phase, but *not* if it is given in the
  next nerve-independent phase.
- Like mammalian embryos, the amphibian reaction is phocomelia
  (which indicates sensory nerve injury, as we have seen in Chapters
  6–12).
- The results point to a common mechanism shared by amphibian
  regeneration and vertebrate embryogenesis.
- The thalidomide-sensitive periods in the embryo and in regenerating amphibia are equivalent. Both precede differentiation. Both are
  nerve-dependent.
- In passing, one should take practical note that amphibian limb
  regeneration provides a potentially effective and cheap animal
  model for screening out sensorineural teratogens like thalidomide.

After its publication, Bazzoli, Manson and Scott sought my opinion
on their paper at a birth defects conference in Storrs, Connecticut;
they were clearly perplexed by their findings. In that discussion, I
volunteered some facts underpinning the laws of regeneration,
clinical neurology and the radiology of phocomelia. It was disappointing that these teratologists did not pursue further work on
what seemed a promising line of research and a beautifully designed
experiment.

Even faced with evidence, scientists are reluctant to jettison the old
dogma that there are no nerves in the embryonic limb bud. The
survival of that notion is a core problem. It is the root cause of the
scientific impasse addressed in this chapter.

The 1998 reviews by Gardiner and Bryant[2] and by Carlson[3]
summarize new evidence of molecular and genetic similarities, but do
not reference the paper by Bazzoli et al.[20] A revised interpretation of
the latter work, integrated with the more recent work in amphibia
cited by Gardiner and Bryant,[2] can finally close this gap in the
comparative biology of the two systems, as follows.

Where does thalidomide act in limb regeneration?

- Knowing that the early phase of limb regeneration in amphibia is
  governed by sensory neurotrophism, the phocomelic malformations produced by Bazzoli et al[20] show that thalidomide
  interferes with the nerves and/or the neurotrophic process during

that nerve-dependent phase. After the nerve-dependent phase, administration of thalidomide does not induce phocomelia.

- Deformity is linked to nerve-dependency in amphibia.
- Thalidomide causes phocomelic amphibian regenerates – the same dysmorphology induced by thalidomide exposure of embryos in humans and experimental animals.
- The early, nerve-dependent phase of limb formation is the time and place at which thalidomide acts, whether in amphibian regeneration or in mammalian embryogenesis.

How does thalidomide act in limb regeneration?

- Thalidomide induces phocomelia in amphibia when administered during the known nerve-dependent stage of regeneration.
- It induces phocomelia (embryonic sensory neuropathy) in human infants exposed during the known 'thalidomide-sensitive period' of embryogenesis.
- That is, the same sensory neuropathic response occurs in the amphibian regenerate and the vertebrate embryo after exposure to this sensory neurotoxin at an equivalent phase.
- This proves the presence of one common underlying mechanism, namely sensorineural damage, in both instances.

Neurotrophism and embryogenesis – a new proposal

A nerve-dependent phase exists in normal embryogenesis

The existence of an early nerve-dependent phase of embryogenesis has not been recognized to date. This may explain why the pathogenesis of many birth defects has remained a mystery.

Most embryology texts dismiss the emergence of the limb bud in a sentence or two, and concentrate on the later and much longer phase of complex differentiation. Yet the period before and during the advent of the limb bud is precisely that of thalidomide's teratogenicity.

Now that the presence of nerves in embryonic limb buds has been proved, other similarities become clear. The thalidomide-sensitive period for thalidomide's limb defects[15] is equivalent to the nerve-dependent phase of limb regeneration in amphibia.[21] The nerve-dependent phase of human embryogenesis is 21–42 days' gestation – the thalidomide-sensitive period.

Neurotrophism operates in the nerve-dependent phase

Regeneration is known to be biphasic, with the *early nerve-dependent phase* of regeneration being responsible for simple cell division, and a subsequent *nerve-independent phase* being responsible for differentiation and organogenesis.

In regeneration, mitosis in early limb buds is driven by neuro-trophism, and growth is said to be nerve-dependent in this early phase:

Normal neurotrophism → normal number of cell divisions
           → normal number of undifferentiated cells in the limb bud in both cases
           → normal size and shape of final limb

Failure of neurotrophism is expressed in this phase

Injury always disturbs nerve function. It is highly unlikely that a damaged nerve could continue to carry out its neurotrophic function. In accordance with accepted neurological principles, we would expect neurotrophism to be disordered in proportion to the extent of nerve damage. A neurotoxic insult to an embryo in the nerve-dependent phase will first damage its function (e.g. neurotrophism), leading to a secondary reduction in the number of mitoses downstream. Thirdly, later, there is a visible reduction in the mesenchymal cell mass in the distal field of that nerve's supply. This can be summarized as follows:

Failure of neurotrophism → reduced number of mitoses
           → reduction in cell mass of bud
           → reduction defect in the field of that nerve's supply

Conclusion

Limb regeneration and limb embryogenesis react to the same neuro-toxin, at the same stage, in the same way (i.e. by neuropathy) and therefore through the same mechanism (damage to nerve/failure of neurotrophism).

Demonstration of nerves in the embryonic limb buds eliminates the only difference between embryogenesis and regeneration. Their presence removes the impasse that has blocked resolution of this issue, by providing the one missing link in the otherwise-identical comparison of regeneration and embryogenesis.

Regeneration and embryogenesis are thus alike in all respects, and are two similar expressions of one and the same basic biological process – nerve-dependent growth, or neurotrophism. A longstanding biological discussion can finally be closed.

A previously unrecognized 'nerve-dependent' phase of early embryogenesis emerges.

References

1. Faber J. Vertebrate limb ontogeny and limb regeneration. *Adv Morphogen* 1971; **9**: 127–47.
2. Gardiner DM, Bryant SV. The tetrapod limb. In: Ferretti P, Géraudie J, eds.

Cellular and Molecular Basis of Regeneration: From Invertebrates to Humans. Chichester: Wiley, 1998: 188–205.

3. Carlson BM. Development and regeneration, with special emphasis on the amphibian limb. In: Ferretti P, Géraudie J, eds. *Cellular and Molecular Basis of Regeneration: From Invertebrates to Humans.* Chichester: Wiley, 1998: 45–61.

4. Bowman BH, Yang F, Adrian GS. Transferrin, evolution and genetic regulation of expression. *Adv Genet* 1988; **25**: 1–88.

5. Dollé P, Dierich A, LeMeur M et al. Disruption of *hoxd-13* gene induces localised heterochrony leading to mice with neotenic limbs. *Cell* 1993; **75**: 431–41.

6. Small KM, Potter SS. Homeotic transformations and limb defects in *HoxA-11* mutant mice. *Genes Dev* 1993; **7**: 2318–28.

7. Davis AP, Capecchi MR. Axial homeosis and appendicular skeleton defects in mice with a targeted disruption of *hoxd-11*. *Development* 1994; **120**: 2187–98.

8. Gardiner DM, Blumberg B, Komine Y, Bryant SV. *Development* 1995; **121**: 1731–41.

9. Ferretti P, Géraudie J, eds. *Cellular and Molecular Basis of Regeneration: From Invertebrates to Humans.* Chichester: Wiley, 1998.

10. Singer M. The nervous system and regeneration of the forelimbs of the adult *Triturus*. The influence of the number of nerve fibres. *J Exp Zool* 1946; **101**: 299–337.

11. Bardeen RB, Lewis WH. Development of the limbs, body wall and back in man. *Am J Anat* 1901; **1**: 1–36.

12. Cameron J, McCredie J. Innervation of the undifferentiated limb bud in rabbit embryo. *J Anat* 1976; **134**: 795–808.

13. Yntema CL. Regeneration in sparsely innervated and aneurogenic forelimbs of *Amblystoma* larvae. *J Exp Zool* 1959; **140**: 101–23.

14. Egar MW, Yntema CL, Singer M. The nerve fiber content of *Amblystoma* aneurigenic limbs. *J Exp Zool* 1973; **186**: 91–6.

15. Nowack E. The sensitive phase of thalidomide embryopathy. *Humangenetik* 1965; **1**: 516–36.

16. Vickers TH. Concerning the morphogenesis of thalidomide dysmelia in rabbits. *Br J Exp Pathol* 1967; **48**: 579–91.

17. Barrow MV, Steffek AJ, King CT. Thalidomide syndrome in Rhesus monkeys. *Folia Primatol Basel* 1969; **10**: 195–203.

18. Neubert R, Merker HJ, Neubert D. Developmental model for thalidomide action. *Nature* 1999; **400**: 419–20.

19. Salzgeber B, Salaun J. Action of thalidomide on the chick embryo. *J Embryol Exp Morphol* 1965; **13**: 159–70.

20. Bazzoli AS, Manson J, Scott WJ, Wilson JG. The effects of thalidomide and two analogs on the regenerating forelimb of the newt. *J Embryol Exp Morphol* 1977; **41**: 125–35.

21. Wallace H. *Vertebrate Limb Regeneration.* Chichester: Wiley, 1981

CHAPTER 17

Neural crest ablation and limb morphogenesis

Chapter Summary
- Aim
- Materials and method
- Results
- Discussion
- Conclusion
- References

Does experimental injury to the neural crest cause malformations? In order to answer this question, I needed the help of a laboratory scientist with skills in chick embryology, tissue preparation and light microscopy. Rose Shoobridge MSc, assisted by Damaras Velkou, performed the following experiment in the Department of Surgery, University of Sydney, with assistance from neurologists and scientists in the Departments of Neurology and Zoology. Funding was from the National Health and Medical Research Council of Australia, and from the Ramaciotti Foundations, NSW. This work was published in *The Lancet* in 1978,[1] and in the *Journal of Experimental Zoology* in 1983,[2] from which this chapter is derived.

In addition to the radiological evidence of a link between limb development and the neural crest, there were two other papers in the literature that lent support to the hypothesis. Hamburger and Waugh[3] discussed a possible trophic effect of the nervous system on limb skeletal growth. This was before publication of Singer's work on neurotrophism. Kieny and Fouvet[4] later suggested that the influence of the nervous system on limb development 'is open for further investigation'.

Aim

The aim of the experiment was to test whether or not injury to the neural crest affects limb morphogenesis.

Materials and method

The chick embryo was chosen as the experimental model because of its ready accessibility to surgery. It was necessary to window the shell and stain the embryo. Two groups of 100 controls each for these two steps were set up in parallel. A third control group of 100 eggs were unoperated normal controls.

At 48 hours' incubation, the caudal end of the neural tube and crest is still unfused at the level of the presumptive sciatic innervation, i.e. at the level of future dorsal root ganglia 26–30.[5]

This provides an opportunity to inflict a unilateral injury upon the caudal neural crest, with the opposite side as an internal control (Figures 17.1 and 17.2). At this stage, no limb buds are visible. Because Rose Shoobridge is left-handed, she chose to cauterize by diathermy the left side of the caudal neural crest, using a minimal current of 100 mA at 8 V for 0.5 s through a single-thread tungsten wire elec-

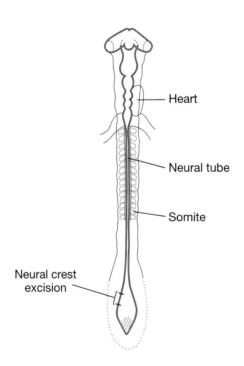

Figure 17.1 *Dorsal view of chick embryo, showing site of diathermy ablation to left neural crest at levels 26–30.*

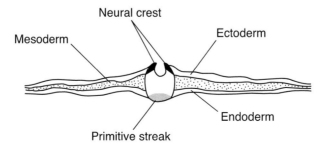

Figure 17.2 *Diagram of transverse section through unfused neural groove, showing site of neural crest to be diathermied.*

trode of 10 µm diameter. The operation was done under an operating microscope with a 3D micromanipulator to position the electrode. The effect of this thermal injury upon neural crest, neural tube, adjacent somitic mesoderm, and subsequent limb morphogenesis was investigated at three stages: immediately, at 24 hours and at 14 days after operation. One hundred embryos were operated on and scheduled for harvest at 14 days after surgery.

Results

Immediate group

All six operated embryos examined immediately after diathermy showed microscopic evidence of damage to the left neural tube and crest over a length of 50–175 µm (Figures 17.3–17.5). Three also had damage to the right tube and crest over a shorter distance. Only one of the six had concurrent damage to the left side of the mesoderm (somite).

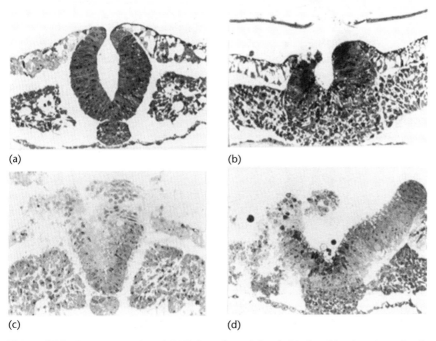

(a)

(b)

(c)

(d)

Figure 17.3 *Transverse sections (×200) through caudal end of 2-day old embryo immediately after injury: (a) control; (b) ablated crest with damage to left neural tube as well; (c) bilateral tube/crest damage; (d) ablation damage to left crest, tube and somite.*

Figure 17.4 *Diagram illustrating length of damage in six embryos immediately after ablation. Damage is white; neural tube/crest is grey; somitic mesoderm is striped. Chicks A–C show bilateral damage in tube/crest. Chicks D and F show localized damage to tube/crest on left side. Chick E shows left-sided damage to tube/crest and somite.*

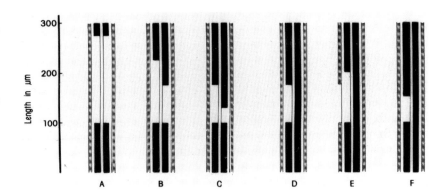

Figure 17.5 *Areas of damage immediately after crest ablation: ratio of left to right cross-sectional areas of neural tube/crest and somitic mesoderm. Black dots represent sections in which either no damage or bilateral damage was found. White dots represent unilateral damage visible microscopically.*

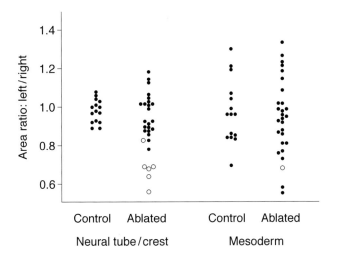

24 hours after ablation

Survival rate

This was 70%.

Extent of damage

All seven operated embryos had bilateral damage to the neural crest, with four being more extensive on the left than the right (Figures 17.6 and 17.7). Most had damage to the neural tube as well. In four, the tube was absent over a short length, and was more reduced on the left than the right in the other three. Three of the seven had normal somitic mesoderm. Another appeared undamaged, but had no somitic segmentation in the operated area. Two others had gross bilateral disruption of somitic mesoderm and midline fusion. Another had left-sided somitic damage.

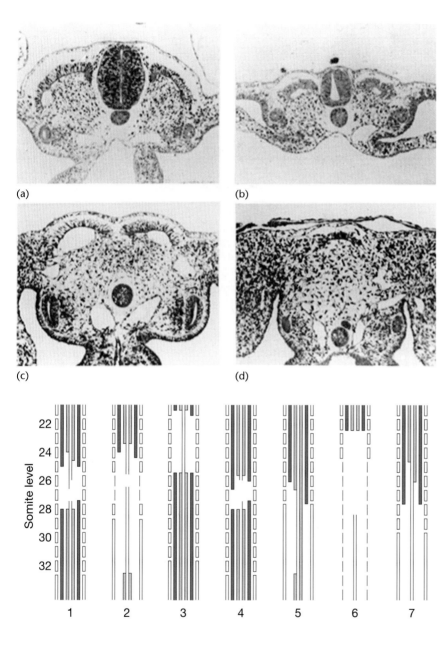

Figure 17.6 *Transverse sections through embryos re-incubated for 20–24 hours after ablation, sampled from area of presumptive leg bud (×100): (a) control; (b) left neural crest ablated; (c) ablation of neural tube but normal somites; (d) gross ablation damage to neural tube with midline somite.*

(a)

(b)

(c)

(d)

Figure 17.7 *Length of damage at 24 hours after ablation: diagrammatic illustration of serial transverse sections of seven chick embryos in dorsal view. Neural crest is dark grey; neural tube is light grey; somitic mesoderm is lateral with varied segmentation. Absence of a structure indicates total destruction by diathermy.*

14 days after ablation

Survival rate

This decreased with each stage of the procedure (Table 17.1): from 85% in the unoperated controls, to 47% in the egg cap controls, to 25% at the stain stage, and finally to 11% (17) of the diathermy ablations. This low survival rate in the operated group was a major problem during the experiment, in that the experimental chicks kept dying.

Table 17.1 Survival and malformation rates in operated and control groups

		Controls		Neural
	Normal	Egg cap stage	Stain stage	crest ablation
Total chicks	100	117	115	143
No. of survivors	85 (85%)	55 (47%)	29 (25%)	17 (11%)
No. with limb malformations	0 (0%)	2 (4.2%)	1 (3.4%)	7 (41.1%)
No. with other defects (non-limb)	0 (0%)	0 (0%)	1 (3.4%)	0 (0%)

Malformation rate

The malformation rate in survivors was 7 of 17 (47%), which is 10 times greater than in the other groups. Of the 17 survivors, 10 showed no limb malformations. Seven had left-leg deformities. One had sirenomelia (fusion of the legs like a mermaid). The left foot was absent in five chicks, with the left tibiofibula ending in a tapered stump as shown in Figure 17.8. Three of these five had a normal right leg and foot, two had digital defects on the right side as well. One chick had absence of the left 4th digital ray and subluxation of the left ankle joint without reduction of the tibiofibula. All were X-rayed in a Faxitron (used for pathology specimens and soft tissues) (Figures 17.9 and 17.10).

Dorsal root ganglia

The mass of the dorsal root ganglia on the left side of the deformed chicks was significantly reduced in comparison with the right side,

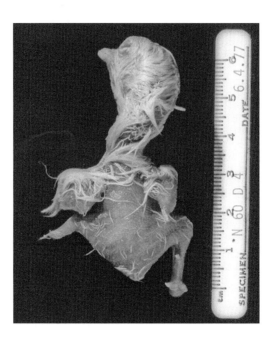

Figure 17.8 *Bilateral leg defects: left foot is absent, with tapered tibia; right foot is partly absent.*

and also in comparison with the controls and the ablated but not deformed group (Figure 17.11).

Spinal cord

There was no significant difference in spinal cord area between the two sides in the deformed group, or in comparison with the 'ablated but not deformed' group or the controls (Figures 17.12 and 17.13). Two ablated chicks with no limb defect had scarred reductions of the spinal cord.

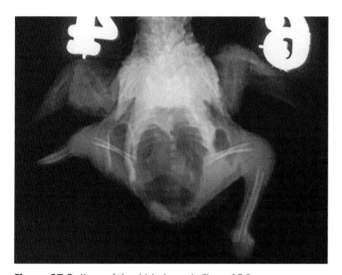

Figure 17.9 *X-ray of the chick shown in Figure 17.8.*

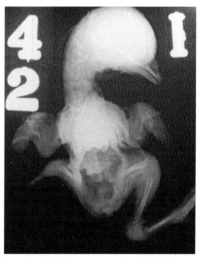

Figure 17.10 *X-ray of unilateral leg defeat. (Reprinted with permission from* The Lancet.*)*

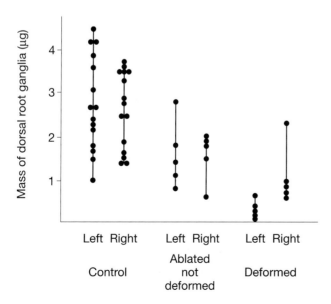

Figure 17.11 *Mass of dorsal root ganglia at 14 days after ablation: comparison between mass of ganglia on left and right sides in each experimental group.*

Figure 17.12 *Spinal cords at 14 days after ablation. Transverse sections (×45): (a) control; (b) ablated but not deformed; (c) local short-segment damage to spinal cord, chick not deformed; (d) deformed embryo with absent dorsal fissure.*

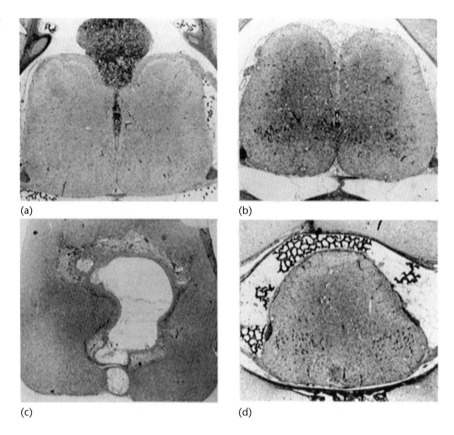

(a)   (b)

(c)   (d)

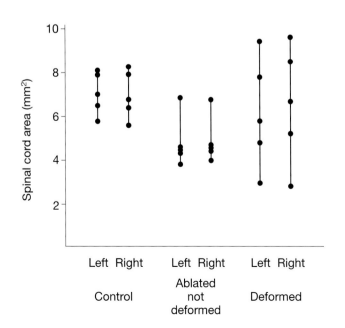

Figure 17.13 *Reduction in spinal cord areas at 14 days after ablation. Each spot corresponds to one chick, and represents the sum of the areas of five transverse sections of spinal cord in that chick. There is no correlation between deformity and spinal cord area.*

Discussion

Accuracy of injury

The aim of diathermy ablation was to injure one side of the neural crest in the region of the future hind limb innervation. It was also intended that only the neural crest should be injured, and that deeper and adjacent tissues such as neural tube and somite should be spared. The immediate and 24-hour results show that this was not achieved. The nature of the diathermy injury was a sphere of coagulation necrosis centred at the tip of the tungsten thread, and it was virtually impossible to confine damage to the crest. The diathermy ablation method proved to be too crude for the requirements of the experiment. A good case exists for repeating this experiment with more precise instruments when these are invented. Conclusions from this experiment are limited by technical problems, but some facts can be extracted from the data.

Survival rate

The steeply decreasing survival rate to only 11% of the operated embryos at 14 days after surgery meant that those that did survive were unlikely to be representative of the original group. Therefore it is not possible to relate the results in the three samples to one another. While it is impossible to predict which embryos in the first two series would survive to 14 days, a logical hypothesis would be that the most extensively damaged embryos would perish first, and that the survivors at 14 days would be those with the least severe original injuries. This hypothesis implies that embryos at 24 hours with absence of the spinal cord plus disruption of mesoderm would be more likely to succumb than those with lesser damage. Certainly there was no 14-day survivor with a long segment of absent cord, although two survived with short segmental cord depletions.

Malformation rate

It is also impossible to predict which, if any, of the embryos in the two early series would have gone on to a limb deformity after 14 days. Using the above hypothesis, it is possible that deformed survivors to 14 days incurred a less severe injury than those that died during that period, but a slightly more severe injury (or damage to a different tissue) than those chicks that survived without limb defects.

Explanation of leg deformities at 14 days after ablation

The presence of leg deformities in 7 of 17 surviving chicks (41% of survivors) is a phenomenon that demands explanation. Table 17.1 shows that the percentages of survivors with limb defects in the three control groups were 0%, 4.2% and 3.4% respectively. A 10-fold increase to 41% followed the ablation procedure. Expressed as a proportion of the original total number of embryos in each group, the incidence of limb defects in ablated chicks is still 3–5 times the incidence in any control group. It follows that the leg defects result from the diathermy injury itself and not from any of the preliminary steps.

It is striking that five leg defects were left-sided and morphologically similar. This also indicates that the limb deformity related to and possibly resulted from the diathermy injury.

On the other hand, since 10 chicks survived the ablation insult without limb defects, it can be argued that deformity is not inevitable after ablation, and that some other modifying factor must be involved. There may be a quantitative explanation for this. *The evidence suggests that it may be a question of how much of which tissue is lost.* We found limb deformity to be associated with reduced mass of dorsal root ganglia related to that limb, but not with depletion of spinal cord. Two chicks actually had scarring and short segmental reductions in spinal cord but no limb defects. Our data point to a relationship between limb morphogenesis and dorsal root ganglia, but not between limb morphogenesis and spinal cord. We concluded that there appears to be a quantitative relationship between neural crest derivatives and normal morphogenesis of a limb.

Evidence from the literature and some theoretical considerations

The neural crest is undoubtedly capable of self-replacement, known as 'regulation'.[6–9] Weston[9] concluded that:

> 'partial ablations (i.e., unilateral removal of neural folds, removal of short lengths of neural crest, or ablations performed after migration has already begun) do not exclude the possibility that replacements can occur by migration, proliferation and phenotypic regulation of the remaining crest cells'.

Migration of crest cells across the midline is known to occur when the neural folds meet. There is also migration of normal crest cells from adjacent levels of the crest on the same side, above and below the operated area. It is characteristic of crest cells to tumble into any defect and heal the breach (Johnston MC, personal communication) – a trait that makes it difficult to secure an intentional surgical deficit.

It is therefore probable that the neural crest tended to repair itself in our ablation experiment. The final outcome would theoretically depend upon the amount of neural crest ablated in the first instance, and its subsequent capacity to replace that amount. Allowing for variations in the amount of crest destroyed, and for variations in regenerative capacity between individual embryos, a spectrum of final

Table 17.2 Review of extirpation experiments in the literature

Authors	H & H[a] stage	No. of somites	Estimated posterior level of neural crest migration[b]	Level of operation in somites	Amount of neural tube taken	No. of limb deformities in surviving embryos	Authors' explanation for cause of limb deformities
Castro[12]	10–14	(10–22)	8–20	17–21	Partial	2/11 wing	No explanation
Hamburger et al[13]	15–17	(24–32)	22–31	23–27 27–tailbud	Total Dorsal Half	34/44 leg	'These defects are probably non-specific effects of the operation'
Kieny et al[14]	(12–15)	14–26	12–24	8–26	Total	37/105 wing and leg	The results did not permit questions relating to causation to be answered
Kieny and Fouvet[4]	(12–14)	18–23	16–23	17–25	Total	90/(265) leg and wing	'The question of the influence of the nervous system in limb development [is] open for further investigation'
Schoenwolf[15]	13–17	(19–32)	17–30	Tailbud	Total	(18)/44 leg	Compression of lateral plate mesoderm; injury
Present authors	11–13	13–19	11–17	26–32	Left dorsal quarter	7/17 leg	Results suggest neural crest injury

[a] Hamburger and Hamilton.
[b] From Weston and Butler (1966).
Figures in parenthesis are calculations from the authors' published data, where the figures were not supplied.

outcomes is to be anticipated for the total ultimate amount of neural crest in the survivors. It is possible that a threshold exists, and that when reconstitution or regulation is insufficient to reach that threshold, a limb defect results.

The contribution of somitic mesoderm to limb formation, especially musculature, is not disputed. Our experiment suggests that the neural crest may also be necessary for limb development. There is no question that distal amputations result in hypoplasia of sensory neurons[10,11] – but that mechanism does not explain how damage to the neuraxis, before limb bud formation, can result in limb deformity.

The effect of damage to the neuraxis by extirpation experiments has been documented by Castro,[12] Hamburger et al,[13] Kieny et al,[14] Kieny and Fouvet,[4] and Schoenwolf.[15] After ablation of the neural tube, all of these authors recorded limb deformities in a proportion of surviving embryos, and most of these papers equate neural damage with neural tube injury. The neural crest was not examined separately. Judging by the methods used, it is almost certain that neural crest was excised with neural tube.

Table 17.2 shows that the operations recorded in all of these papers included parts of the neural crest in different stages of its migration. The authors' conclusions as to the cause of the limb deformities range from no explanation to the suggestion that the nervous system is 'open for further investigation', with which we concur. Despite the limitations of diathermy ablation, our results at 14 days show that a role for the neural crest in limb morphogenesis does deserve further investigation.

Conclusion

Our results align with the principles of neurotrophism, where the first principle is that sensory denervation prevents limb regeneration. In our experiment, partial sacral neural crest ablation (sensory denervation) prevented embryogenesis of the related distal leg.

References

1. McCredie J, Cameron J, Shoobridge R. Congenital malformations and the neural crest. *Lancet* 1978; **ii**: 761–3.

2. Shoobridge R, Velkou D, McCredie J. Neural crest ablation and limb morphogenesis. *J Exp Zool* 1983; **225**: 73–87.

3. Hamburger V, Waugh M. The primary development of the skeleton in nerveless and poorly innervated limb transplants of chick embryos. *Physiol Zool* 1940; **13**: 367–80.

4. Kieny MA, Fouvet B. Innervation et morphogenèse de la patte chez l'embryon de poulet. II Anomalies consécutives a l'excision d'un tronçon de tube neural a deux jours d'incubation. *Arch Anat Microsc Morphol Exp* 1974; **63**: 281–98.

5. Fouvet B. Innervation et morphogènese de la patte chez l'embryon de poulet. 1. Mise en place de l'innervation normale. *Arch Anat Microsc Morphol Exp* 1973; **62**: 269–80.

6. Lehman HE, Youngs LM. An analysis of regulation in the amphibian neural crest. *J Exp Zool* 1952; **121**: 419–47.

7. Bodenstein D. Studies on the development of the dorsal fin in amphibians. *J Exp Zool* 1952; **120**: 213–45.

8. Chibon P. Marquage nucléaire par la thymidine tritée des dérivés de la crête neurale chez l'amphibien urodele *Pleurodeles waltlii Michah. J Embryol Exp Morphol* 1967; **18**: 343–58.

9. Weston JA. The migration and differentiation of neural crest cells. *Adv Morphogen* 1970; **8**: 41–114.

10. Hamburger V, Levi-Montalcini R. Proliferation, differentiation and degeneration in the spinal ganglia of the chick embryo under normal and experimental conditions. *J Exp Zool* 1949; **111**: 457–502.

11. Carr VMcM, Simpson FB Jr. Proliferative and degenerative events in the early development of chick dorsal root ganglia. II Responses to altered peripheral fields. *J Comp Neurol* 1978; **182**: 741–56.

12. Castro G. Effects of reduction of nerve centres on development of residual ganglia and on nerve patterns in the wing of the chick embryo. *J Exp Zool* 1963; **152**: 279–95.

13. Hamburger V, Wenger E, Oppenheim R. Motility in the chick embryo in the absence of sensory input. *J Exp Zool* 1966; **162**: 133–60.

14. Kieny MA, Mauger A, Thevenet A. Influence du système nerveux axial sur le morphogenèse des membres, chez l'embryon de poulet. *C R Acad Sci Hebd Seances Acad Sci D* 1971; **272**: 121–4.

15. Schoenwolf GC. Effects of complete tail bud extirpation on early development of the posterior region of the chick embryo. *Anat Rec* 1978; **192**: 289–96.

CHAPTER **18**

Thalidomide deformities and their nerve supply: First morphometric study in rabbits

Introduction

If thalidomide causes embryonic neuropathy through toxic damage to the neural crest, what is the condition of the nerves supplying the deformed limbs?

In order to address this question, we needed to induce thalidomide deformities in an animal model and look at the peripheral nerves supplying those deformities. For this purpose, the rabbit was an ideal model, being cheap and plentiful in Australia, and a reliable mimic of thalidomide embryopathy in humans. Previous researchers had established dose regimes, and I had conducted unpublished pilot studies prior to the one reported here. Originally, a mystique had arisen in thalidomide research over New Zealand White rabbits, the first breed to yield the defects in Somers' laboratory at the Distillers Company in the UK. New Zealand Whites had become the essential model. But we had access to a motley array of rabbits in the animal house of Sydney University, and we had easily induced deformities in black, white and brindle rabbits. For the present experiment, we used the standard strain bred in our animal house at Castle Hill, Sydney. The strain has been free of any record of congenital malformations for over 10 generations.

We were fortunate to be able to work with Professor McLeod and his team in the Neurological Laboratory, which is fully equipped to investigate clinical peripheral neuropathies by quantitative methods. Many clinical peripheral neuropathies are due to reduction in numbers or sizes of nerve fibres or nerve cells, and are diagnosed by quantitative neuropathology (counting and measuring of nerve fibres). There is an extensive array of different neuropathies in clinical neurology, and a corresponding range of quantitative changes affecting motor and sensory modalities and cell/fibre sizes and functions. The pathology of peripheral neuropathy is often quantitative rather

Chapter Summary
- Introduction
- Aims
- Materials and methods
- Results
- Discussion
- Conclusions
- References

than qualitative, with normal cells and axons but abnormal numbers of them.

This definitive study was carried out by Kathryn North MB BS BSc Med (now MD, and Professor and Head of Paediatrics at Sydney University). She was assisted by Robbert de Iongh MSc (now PhD). It was conducted in the Departments of Pathology, Medicine and Surgery at the University of Sydney, funded by the National Health and Medical Research Council of Australia. Joy Mahant and Damaras Velkou provided technical assistance in radiography and histology respectively. Anne Kricker BA, MPH (now PhD) assisted with research and Margaret Murray BA typed the manuscript. Critical discussion and advice was obtained from a wide range of academics: Professor Susan Dorsch (Pathology), Professor James McLeod (Neurology), Professor Patricia Armati (Zoology), Professor Marcus Singer and Dr Margaret Egar (Developmental Biology, Case Western Reserve University, Cleveland, Ohio), Professor Jacqueline Géraudie (Regeneration Biologist, Paris), Dr Philip Baird (Pathologist), and a number of Australian surgeons, radiologists, neurologists and paediatricians.

The following is extracted from the publication 'Thalidomide deformities and their nerve supply' in the *Journal of Anatomy*,[1] with permission.

Aims

Two questions were addressed:

1. *Is there any difference between the peripheral nerves that supply limb deformities and those supplying normal limbs?* If not, the neural crest hypothesis is refuted. Even if there is a difference, the neural crest hypothesis is not proven, since it might be argued that a neural difference is secondary to deformity in the limb. A more important question concerns the innervation of thalidomide-exposed but anatomically normal limbs. Within any thalidomide-treated litter of laboratory rabbits, some young are born with and others without limb deficiency. Thus the second question arises:

2. *Is there any difference between the peripheral nerves of untreated controls and those of thalidomide-exposed rabbits born without deformity?* In other words, *does neural abnormality precede the limb defect, or does the limb defect come first?* A difference between nerves of untreated animals and those of treated animals with normal limbs would support the neural crest hypothesis of a primary neurotoxic action of the drug. Conversely, if no difference were found, this would favour primary drug action upon the peripheral mesenchyme from which limb structures develop.

The aim of this study was to examine these two questions by means of a quantitative histological comparison of peripheral nerve trunks in control and thalidomide-treated rabbits.

Materials and methods

Twenty-one female laboratory-bred rabbits of the Castle Hill White strain were mated naturally at time zero of gestation. After mating, the does were placed in separate cages, with free access to water and rabbit pellets.

Sixteen does were given oral thalidomide from days 7 to 11 of gestation at a dose of 150 mg/kg/day. Thalidomide powder in olive oil was mixed with rabbit food pellets. Food was withheld on the 6th day of gestation in order to increase consumption of the drug on the 7th day. The amount of thalidomide ingested was estimated to be 300–500 mg/day for each rabbit.

Five control does were subjected to a similar regime, but with no thalidomide in the olive oil. On day 29 of gestation, all fetuses were removed by laparotomy under general anaesthesia. In the rabbit embryo, rapid organogenesis follows implantation on the 6th day, rendering it difficult to predict consistent malformations. In this experiment, all females treated with thalidomide produced litters in which some offspring were anatomically normal and some had lower limb defects (Figures 18.1–18.6).

Each fetus was anaesthetized and perfused through the left ventricle with Karnovsky's fixative,[2] eviscerated and stored in Karnovsky's fixative at 4°C. After 24 hours, they were transferred to sodium cacodylate buffer, pH 7.4 at 4°C. Each specimen was measured, photographed and radiographed to demonstrate the extent of any skeletal malformation.

The crown–rump length was recorded, as were the number, type and degree of limb deformities, radiographs of which were graded according to the pattern of dysmelia in humans.[3] The anatomical similarity

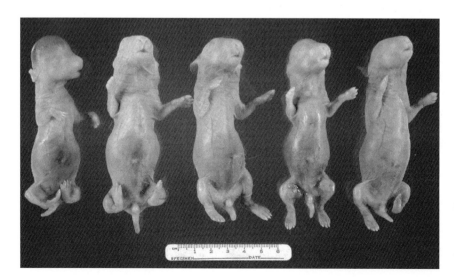

Figure 18.1 *A typical litter with two bilateral and one unilateral leg deformities. Two littermates have no leg deformities in spite of thalidomide exposure (TND).*

Figure 18.2 *(a) Control, untreated. (b) Bilateral hind limb reductions in thalidomide-exposed rabbit.*

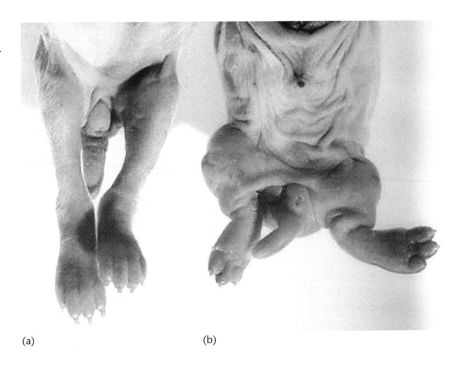

(a)   (b)

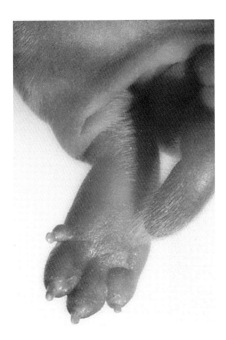

Figure 18.3 *Hypoplastic pedunculated digit after thalidomide.*

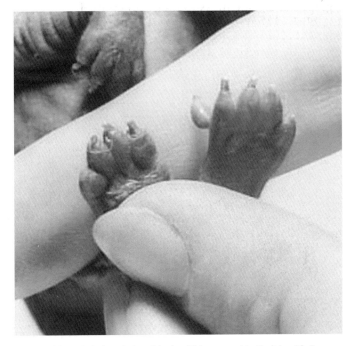

Figure 18.4 *Polydactyly in a black rabbit exposed to thalidomide in a pilot study.*

of thalidomide embryopathy in humans and rabbits has been well documented.[4–6] From the radiographs of deformed fetal rabbits, partial or total absence of the tibia was ascertained. The fetuses were then classified as follows: control (C); thalidomide-treated but not deformed (TND) and normal radiologically; moderately deformed (M), with partial loss or hypoplasia of tibia, with or without decrease in size of the fibula; and severely deformed (S) with absence or aplasia of the tibia.

For quantitative comparison, 4 controls and 13 treated fetuses were selected on the basis of equivalent crown–rump lengths (Table 18.1). Six of the treated group were not deformed (TND). Seven had gross clinical and radiological deformities of the hindlegs, two of moderate degree (M), and five of severe degree (S).

The hindquarters of these 17 fetuses were dissected from the trunk en bloc with the lumbar spine and sacrum. All hindquarters were taped firmly to a cassette and radiographed in the lateral position with the long bones parallel to the film, using a Faxitron for soft tissue exposure (Figures 18.7 and 18.8). The foot was turned towards the anteroposterior position to display the metatarsal and digital rays.

From the radiograph, the length of each femur, tibia and fibula was measured and recorded with a description of any skeletal defects present (Table 18.1). Comparison of radiographs and bone measurements of controls and TND rabbits established that there was no difference in skeletal morphology between these two groups, which validated the designation of 'treated not deformed (TND)' for these six fetuses.

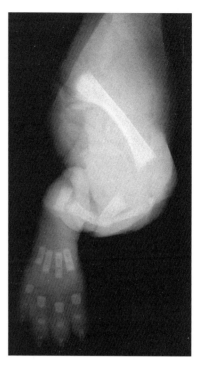

Figure 18.5 *Distal tibial aplasia. Note the triangle of proximal tibia.*

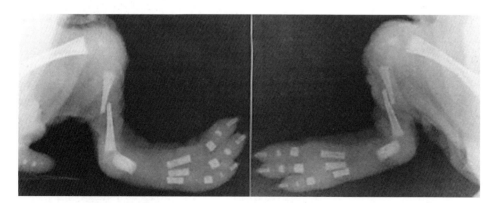

Figure 18.6 *Total tibial aplasia in two rabbits with absence of one digital ray. The fragile fibula has fractured and the baby will die, unable to compete for its mother's milk against its non-deformed littermates.*

Table 18.1 Results of morphometric study

Sciatic nerve[a]	Crown-rump length (mm)	Radiological anatomy	Bone lengths (mm)			Total number of myelinated axons	Total fascicular area (mm²)	Axon diameter distribution (µm)	
			Femur	Tibia	Fibula			Range	Mean
C1	92	Normal	10.35	12.25	12.40	5302	0.1800	0.8–9.4	1.8
C2	87	Normal	11.75	12.60	13.30	5398	0.2196	0.8–8.0	2.0
C3	97	Normal	10.95	11.45	11.80	5373	0.2127	0.8–8.0	2.1
C4	94	Normal	11.60	12.90	13.50	6088	0.1946	0.8–6.7	1.7
Mean±S.D.	92.5±4.2		11.16±0.64	12.10±0.59	12.75±0.79	5540±367	0.2017±0.0179		1.90±0.18
TND 1	96	Normal	11.90	12.60	13.00	5414	0.1664	0.8–5.8	2.2
TND 2	92	Normal	11.60	13.00	13.20	4636	0.1652	0.8–6.3	2.3
TND 3	93	Normal	11.00	12.00	12.00	5339	0.1284	0.8–4.2	2.1
TND 4	96	Normal	11.30	11.10	11.70	5236	0.1202	0.6–3.1	1.9
TND 5	100	Normal	11.20	12.05	12.20	4462	0.1774	0.5–4.3	1.7
TND 6	100	Normal	11.25	12.05	13.00	4797	0.1669	0.6–5.6	2.1
Mean±S.D.	96.2±3.4		11.38±0.32	12.13±0.64	12.52±0.63	4981±401	0.1541±0.0236		2.05±0.22
M1	84	Absence of distal tibia	10.55	7.45	8.75	4220	0.1167	0.8–4.6	1.9
M2	92		11.50	3.50	9.50	4087	0.1555	0.8–3.7	2.1
Mean±S.D.	88.5±5.0		11.02±0.48	5.48±1.97	9.13±0.37	4154±94	0.1361±0.0274		2.00±0.14
S1	85	Absent tibia	10.75	—	9.15	4349	0.1156	0.8–3.2	2.1
S2	91	Absent tibia	10.35	—	9.05	3478	0.0841	0.9–3.2	2.0
S3	91	Absent tibia	10.40	—	8.85	3663	0.0828	0.9–3.6	1.6
S4	93	Absent tibia	10.90	—	9.50	4220	0.1048	0.8–4.1	1.9
S5	96	Absent tibia	10.10	—	10.40	3646	0.0951	0.6–2.3	1.5
Mean ± S.D.	91.2±4.0		10.50±0.32	—	9.39±0.61	3871±387	0.0965±0.0239		1.82±0.26

[a] C, controls; TND, treated not deformed; M, moderately deformed; S, severely deformed.

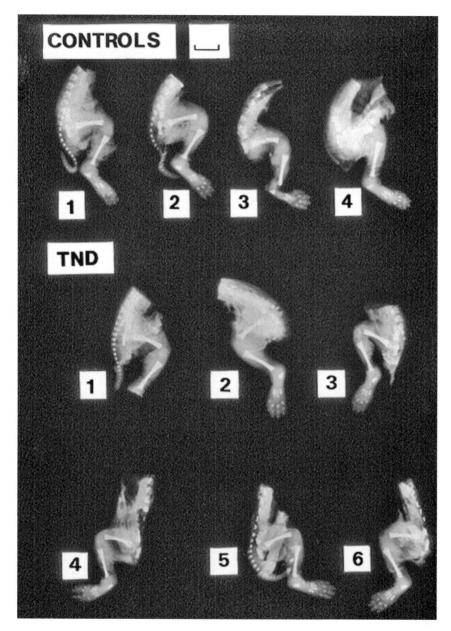

Figure 18.7 *Radiographs of untreated controls and treated, not deformed (TND).*

Sciatic nerves were dissected from the hindlimbs of the four controls and the 13 thalidomide-exposed fetuses (Figure 18.9). Proximally, each nerve was sectioned transversely, above the knee but below the branches to the thigh muscles. Distally, the nerve was sectioned obliquely at the level of the knee joint. This unbranched segment of sciatic nerve was transferred to 0.1 M cacodylate buffer at 4°C, and labelled.

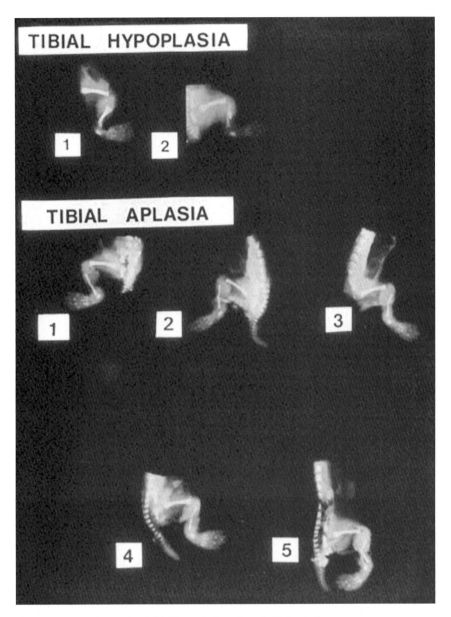

Figure 18.8 *Radiographs of tibial hypoplasia and total tibial aplasia.*

Each nerve was postfixed in 1% Dalton's chrome osmium tetroxide,[7] stained en bloc with aqueous uranyl acetate, and dehydrated through graded ethanol solutions. After embedding in Spurr's resin,[8] a transverse section 0.5 μm thick was taken from each nerve. The sections were stained with 1% toluidine blue in 1% borax. Sections were photographed, enlarged ×1300, and a montage of each nerve was constructed.

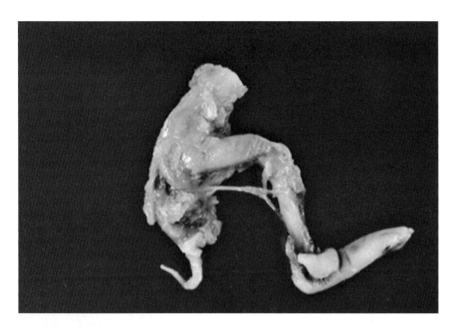

Figure 18.9 *Dissection of sciatic nerve for biopsy.*

The number of myelinated axons per nerve, and the frequency distribution of axon diameters, was determined using a Zeiss TGZ-3 particle size analyser. Measurements were taken from the inner edge of the myelin sheath of each axon. For ovoid fibres, the lesser axis was considered to represent the correct diameter.[9] A Hewlett-Packard digitizer was used to trace the intraperineurial outline of each fascicle and thus to compute the fascicular area.

The following quantities were measured in each sciatic nerve:

- *Total fascicular area:* this was the sum of areas of all fascicles in the nerve.
- *Myelinated axon density per fascicle:*

$$\text{myelinated axon density/fascicle} = \frac{\text{total myelinated axons per fascicle}}{\text{area of fascicle}}$$

- *Total number of myelinated axons per sciatic nerve (N):* since for one fascicle, the number of myelinated axons (*n*) is equal in the myelinated axon density multiplied by the area of the fascicle (*E*), in each sciatic nerve, *N=En*.
- *Axon diameter distribution curve:* a frequency distribution curve of axon diameters was constructed for each nerve using the Hewlett-Packard 9830 computer and 9862A Calculator Plotter.

The results within each group (C, TND, M and S) were compared, using the two-tailed Student's *t*–test; $p < 0.05$ was considered to be of significance.

Results

Each sciatic nerve comprised from two to seven fascicles – usually one large and several smaller ones. Most fascicles contained a large number of well-myelinated fibres. However, in both control and treated groups, some of the smaller fascicles and isolated areas of the larger fascicles contained areas with a low density of myelinated fibres.

The only histological abnormality seen with the light microscope was a reduction in the total fascicular area of sciatic nerves in fetuses treated with thalidomide compared with controls. There was no evidence to suggest the presence of damaged nerve fibres by light microscopy.

The results of the morphometric study are recorded in Table 18.1, and findings for the specific parameters are as follows.

Total fascicular area

There was a significant decrease ($p<0.05$) in the total fascicular area of sciatic nerves in all thalidomide-treated fetuses (Figure 18.10). The decrease was apparent in

- TND fetuses (0.1541 ± 0.0236 mm^2)
- moderately deformed fetuses (0.1361 ± 0.0274 mm^2) and
- severely deformed fetuses (0.0965 ± 0.0239 mm^2)

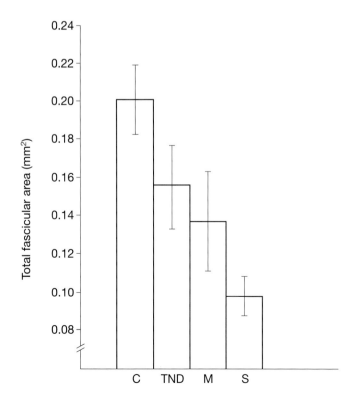

Figure 18.10 *Histogram of total fascicular areas of sciatic nerves. C, control untreated; TND, treated but not deformed littermate; M, moderately deformed with tibial hypoplasia; S, severely deformed with tibial aplasia.*

when compared with

- control fetuses (0.2017 ± 0.0179 mm^2)

Myelinated axon density per fascicle

A wide range of density values was observed in all groups examined. There was no significant difference between these values in control and thalidomide-treated groups (Figure 18.11).

Total number of myelinated axons

There was no significant difference in the total number of myelinated fibres in sciatic nerves from TND fetuses and from controls (Figure 18.12):

- The control value (5540 ± 367 mm^2)

was significantly higher than the value from

- moderately deformed fetuses (4154 ± 94 mm^2) and
- severely deformed fetuses (3871 ± 387 mm^2)

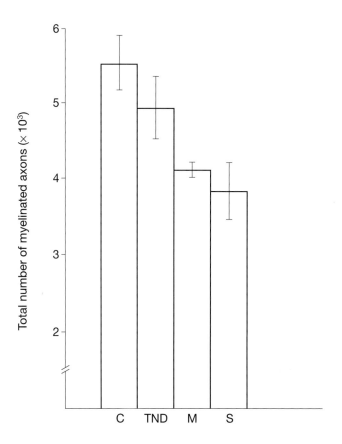

Figure 18.11 *Histogram of total number of myelinated fibres in sciatic nerves. C, control untreated; M, moderately deformed hindlimb; S, severely deformed hindlimb.*

Figure 18.12 *Light microscopy of sciatic nerves. Scale bar = 20 μm. C, control; TND, treated but not deformed; M, moderately deformed; S, severely deformed.*

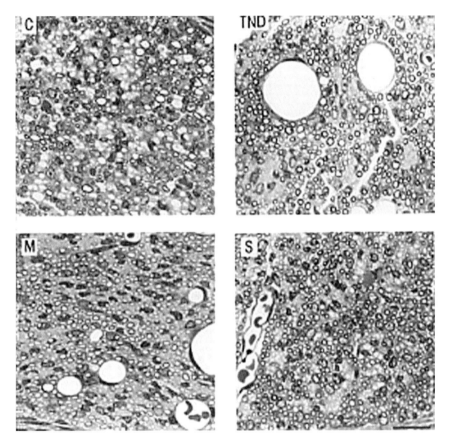

Distribution of myelinated axon diameters

The distribution of diameters of myelinated axons in each nerve was plotted as a function of the frequency of axons of that size per square millimetre (Figure 18.13):

- Each nerve exhibited a unimodal distribution.
- However, there was a difference in the range of diameters between each group, with fewer large-diameter axons in all thalidomide-exposed groups, including TND fetuses.
- The diameters of the largest fibres present in the control group exceeded those in the other three groups.
- These features indicate loss of large-diameter axons in all thalidomide-exposed fetuses.
- The more severe the deformity, the more apparent was the deficit of large-diameter axons.

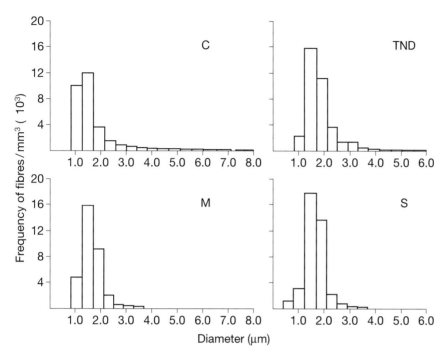

Figure 18.13 *Frequency distribution curves of sizes of myelinated axons in sciatic nerves. Each histogram is a mean for the group, derived from myelinated fibre counts of all rabbits in that group. C, controls (n = 4), TND, treated but not deformed (n = 6), M, partial tibial aplasia (n = 2); S, total tibial aplasia (n = 5).*

Discussion

The absence of qualitative histopathological changes on light microscopy does not refute the neural crest hypothesis. On the contrary, normality of surviving axons would be anticipated in fetuses at this stage of development, because the drug had acted 18–22 days earlier, when no axon was long enough to be present in the sciatic nerve biopsy. The axons visible in sciatic nerves at 29 days' gestation should theoretically be those that had escaped the damaging effect of the drug. According to the neural crest hypothesis, a toxic disruption in the development or function of a segment of neural crest should affect and possibly halt the growth of the related axons. This would delete a whole group of axons, while those unaffected would continue to grow and should be histologically normal. Therefore quantitative rather than qualitative changes were to be anticipated, and are indeed displayed in the results of this morphometric study.

The decrease in total fascicular area of sciatic nerves in all animals exposed to thalidomide is significant in all groups, even in the TND animals. This is not a function of the size of the fetuses, because they were selected for the study on the basis of equal size (crown–rump length) and had similar lengths of long bones, as shown in Table 18.1. Nor can it be explained as a phenomenon secondary to a primary insult to the peripheral mesenchyme, for there is no anatomical defect measurable, either clinically or radiographically, in the TND rabbits (Table 18.1; Figures 18.1 and 18.7). This result supports the concept of a primary neurotoxic action of thalidomide, with a reduction of total neurofascicular area occurring before any defect in the peripheral skeleton is apparent.

The graduated reduction in total fibre number and total fascicular area in the four groups (Figures 18.10 and 18.11) suggests that a threshold effect may exist in the mammalian embryo, whereby a minimum amount of axoplasm must be available before limb structures such as the skeleton will develop. Such a threshold is well documented with respect to limb regeneration in amphibia.[10–17] For limb regeneration to occur after amputation, Singer has shown that a minimum amount of axoplasm per unit area of the amputation wound must be present. The threshold is a band rather than a single line. Below its lower limit, there is insufficient axoplasm to support regeneration, and the limb fails to regrow. Above the upper limit of the threshold, regeneration takes place in an all-or-none type of response to a quantitatively adequate nerve supply. Within the threshold band, positive and negative cases of regeneration occur, in proportion to the number of fibres.[14] This suggests a sliding scale within the threshold range.

The important principles of neurotrophism have been laid out in Chapter 14, and are relevant to interpretation of the results of this experiment. In particular, the third principle states that neurotrophism is quantitative, in that the size of a limb regenerate is directly proportional to the amount of its nerve supply (i.e. cross-sectional area of axoplasm) and that thresholds apply to regeneration.

Our results suggest that failure of limb growth in the embryo is due to drug-induced reduction in the quantity of nerve tissue within the limb bud. This is supported by our previous experiment showing the presence of axons in the undifferentiated early limb bud of rabbit during the thalidomide-sensitive period (Chapter 15). In theory, a threshold gradient for the minimum amount (in transverse section) of axoplasm necessary for limb formation in rabbit embryo would lie somewhere between the values for the TND and the moderately deformed groups in Figures 18.10 and 18.11. It follows that neurotrophism, as defined by studies of limb *regeneration* in amphibia, plays an important role in *embryonic development*.

An alternative explanation (for the decreased numbers of myelinated fibres in nerves to deformed limbs) is that neuronal cell death is induced by absence of peripheral structures.[18–20] That explanation does not fit these circumstances, although it may explain the neural response to distal amputation at a later age. If an explanation based on secondary neuronal cell death were valid, there would be no neural changes in the TND group compared with controls. The observed changes in fibre size and fascicular area in the TND rabbits make the explanation of secondary cell death of neurons unlikely.

Loss of large-diameter fibres in treated animals compared with controls is a striking phenomenon that demands an explanation. This histopathological change is identical with the changes reported in adult human nerves with thalidomide-induced sensory peripheral neuropathy. Selective loss of large-diameter fibres was recorded in sural nerve biopsies of six British patients with sensory polyneuropathies due to use of thalidomide as a sedative, when examined 4–6 years after stopping the drug treatment.[21] There was no segmental demyelination. In two of the six, a marked increase in number of small fibres was thought to indicate regeneration.

Krücke et al[22] examined sural nerve biopsies of four German patients with well-established thalidomide polyneuropathy, and compared the histological appearances with four sural nerve biopsies from normal controls, using light and electron microscopy. They observed a loss of large myelinated axons, an increase in the absolute number of small myelinated axons, and a shift to the left in the 'calibre spectrum' of fibre diameters within the nerves affected by thalidomide. They found no evidence of demyelination, but substantial ultrastructural evidence of axonal degeneration of large myelinated fibres and non-myelinated axons. The increase in the population of small myelinated axons, some of them still not mature, led Krücke et al[22] to conclude that the subsequent regeneration of damaged fibres is histologically incomplete, which they correlated with incomplete clinical recovery.

Klinghardt[23] examined nerves and spinal cords of two patients with thalidomide embryopathy who died from other causes (Chapter 4). He found axonal degeneration in peripheral nerves, destruction of some spinal ganglion cells, and severe degeneration in the posterior (sensory) columns of the spinal cord. Failure of clinical recovery in thalidomide neuropathy in adults is thought to be related to Klinghardt's pathological finding of loss of spinal ganglion cells – an indication that some neurons are totally destroyed by the drug.[24]

In our experiment, sciatic nerves of all embryos treated with thalidomide display a shift to the left in the frequency distribution curve of axonal diameters (Figure 18.13), similar to the quantitative changes described in human polyneuropathy due to this drug (Chapter 4). This could be explained by a replacement of damaged large fibres by small fibres, similar to the process suggested by Klinghardt,[23] Fullerton and O'Sullivan,[21] and Krücke et al[22] in adult thalidomide neuropathy. In the spectrum of thalidomide-exposed nerves in our study, those least affected by the drug (the TND group) appear to maintain normal fibre numbers, but with loss of the largest axons and an increase in the smaller ones, and with some reduction in total fascicular area. The greater the damage caused by the drug in the two deformed groups, the less adequate is the axonal regeneration, and the more probable that numbers of axons and neurons are irreversibly destroyed and deleted. Since this quantitative neurohistological response in thalidomide-exposed embryos of the rabbit so closely approximates that described in human adults with thalidomide polyneuropathy, it is highly probable that the underlying process corresponds. The evidence indicates a primary process of toxic damage to sensorineural tissues in both instances.

Conclusions

- Thalidomide acts upon embryonic *nerves not mesenchyme*.
- Dysmelic deformities of the limbs are secondary to toxic embryonic neuropathy.
- It is suggested that skeletal defects result when irreversible damage to nerves reduces the transverse fascicular area below a *critical minimum threshold*.
- The results of this application of neuro-quantitation to congenital malformations has confirmed a site of action and *a quantitative lesion* within the peripheral nervous system.
- Thus thalidomide embryopathy is shown to be an extension of a large group of *neurological diseases*, collectively known as sensory peripheral neuropathy.
- Thalidomide embryopathy can be better understood if it is recognized as '*embryonic sensory peripheral neuropathy*'.

References

1. McCredie J, North K, de Iongh R. Thalidomide deformities and their nerve supply. *J Anat* 1984; **139**: 397–410.
2. Karnovsky MJ. A formaldehyde–glutaraldehyde fixative of high osmolality for use in electron microscopy. *J Cell Biol* 1965; **27**: 137a.
3. Henkel H-L, Willert H-G. Dysmelia: a classification and a pattern of malformation in a group of congenital defects of the limbs. *J Bone Joint Surg* 1969; **51**: 399–414.
4. Somers GF. Thalidomide and congenital abnormalities. *Lancet* 1962; **i**: 912.
5. Vickers TH. Concerning the morphogenesis of thalidomide dysmelia in rabbits. *Br J Exp Pathol* 1967; **48**: 579–91.
6. Vickers TH. The thalidomide embryopathy in hybrid rabbits. *Br J Exp Pathol* 1967; **48**: 107–17.
7. Dalton AJ. Chrome osmium fixative for electron microscopy. *Anat Rec* 1955; **121**: 281.
8. Spurr AR. A low viscosity epoxy resin embedding medium for electron microscopy. *J Ultrastructure Res* 1969; **26**: 31–43.
9. Dyck PJ. Pathologic alterations of the peripheral nervous system of man. In: Dyck PJ, Thomas PK, Lambert EM, eds. *Peripheral Neuropathy*, Vol 1. Philadelphia: WB Saunders, 1975: 296.
10. Singer M. The nervous system and regeneration of the forelimb of the adult *Triturus*. The influence of number of nerve fibres. *J Exp Zool* 1946; **101**: 299–337.

11. Singer M. Induction of regeneration of the forelimb of the postmetamorphic frog by augmentation of the nerve supply. *J Exp Zool* 1954; **126**: 419–71.

12. Singer M. Induction of body parts in the lizard *Anolis*. *Proc Soc Exp Biol Med* 1961; **107**: 106–8.

13. Singer M. A theory of the trophic nervous control of amphibian limb regeneration including a re-evaluation of quantitative nerve requirements. In: Kortsis V, Trampusch HAL, eds. *Regeneration in Animals and Related Problems*. Amsterdam: North-Holland, 1965: 20–32.

14. Singer M. *Limb Regeneration in the Vertebrates* (Addison-Wesley Module in Biology No. 6). Reading, MA: Addison-Wesley, 1973.

15. Singer M. Neurotrophic control of limb regeneration in the newt. *Ann NY Acad Sci* 1974; **228**: 308–22.

16. Singer M. On the nature of the neurotrophic phenomenon in *Urodele* limb regeneration. *Am Zool* 1978; **18**: 829–41.

17. Ferretti P, Géraudie J, eds. *Cellular and Molecular Basis of Regeneration: From Invertebrates to Humans*. Chichester: Wiley, 1998.

18. Hamburger V, Levi-Montalcini R. Proliferation, differentiation and degeneration in the spinal ganglia of the chick embryo under normal and experimental conditions. *J Exp Zool* 1949; **111**: 457–500.

19. Prestige M. Evidence that at least some of the motor nerve cells that die during development have first made peripheral connections. *J Comp Neurol* 1967; **170**: 123–4.

20. Hamburger V. Cell death in the development of the lateral motor column of the chick embryo. *J Comp Neurol* 1975; **160**: 535–546.

21. Fullerton PM, O'Sullivan DJ. Thalidomide neuropathy – a clinical, electrophysiological and histological follow-up study. *J Neurol Neurosurg Psychiatr* 1968; **31**: 543–51.

22. Krücke W, von Hartrott H-H, Schröder JM et al. Light and electron microscope studies of late stages of thalidomide polyneuropathy. *Fortschr Neurol Psychiatr Grenzgeb* 1971; **39**: 15–50.

23. Klinghardt GW, Ein Betrag der experimentallen Neuropatholgie zur Toxizitätsprüfung neuer Chemotherapeutica. *Mitt Max-Planck Gesell* 1965; **3**: 142–55.

24. Le Quesne PM. Neuropathy due to drugs. In: Dyck PJ, Thomas PK, Lambert EH, eds. *Peripheral Neuropathy*, Vol 2. Philadelphia: WB Saunders, 1975: 1273–5.

CHAPTER 19

Thalidomide deformities and their nerve supply: Second morphometric study in rabbits

Introduction

In order to check the findings of the experiment described in Chapter 18, and to look at nerves closer to the affected bone, we performed another similar experiment using quantitative neuropathology. This was carried out by Dr Gillian Dunlop MB BS BSc Med, with assistance from Mr Robbert de Iongh MSc (now PhD), Mrs Joy Mahant and Mrs Kerry Dowsett. Lilly Industries provided a grant in aid to Dr Dunlop. The paper was published in the Proceedings of the Sixth Marcus Singer Symposium[1] and in Dr Dunlop's thesis.[2] This chapter is based on her paper.

Aims

The aims of this investigation were:

1. To confirm or refute the previous findings[3] (Chapter 18).
2. To address the question 'What is the relationship between thalidomide exposure, skeletal deformity and changes in the nerves that normally supply the absent/deformed bone?'

Materials and methods

As in the study described in Chapter 18, the approach was to compare quantitative neurohistological parameters of rabbit fetuses with thalidomide-induced tibial aplasia, of littermates without deformities and of untreated controls. This time, the tibial nerve rather than the sciatic nerve was examined.

Chapter Summary
- Introduction
- Aims
- Materials and methods
- Results
- Discussion
- Conclusions
- References

Animal breeding

Animal breeding methods were almost identical with these described in Chapter 18,[3,4] with certain modifications of dosage. Seventeen does were mated. Two were used as untreated controls. Fifteen were given oral thalidomide 800 mg/day from days 6 to 10 of gestation, administered as described in Chapter 18.[3,4]

Tissue preparation

Tissue was prepared as in Chapter 18; the references used were the same, and will not be repeated here. The fetuses were divided into three groups: control, treated but not deformed (TND), and DEF. The latter deformed group included both hypoplasia and aplasia of the tibia, confirmed radiologically. All fetuses in the study were matched for crown–rump length.

A 5 mm length of the tibial nerve was removed distal to the knee joint and distal to the leash of muscular branches supplying the proximal calf muscles. The selected nerve contains fibres to the tibia.

The specimens were fixed and embedded as described before, and photographed and montaged at × 1250 enlargement.

Quantitation

Myelinated axons were counted on a Zeiss TGZ-3 Particle Size Analyser, which measures axon diameters and groups them into graded bins according to size.

The perimeter of each transverse section of tibial nerve trunk was traced at a constant magnification of × 560, using a camera lucida drawing attachment mounted on an Olympus microscope. The area of each nerve was computed from the perimeter measurement using a Hewlett-Packard digitizer interfaced with a Hewlett-Packard table top computer/calculator. The area of blood vessels within the fascicles was measured and subtracted in order to measure more accurately the amount of axonal tissue within the peripheral nerve. This measurement of transverse fascicular area includes cross-sections of myelinated axons, unmyelinated axons, Schwann cells and connective tissue.

Results

Animal breeding

The two control rabbits yielded litters of eight and nine fetuses with one resorption site. None of the progeny was deformed on external appearance or on radiographs.

Of the 15 treated does, 9 had no fetuses on palpation or on abdominal radiographs at day 29, and they were not submitted to laparotomy but returned to the animal house. The number of resorption sites is unknown.

Six treated does bore litters of between 1 and 5 live fetuses, totalling 18, with a total of 20 resorption sites. On physical examination, the hindlimbs of the treated fetuses without deformity (TND) were indistinguishable from those of the controls. On dissection, the muscles and other soft tissues were anatomically normal.

Four of the 18 treated fetuses had hindlimb malformations. Radiographs showed three to be aplasia and one to be hypoplasia of the tibia. On dissection of the calf, there was gross disorganization of the muscle anatomy and diminished muscle bulk.

Quantitative analysis

Total number of myelinated fibres

The total number of myelinated fibres in the tibial nerves of deformed fetuses was significantly reduced in comparison with both the control and TND values. Although there was a reduction in the total number of myelinated fibres of TND rabbits compared with controls, this did not reach statistical significance (Figure 19.1).

Total fascicular area

The total fascicular area of each group of the tibial nerves differed significantly from the other two (Figure 19.2).

Fibre size distribution

There was no significant difference between any of the three groups in the distribution of axon diameter. In all groups, there was a similar unimodal distribution ranging up to 3 µm diameter, with the peak at 1 µm diameter.

Length of hindlimb bones

There was no difference between control and treated fetuses with radiologically normal skeletons in terms of the length of the major long bones, which supports their classification as 'treated but not deformed (TND)'. There was measurable reduction in length of all major long bones within the hindlimbs of animals with dysplasia of the tibia.

Discussion

The slightly increased dose of thalidomide administered 1 day earlier than in the sciatic nerve study showed the typical features of a teratogen. Timing and dosage interact in the schedule of embryology

Figure 19.1 *Histogram of total number of myelinated fibres in tibial nerves. C, control untreated; TND, treated but not deformed; DEF, deformed.*

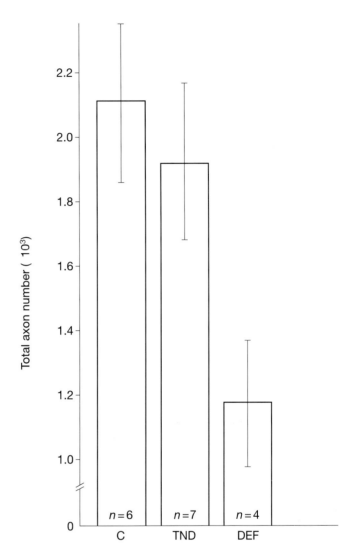

so that both must be finely tuned to target the embryonic window and create deformities. Too much too soon causes death of the embryo and abortion (or resorption sites in animals). The high proportion of failed pregnancies and small litters with several resorption sites shows that we were pushing the timing and dosage of the drug towards its limits. Conversely, giving too little too late misses the sensitive period and fails to induce birth defects.

Two findings in the tibial nerves corroborate those in the sciatic nerves – namely reductions in total fascicular area and total fibre number. However, the tibial nerves did not show the loss of large-diameter fibres seen in the treated sciatic nerves, nor did the control tibial nerves contain such large-diameter fibres. The explanation for this probably lies in the anatomy of the subdivision of the sciatic nerve, of which the tibial nerve is the terminal branch. Another

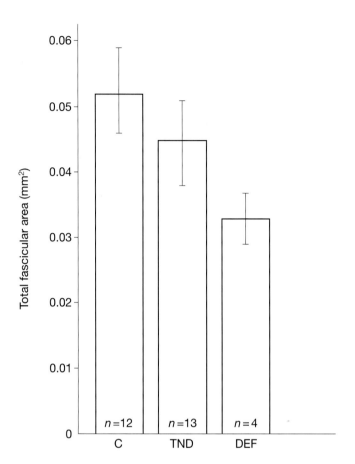

Figure 19.2 *Histogram of total fascicular areas of tibial nerves. C, control untreated; TND, treated but not deformed; DEF, deformed.*

higher branch of the sciatic nerve is the medial sural cutaneous nerve, which unites with the peroneal communicating branch of the peroneal nerve to form the sural nerve, which is purely sensory and normally rich in large-diameter axons. Our sections of tibial nerve were taken distal to this sensory branch and therefore did not include the large-diameter fibres seen in the sciatic nerve above that branch. The different findings are a function of the site examined. Because of its high proportion of large sensory axons, the sural nerve is an important biopsy site in neurology for establishing the diagnosis of sensory peripheral neuropathy. Fullerton and O'Sullivan[5] recorded a selective loss of large-diameter fibres in sural nerve biopsies of six adult patients with sensory polyneuropathy due to thalidomide, confirmed by other neuropathologists.

The results of other parameters reproduce those of the sciatic nerve study and validate the previous findings.

In the tibial nerve study, the total number of fibres in the deformed group differed significantly from both the control and TND values. Although there was a reduction in total fibre number in TND fetuses compared with controls, the difference was not statistically significant.

However, the total fascicular areas (TFAs) of each of the three groups were significantly different from one another. It appears that, as a parameter, TFA is best able to differentiate between the three groups in the study. TFA appears to be the most sensitive indicator of nerve reduction by thalidomide.

Significant reduction in TFA in the tibial nerves of TND fetuses compared with untreated controls means that nerve injury occurs after thalidomide exposure, even without skeletal defect. Therefore there is probably a threshold TFA above which there is mild nerve depletion, insufficient to reduce the dependant skeleton, but below which skeletal defects result. The presence of a threshold TFA would explain why some exposed animals are born without skeletal defects. Their exposure was insufficient to reduce the TFA below the threshold level. In our study, the threshold value of TFA must lie between the TFA values for the TND and deformed groups. A toxic insult to the presumptive peripheral nerve supply (reflected as reduction in total fibre number or TFA or both) may conceivably stop limb morphogenesis if the damage is enough to reduce these parameters below their teratogenic thresholds.

A threshold concept is well established in the literature about limb regeneration. In 1946, Singer[6] proposed that a threshold number of nerve fibres was necessary for limb regeneration after amputation, and that, below this threshold, limb regeneration did not occur. Singer et al[7] related trophic activity to the total amount of nerve substance at the amputation site rather than the number of axons. They noted that in the frog *Xenopus*, the number of nerve fibres at the amputation site was well below the threshold number required for limb regeneration in a lower species, the newt *Triturus*, and yet limb regeneration in *Xenopus* was possible. A histological study revealed that the nerve fibres of *Xenopus* make up in individual size what they lack in numbers. Their axons are very large, but there are fewer of them. The supply of axoplasm in terms of volume is equivalent to the newt with its host of small-diameter axons. Singer[6,7] advocated the concept of cross-sectional area of axoplasm presenting at the amputation site, in order to stress the volumetric rather than the numerical requirement. The threshold required for amphibian limb regeneration is a function of the 'cross-sectional area of axoplasm'.

Its equivalent in our experiment is the TFA. The TFA is a realistic measurement of the volume of axoplasm in the tibial nerve, since it includes all myelinated and unmyelinated fibres. Only myelinated fibres are included in the total count of fibres. TFA is therefore a true index of the total volume of axoplasm, and approximates Singer's concept more closely than does fibre number. Our finding that changes in area rather than in number of fibres are a better index of a teratogenic threshold seems to provide another example of the biological principle that the amount or volume of nerve tissue is more important than the fibre number, as far as neurotrophism is concerned.[6,7]

Using the threshold principle, limb regeneration has been artificially induced by nerve augmentation in animal species that do not normally regenerate their limbs (Chapter 14). The nerve supply was augmented by deviation of other nerves[8,9] or by implants of nervous tissue to the amputation site,[10] thus lifting the TFA above the threshold.

Thalidomide works in the opposite sense: it depresses the TFA through a range of values. Moderate depression of TFA, below normal but above the threshold for deformity, allows some offspring to avoid deformity (our TND group). If thalidomide reduces the nerve supply severely – to levels below the threshold for deformity – the animals are born with reduction deformities.

Conclusions

The findings of the previous experiment (Chapter 18)[3] were confirmed.

- *Evidence for the presence of thresholds.* Thalidomide exposure resulted in some fetuses with skeletal deformities (reduction of tibia) and some apparently normal littermates. There was significant reduction in the TFAs of the tibial nerves of both these groups – most marked in the deformed fetuses. The results suggested that a threshold TFA was operating, whereby skeletal defects occurred below the threshold, and non-deformed littermates fell into the range above the threshold but below the normal controls. Even without skeletal deformity, the tibial nerves of exposed fetuses were depleted below normal, showing that the primary action of thalidomide is on the nerves; reduction of the skeleton is secondary to more profound nerve reduction.
- *Results obey principles of neurotrophism.* These results obey the principles established in experiments on neurotrophism in amphibia (Chapter 14). Thus thalidomide is a chemical that mimics the experimental manipulation of neurotrophism.

References

1. Dunlop G, McCredie J. Thalidomide, tibial nerves and the threshold concept. In: Inoue S, ed. *Proceedings of 6th Marcus Singer Symposium*, 1988: 233–50.

2. Dunlop G. Studies of the pathogenesis and the anatomy of congenital limb defects. BSc Med Thesis, University of Sydney, 1984.

3. McCredie J, North K, de Iongh R. Thalidomide deformities and their nerve supply. *J Anat* 1984; **3**: 397–410.

4. North K. Teratogenic mechanisms in the embryo. BSc Med Thesis, University of Sydney, 1982.

5. Fullerton PM, O'Sullivan DJ. Thalidomide neuropathy – a clinical, electrophysiological and histological follow-up study. *J Neurol Neurosurg Psychiatr* 1968; **31**: 543–51.

6. Singer M. The nervous system and regeneration of the forelimbs of adult *Triturus*. The influence of number of nerve fibres. *J Exp Zool* 1946; **101**: 299–337.

7. Singer M, Rhezak K, Maier C. The relation between the calibre of the axon and the trophic activity of the nerves in limb regeneration. *J Exp Zool* 1967; **166**: 89–98.

8. Simpson SB. Induction of limb regeneration in the lizard *Lygosoma laterale*, by augmentation of the nerve supply. *Proc Soc Exp Biol Med* 1961; **107**: 108–11.

9. Singer M. induction of regeneration of the forelimb of the postmeta-morphic frog by augmentation of the nerve supply. *J Exp Zool* 1954; **126**: 419–71.

10. Fowler I, Sisken BF. Effect of augmentation of the nerve supply upon limb regeneration of the chick embryo. *J Exp Zool* 1982; **221**: 49–59.

CHAPTER 20

The sensory nerve supply of bone

Introduction

Do bones have a nerve supply? Clinically, the unequivocal answer is yes, but objective proof been difficult to obtain, and the real picture has been slow to emerge over the past 160 years.

Clinical evidence

In clinical practice, the intense pain caused by trauma, inflammation or neoplasm in bone is proof that sensory nerves exist within bones and joints. Clinical neurologists were prepared to deduce their presence from clinical observations. For instance, Bohler's 1929 technique of a single large injection of local anaesthetic agent between the ends of a fractured bone induced relaxation of local spasm and anaesthesia, which enabled relatively painless reduction of the fracture to be achieved. The deep injection leaves the overlying skin sensitivity unaltered, and the French neurologist Leriche[1] endorsed this as evidence of the presence of pain fibres within bone.

Diseases of nerves such as neurofibromatosis can involve bones, which is further clinical evidence that there are nerves in bones.

Clinical observations predated the anatomical and microscopic demonstration of nerves within bone, and historically it has proved difficult to demonstrate their presence by either dissection or histology.

Anatomical dissection

The history of the anatomical search for nerves in bone is littered with failures. The textures of the two tissues lie at opposite extremes: bone is the toughest tissue in the body, whereas unmyelinated nerve axons, mere threads of protein, are the most fragile.

Chapter Summary
- Introduction
- Clinical evidence
- Anatomical dissection
- Microscopic histology
- Modern advances in neurohistopathology
- What are the functions of nerves at these sites?
- Conclusion
- References

According to Leriche,[1] a French anatomist in 1846 demonstrated a nerve accompanying the nutrient artery into the femur of a horse. Small branches were given off to the periosteum. Attempts to trace the nerves into bone by gross dissection failed, and interest by anatomists languished for over a century. Nerves were seen in bone marrow by Kuntz and Richins[2] in 1945, but their presence within Haversian canals was less convincing and remained debatable.

'Many articular twigs are so delicate that they escape detection by gross dissection' said Gardner[3–5] in the late 1940s. Stilwell[6–8] in the 1950s showed 'undissectable threads' of nerve fibres entering periosteum from adjacent muscles.

The scant treatment afforded the subject of innervation of bone in standard texts on the skeletal and nervous systems has been remarked in the past[3]. Sherman[9] in 1963 stated 'there has been so little interest in the nerve supply of bone that most textbooks of anatomy, even books devoted solely to bone, scarcely mention the subject' and cited eight references. Uncertainty led one author[10] to declare in 1971 that the nerve supply of bone was 'unfortunately terra incognita'.

Microscopic histology

Cortex

Histology originally presented the same difficulties: the contrasting textures. To show delicate unmyelinated axons histologically, especially within hard bony cortex, challenged routine laboratory techniques. We know from neurology that in adults, many nerve endings that subserve pain sensation are fine, bare, unencapsulated filaments of 2–5 μm diameter. The most delicate of all sensory terminals, they branch widely and overlap with their neighbours, penetrating between other cells. Axons are protein filaments that retract and snap when heat is applied. They are easily destroyed by routine formalin fixation and hot-paraffin embedding methods, even in soft tissues. But within bone cortex, the hardest of all tissues, axons are at even greater risk, because routine decalcification procedures (to soften bone for cutting) simultaneously damage axons. Preparation of one destroys the other.

Routine laboratory methods to fix and stain bones for light microscopy have consistently failed to show axons. This has been interpreted as absence of nerves in bones, rather than inability to demonstrate nerves in bones. Again, absence of evidence is not evidence of absence!

Bone marrow

Early studies of bone marrow rather than cortex met with more success.[2] In 1881, Variot and Remy[11] studied bone marrow treated with gold chloride, osmic acid or picrocarmine, and found an extraordinarily rich supply of both myelinated and unmyelinated fibres.

Interest lapsed until the 1920s. Based upon the discovery that axoplasm has an affinity for heavy metals (silver, gold, lead, osmium and uranium) – De Castro[12] (as quoted by Hurrell[13]) evolved a method for silver impregnation of nerves, showing them as black threads in decalcified tissues. He described the nerve supply to growing bones, and traced nerves entering bone (with a nutrient artery) to their endings, which he observed to contact the protoplasm of osteoblasts. De Castro believed these nerves to be autonomic. He described both myelinated and non-myelinated fibres within adult bone, terminating on the walls of blood vessels.

Periosteum, matrix and Haversian canals

Miskolczy[14] (again as quoted by Hurrell[13]) studied periosteum by similar methods, and observed nerve fibres entering the bone surface at Haversian canals and other points. He did not follow them any more deeply.

Hurrell[13] went further. He traced nerve fibres into and along Haversian canals of adult bones and into the bone matrix, and described their distribution and endings, noting that some fibres terminated in close relation to osteoblasts. He observed that nerve fibres entering bone with the main nutrient artery seemed to be destined for the marrow, whereas fibres destined for the bone matrix accompanied smaller vessels that entered the Haversian canals here and there over the surface of the bone. These unmyelinated nerve fibres ran parallel to one another within Haversian canals, and maintained this relationship even in the depths of the bone. They branched and overlapped in a free and irregular manner 'covering well over half the distance to the next adjacent canal'. Occasionally, the nerves of adjacent canals appeared to communicate. In many places, the fibres were thickly intertwined and gave off terminal twigs. Nerve endings within bone matrix had an appearance similar to nerve terminals seen in periosteum. Hurrell[13] made the tentative suggestion that the nerve fibres he had shown 'may be the two ends of a reflex arc governing bone growth and maintenance'. This hypothesis has not been pursued, but it remains a seminal scientific idea.

Leriche[1] stated that bone contained nerves that mediated both pain perception and proprioception. Kuntz and Richins[2] confirmed the presence of unmyelinated sympathetic fibres anatomically and functionally related to blood vessels, and afferent myelinated fibres partly related to blood vessels. Some fibres connected with receptors in the bone marrow were thought to be pain conductors, since the range of their axonal calibre was consistent with that of pain fibres elsewhere.

Ligaments, tendons, synovium and fasciae

Ralston et al[15] used amputation specimens to search for nerve endings in human fasciae, tendons, ligaments, periosteum and joint synovial membranes. They showed three main varieties of nerve endings similar to those already recognized as sensory receptors in the skin. It seemed likely that these conveyed the same modalities of sensation. Periosteum was particularly richly innervated, especially at the sites of insertion of ligaments, tendons or capsules of joints. The capsules and ligaments of joints receive nerve fibres from neighbouring muscles and nerve trunks.[15,16]

Vertebrae

The innervation of the vertebrae and associated structures was studied in humans by Gardner et al[5] and in monkeys by Stilwell[6,7] with similar results. Somatic sensory fibres were shown to end in longitudinal ligaments, blood vessels, bone marrow, periosteum, joints and dura mater. Furthermore, a one-segment overlap in innervation of the skeletal structures was shown, corresponding to the typical overlap of cutaneous dermatomes.

Joints

The innervation of joints was discussed by Hilton[17] in relation to the nerves of the adjacent muscles and skin. Hilton found that the same nerve trunks supplying groups of muscles that move a joint also furnish a distribution of nerves to the skin over the insertions of the same muscles, and to the interior of the joint beneath, confirmed by Barnett et al.[16]

Meanwhile, Gardner's studies[3–5] between 1944 and 1955 added much information about adult and fetal joint innervation. His serial sections of fetal limbs showed that large joints have a much more extensive nerve supply than is indicated in most textbooks. As already mentioned, he found many of the articular twigs to be so small and delicate that they defy gross dissection. The nerve supply to fetal joints is from multiple sources, such as the local peripheral nerve trunks and neighbouring muscular branches. The territories of supply of particular nerves within the joints were shown to be more or less constant, with overlap of territories of adjacent nerves. Gardner found that the basic pattern of distribution of nerve fibres to the human knee joint was similar to that found in mouse, cat, horse and frog. The overlap of nerves within the joint was considerable. Three or four peripheral nerves might contribute to the innervation of any one particular part of the joint, so that 'no nerve supplies a portion of the capsule that is not reached by another nerve'. The segmental supply was from lumbar 3 to sacral 1, with the greatest representation from the 4th lumbar segment.

Four types of sensory nerve ending were identified. Innervation in the fibrous capsule and ligaments of joints was rich, whereas that of synovial membrane was poor. In 1952, Samuel[18] compared the density of innervation of joints from normal and sympathectomized animals. He concluded that a large number of myelinated fibres in the articular nerves are of somatic sensory origin.

Thus, by 1960, axons and nerve endings had been found in abundance in periosteum, cortex and marrow, and in joint capsules, ligaments, tendons and fascia, especially where these meet the bone. Fetal joints are particularly richly innervated, as are vertebrae and paravertebral structures. Sensory terminals are less dense in spongiosa and bone marrow than in cortical bone, and are relatively sparse in muscles.

Modern advances in neurohistopathology

Histology and neurohistopathology evolved rapidly after 1960. Old harsh preparations such as formalin fixation and hot-paraffin embedding that shrink and snap fine protein filaments such as axons have been replaced by gentle fixatives (e.g. glutaraldehyde) and cold embedding techniques (Araldite or Spurr's medium). Fixative perfusion, where appropriate, can provide undamaged in vivo quality neural tissue for examination. Araldite enables ultrathin sections for electron microscopy, whereby axons become visible where they were not previously seen, their diameters of less than 5 nm being beyond the resolution of the light microscope (magnification $< \times 800$). With magnifications $> \times 70\,000$, electron microscopy reveals internal structures, organelles and details of synaptic junctions. Electron microscopy reveals axons within undifferentiated limb buds of embryos[19] that were previously said to be 'without nerves' on light microscopy[20] (Chapter 15).

Histochemistry evolved from 1960,[21] immunocytochemistry in the 1980s and DNA technology in the 1990s. By 1996, *Carpenter's Human Neuroanatomy*[22] had illustrations of nerves arborizing within human skeletal tissues (Figure 20.1).

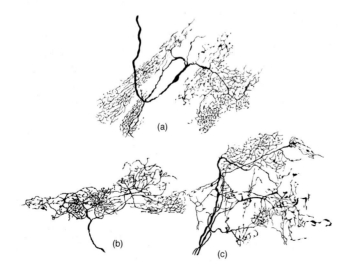

Figure 20.1 *Nerves in human skeletal tissues: (a) patellar ligament; (b) capsule of knee joint; (c) periosteum of femur. (From Parent A, ed.* Carpenter's Human Neuroanatomy, *9th edn. Baltimore: Williams and Wilkins, 1996.[22])*

Old anatomical barriers had given way before these powerful modern tools, and allowed hormones, neurotransmitters and other chemicals to be identified in neural tissue. Labelled molecules can trace the axons in which they are located. Thus previously invisible nerve pathways are being revealed by histochemical mapping. The new science of 'chemical neuroanatomy' confirmed the presence of nerves in skeletal sites discussed above, and also in other sites such as the epiphyseal plate[24] and within the early soft callus of healing fractures.[25]

What are the functions of nerves at these sites?

Transmission of sensations of pain and proprioception are recognized functions. Neurotrophism is another function of nerves in general, and sensory nerves in particular, as discussed in earlier chapters. Growth and repair of limbs and their skeletal parts is subserved by neurotrophism.[26] Evidence is emerging from cell biology that neural signals are involved in remodelling of bone.[27,28]

Conclusion

Innervation exists in the skeleton as in all other organs.

References

1. Leriche R. *Physiologie normale et pathologie du tissue osseux*. Paris: Masson, 1939.
2. Kuntz A. Richins CA. Innervation of the bone marrow. *J Comp Neurol* 1945; **83**: 213–22.
3. Gardner ED. The distribution and termination of nerves in the knee joint of the cat. *J Comp Neurol* 1944; **80**: 11–32.
4. Gardner ED. The innervation of the knee joint. *Anat Rec* 1948; **101**: 109–30.
5. Gardner ED, Pederson HE, Blunck CFJ. The anatomy of lumbosacral posterior primary divisions and sinu-vertebral nerves, with an experimental study of their function. *Anat Rec* 1955; **121**: 297.
6. Stilwell DL. The nerve supply of the vertebral column and its associated structures in the monkey. *Anat Rec* 1956; **125**: 139–69.
7. Stilwell DL. Regional variations in innervation of deep fascia and aponeuroses. *Anat Rec* 1957; **127**: 635.
8. Stilwell DL. The innervation of tendons and aponeuroses. *Am J Anat* 1957; **100**: 289.
9. Sherman MS. The nerves of bone. *J Bone Joint Surg* 1963; **45A**: 522–528.
10. Brookes M. *The Blood Supply of Bone*. London: Butterworths, 1971.
11. Variot G, Remy C. Sur les neufs de la moëlle des os. *J de l'Anat et de la Physiol* 1880: 273–94.
12. De Castro F. *Trab Lab Invert Biol Univ Madrid* 1925; **23**: 429.
13. Hurrell DJ. The nerve supply of bone. *J Anat* 1937; **72**: 54–61.

14. Miskolczy D. Z ges Anat Entw Gesch 1926; **81**: 638.

15. Ralston HJ, Miller MR, Kasahara M. Nerve endings in human fasciae, tendons, ligaments, periosteum and joint synovial membranes. *Anat Rec* 1960; **136**: 137–47.

16. Barnett CH, Davies DV, MacConaill MA. *Synovial Joints*. London: Longmans, 1961.

17. Hilton J. *Rest and Pain. A Course of Lectures*, 2nd edn. Cincinnati: PW Garfield, 1891.

18. Samuel EP. The autonomic and somatic innervation of the articular capsule. *Anat Rec* 1952; **113**: 53–70.

19. Cameron J, McCredie J. Innervation of undifferentiated limb bud in rabbit embryo. *J Anat* 1982; **134**: 795–808.

20. O'Rahilly R, Gardner E. The timing and sequence of events in development of the human embryo. *Anat Embryol* 1975; **148**: 1–23.

21. Panula P, Paivarinta H, Soinila S. eds., *Neurohisto-chemistry: Modern Methods and Applications*. New York: Alan R Liss, 1988.

22. Parent A, ed. *Carpenter's Human Neuroanatomy*, 9th edn. Baltimore: Williams and Wilkins, 1996.

23. McCredie J, Forgotten principles of bone pain. *Osteologie* 1999; **8**: 68–74.

24. Hara-Irie F, Amizuka N, Ozawa H. Immunohistochemical and ultrastructural localization of CGRP-positive nerve fibers at the epiphyseal trabecules facing the growth plate of rat femurs. *Bone* 1996; **18**: 29–39.

25. Hukkanen M, Konttinen YT, Santavirta S et al. Rapid proliferation of CGRP-immunoreactive nerves during healing of rat tibial fractures suggests neural involvement in bone growth and re-modelling. *Neuroscience* 1993; **54**: 969–79.

26. Ferretti P, Géraudie J, eds. *Cellular and Molecular Basis of Regeneration: From Invertebrates to Humans*. Chichester: Wiley, 1998.

27. Eleftheriou F, Ahn JD, Takedas S et al. Leptin regulation of bone resorption by the sympathetic nervous system. *Nature* 2005; **434**: 514–20.

28. Elmquist JK, Strewler GJ. Do neural signals remodel bone? *Nature* 2005; **434**: 447–8.

CHAPTER 21

The sclerotomes

Introduction

Segmental arrangement of sensory innervation

A spinal segmental distribution of innervation in general is common knowledge. Establishing the fact that the skeleton has nerves has been slow; the fact that these nerves shared the general segmental layout was established in 1944, but then lost or overlooked. The key paper of 1944[1] drew upon past work of anatomists[2,3] and neurologists,[4,6] plus a new study of the distribution of pain radiation from skeletal structures, or referred pain. The concept of referred pain is not easy to understand, but the principles are as follows.

General principles of referred pain

Pain provoked by the irritation of tissues deep to the skin has a characteristic persistent, deep and aching quality, and is associated with other reflex phenomena, such as nausea, drop in blood pressure and pulse rate, and local muscle spasm. It radiates diffusely beyond the site of stimulus, and this radiation is termed 'referred pain'.

The possible spinal segmental distribution of referred pain from deep structures had been noted by Lewis.[4,5] He showed by experiment that the quality of pain evoked from somatic structures depends more upon the structure stimulated than upon the nature of the stimulus. At the same time, he noticed that pain arising from muscle tended to be referred to a distance. His colleague Kellgren[6] followed up this observation by systematic analysis of the pain provoked by injection of accessible muscles in normal subjects. Kellgren concluded that the distribution of referred pain arising from muscle follows a spinal segmental pattern but that the pain is deep and diffuse and does not correspond with the sensory segmental innervation of the skin (dermatomes).

Chapter Summary
- Introduction
- Definition of a sclerotome
- Orthodox concept of limb anatomy
- A new unorthodox concept of limb anatomy
- The sclerotome maps
- The laws of neurology applied to the sclerotomes: overlap of innervation between segments
- Sclerotome subtraction
- Conclusions
- References

Referred pain from skeletal structures

In a second study, Kellgren[6] mapped out approximate segmental areas of deep pain sensation referred from injection of interspinous vertebral ligaments, and also from other ligaments, tendons, cartilage and bone in the limbs. He was able to conclude that the pain is fully segmental in distribution when arising from the interspinous ligaments, intercostal spaces, and other structures situated deeply in the trunk and limb girdles. The pain was more local when arising from stimuli in the extremities, the joints, and the less deeply placed structures in the limbs and trunk.

Origin of the sclerotome maps

In the early 1940s, Inman and Saunders[1] of San Francisco investigated the distribution of referred pain from skeletal structures.

Saunders, an anatomist, made 160 observations on 26 volunteers during stimulation of ligaments and periosteum at different sites, by means of mechanical scratching and drilling or by chemical irritation or pressure from injections of weakly acid solutions or isotonic saline.

Inman, an orthopaedic surgeon, recorded the distribution of deep pain sensation in patients suffering from a wide variety of lesions affecting discrete sites in bony and ligamentous structures.

Inman and Saunders[1] found the periosteum to be most sensitive, followed in order by ligaments, joint capsules, tendons, fascia, and, lastly, least sensitive, the muscles. Ligaments and joint capsules were particularly sensitive near their insertions into bone.

In the experimental series, the deep referred pain that radiated from the site of stimulus had five characteristics:

1. It was constant in character, whatever the stimulus, whether physical or chemical. It was often delayed in onset.
2. It was continuous from the local site of injury along a zone of proximal and/or distal radiation.
3. Stimulus of the same anatomical structure always resulted in radiation of pain along the same path and in the same direction.
4. The extent of the pain radiation varied with the intensity of the stimulus. The greater the stimulus, the more extensive the radiation.
5. Pain could radiate either proximally or distally from the point of stimulation, and on occasion persisted for several days, even when the experimental injury was small.

When the experimental and clinical observations were compared, the areas to which pain radiated from a particular site of stimulus 'were found to correspond with surprising regularity' in all instances. Inman and Saunders[1] concluded that the distribution of referred pain from skeletal structures was definitely segmental in character, and that, although approximately similar, this segmental distribution did not correspond exactly with dermatomes of the skin. They designated these segmental areas of skeletal innervation as 'sclerotomes', analogous to the dermatomes and myotomes.

Definition of a sclerotome

A sclerotome was defined as a continuous band of skeletal elements extending from the spine towards the periphery, supplied by one spinal segmental sensory nerve.[1]

The dermatomes are areas of skin supplied by spinal segmental sensory nerves. Their layout is somewhat different – more like a patchwork. They are discontinuous, arranged about the pre- and post-axial lines of the limbs. Each dermatome overlies only a portion of the sclerotome with which it shares its segmental nerve supply.

Inman and Saunders combined their experimental and clinical data, and examined its correspondence with known neuro-segmental anatomy.[4-8] They constructed 'sclerotome maps' of the skeleton, stressing that the sclerotomes as depicted were approximate rather than exact, for several reasons:

1. The maps are two-dimensional representations of three-dimensional structures.
2. Each borderline is approximate, since there is up to one segment of overlap between the territories of adjacent nerves.
3. As can be seen in the maps, variations are possible between anterior and posterior aspects of a limb.
4. Natural variations can occur between right and left sides of the same individual.
5. Natural variations can occur between different individuals.

Orthodox concept of limb anatomy

The accepted concept of the limb skeleton is that each bone is one anatomical unit. The limb is a series of such units hinged together by transverse joints. The arm is described by the shoulder girdle, shoulder joint, humerus, elbow joint, radius and ulna, wrist, and the bones and joints of the hand. The leg is described by its obvious transverse articulations: pelvis, hip joint, femur, knee, tibia and fibula, ankle, and the small bones and joints of the foot.

A new unorthodox concept of limb anatomy

The sclerotomes offer a new way of thinking about limb anatomy and pathology, based upon segmental nerve supply, and indeed based upon their embryogenesis.

Instead of one bone being the unit, one sclerotome is the unit – a segmental neuroanatomical unit. Normal development meshes several adjacent sclerotomes together to achieve the shape and size of the normal skeleton.

This radical reorientation is difficult to envisage for two reasons. First, normal sclerotomes are invisible. Secondly, upright human posture distracts from the fact that neural segments are actually a horizontal series, whereas they appear to be perpendicular in the vertical limbs. Neural segments extend away from the spine at 90° to the midline of the body. Because of elongation of the limbs during evolution, they hang down parallel with the midline. The shoulder and the hip are the sites of a 90° turn downwards.

This disorientation can be corrected by positioning arms and legs horizontally, in the rather ungainly pose shown in Figure 21.1. This places the human dermatomes (segmental sensory innervation of skin) in a stack of serial spinal segmental units.

Instead of dividing the limbs transversely though the joints, we can now divide the limbs longitudinally, along their long axes. In so doing, we ignore the joints, slicing across them as they fall into the path of the horizontal section. Each section relates to a spinal neural segment and is a segmental dermatome. The whole body is a stack of horizontal slices, resembling a stack of pancakes. It is a reminder that our basic anatomical structure evolved from primitive vertebrates, all of which

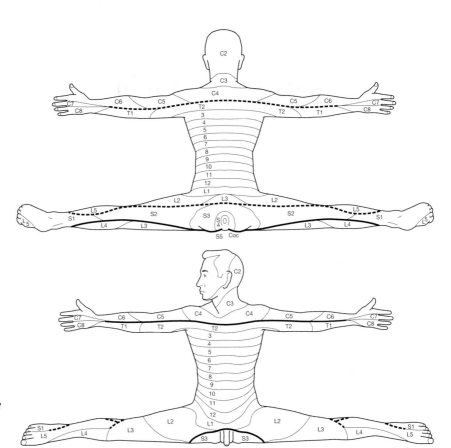

Figure 21.1 *Dermatomes of the body arranged to show the serial neural segments from which they are derived. The horizontal order shown in this posture is obscured when the man stands upright and the dermatomes fall into apparent disarray. Beneath each dermatome is the corresponding sclerotome of the skeleton, with the same segmental level of sensory nerve supply as its dermatome.*

were developed as a series of interlocking spinal neural segments from the central neuraxis of brain and spinal cord. This basic and ancient segmental arrangement is obvious in other vertebrates and also in some invertebrates, but is more obscure in ourselves.

The sclerotome maps

Figures 21.2 and 21.3 show the sclerotome maps of the upper and lower limbs respectively. They are repeated in colour, on the front and back endpapers of this book.

From the diagram of the horizontal dermatomes, one can imagine that, deep to the dermatomes, the sclerotomes of the skeleton are now arranged in their own stack of horizontal segments, each supplied by one spinal segmental sensory nerve. According to Inman and Saunders,[1] each sclerotome extends as a continuous anatomical unit from the spinal neuraxis towards the periphery. It crosses the joints in its path, irrespective of the outlines of individual bones and joints. The sclerotomes are not disconnected from the spinal neuraxis as the dermatomes are. Thus the sclerotomes would form a neater stack of parallel neural segments than do the discontinuous dermatomes.

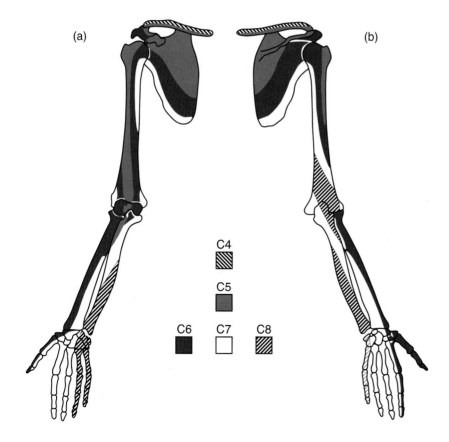

(a)

(b)

C4

C5

C6   C7   C8

Figure 21.2 *Upper limb sclerotomes: (a) anterior view; (b) posterior view. C, cervical innervation.*

Figure 21.3 *Lower limb sclerotomes: (a) anterior view; (b) posterior view. L, lumbar innervation; S, sacral innervation.*

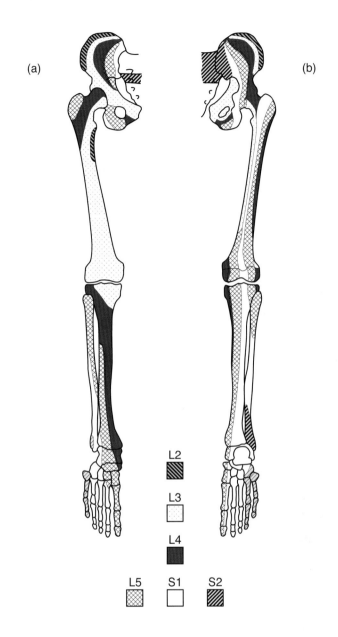

(a)   (b)

L2
L3
L4
L5   S1   S2

The laws of neurology applied to the sclerotomes: overlap of innervation between segments

Overlap between adjacent segments of innervation is well recognized as far as the dermatomes and myotomes are concerned, and is implicit in the sclerotome maps. Stilwell (1956) documented a one-segment overlap of nerve supply of primate bones. More is known about dermatomes than sclerotomes, although both are part of segmental nerve supply. Skin innervation is easier to study, but the principles of spinal segmentation of the peripheral nervous system are common to both, and basic data derived from dermatomes can be applied to the sclerotomes.

From classical neurology, we know that adjacent dermatomes overlap one another, and that they mesh in the skin by sharing innervation of their border territories with their neighbours. The area of shared innervation is considerable – about half the width of a dermatome, as shown in Figure 21.4. This diagram demonstrates that despite the interpolation of plexuses among the main nerve trunks, the segmental nerves remain true to their distal target tissues. It also shows that the central of three dermatomes is supplied by all three nerves, whereas the lateral margins of the structure are supplied by only one nerve. This makes the lateral dermatomes more vulnerable than the central one, in that they have no alternative source of innervation should their single nerve supply fail. In the hand, for instance, if one envisages overlap between C6, C7 and C8 of about one segment then it becomes apparent that parts of the sclerotomes on the margins of the hand have single innervation, while C7, in the middle, has threefold innervation (C6, C7 and C8). This must render the marginal sclerotomes more vulnerable to nerve injury than the central one.

Triple innervation gives that central zone a superlative failsafe device in the event of neurotoxic damage. For this reason, one could

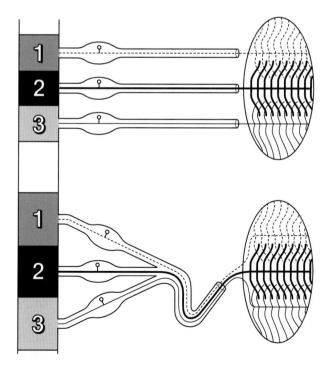

Figure 21.4 *Normal overlap of spinal segmental innervation. Neighbourly support strengthens centre of hand and foot by multiple nerve supply. Margins, with single nerve supply, are more vulnerable than centre.*

argue that the least well-innervated sclerotomes fail first; sclerotomes with greatest supportive innervation should be the most stable, and the last to fail. In Figure 21.2, the hand is supplied by three sclerotomes: cervical 6, 7 and 8. According to the above reasoning, the middle third of the hand is supplied by all three nerves, making it a more stable, less vulnerable structure than the sides of the hand. This would support the interpretation of a hockey-stick or boomerang bone in the arm as a conglomerate of C7 fragments of humerus, radius and ulna, with two or three central fingers remaining.

The foot is also supplied by three sclerotomes: lumbar 5 and sacral 1 and 2 (Figure 21.3). Abnormality of the great toe (L5) is unusual, but loss of the one or two lateral toes (S2) are more frequent than reductions in the central toes. The latter could gain stability from their triple innervation from all three nerves.

Like the dermatomes in Figure 21.4, the sclerotomes are normally inseparable from one another, welded together by the physiological overlap of innervation between adjacent segments. This overlap of innervation provides a powerful locking device. As we have seen in Chapter 20, the infiltration of nerve fibres into shared territories causes a tangle of fibrils that defy dissection. It is impossible to prize the sclerotomes apart by surgical means, even with a hammer and chisel! But it is possible to take them apart *chemically*, with a sensory neurotoxin such as thalidomide. And they are rendered visible in certain *neurological diseases*, such as neurofibromatosis and melorheostosis. The advantage of overlapped nerve supply is that it provides an unseen insurance against injury, because multiple sources of nerve supply provide a relatively strong, fail-safe defence.

One of the qualifications laid down by Inman and Saunders[1] was that the lines drawn upon the bones are not, in fact, exact borders between two sclerotomes, but the approximate midlines of the physiological zone of transition between the overlapping borders. At the borderlines as drawn in the sclerotome maps, the nerve supply overflows each way from one sclerotome to the next, which practically ensures that variability is the rule rather than the exception when sclerotomes are involved in disease. The maps were intended as a general clinical guide to segmental sensory innervation of the skeleton. They were not intended for rigid application, which would be inappropriate in view of the biological variability of the system that they depict. The natural variations inherent in the sclerotome maps must be constantly kept in mind during their application to any anatomical or neurological problem.

Sclerotome subtraction

Whole-segment injury with ablation of sclerotome

Let us suppose that the sclerotomes can be 'unlocked' from one another, and that one of these morphological units may be affected by toxin or disease, while its neighbours remain normal. Subtraction of a whole sclerotome can be imagined by lifting one band out of the maps. Removal of the black sclerotome (C6) from the map of the arm (Figure 21.2) results in removal of radius and thumb. In Figure 21.3, removal of the black (L4) sclerotome results in tibial aplasia. These were the most common malformations in thalidomide embryopathy.

The separation of one sclerotome from its neighbours will demonstrate the segmental nerve supply of that unit. But some residual variation or irregularity of the final outline will probably persist to mark the site of separation, because of the zone of overlap with its neighbour, with attempted retrieval of tissue in the zone of overlapping supply.

Partial or multiple segments involved

Sometimes, the missing segment is longitudinal, but does not neatly fit one sclerotome, or it has two possible interpretations, or is more complex than one sclerotome. Such cases are variations of the standard sclerotome pattern as defined in the maps, equivalent to standard deviations around an anatomical mean. There are numerous possible explanations. In reading the sclerotomes against actual malformations, the inherent variability of the sclerotomes must be respected. Some defects fit neatly into the outlines as defined on the maps. Others deviate in some respects, and this deviation must be allowed, in order to keep in focus the confluent process of the underlying pathology. This point cannot be emphasized too strongly, if the pitfalls that obscure the truth are to be avoided. A rigid application of the given maps is ridiculous neurologically, because, according to their authors, the maps are only approximate at best.

The sclerotomes are more plausible as a biological concept because of the presence of variations, rather than the reverse.

Variables inherent in the neural crest

Furthermore, as described in Chapters 12 and 13, the neural crest in the embryo is a continuous ribbon of tissue that is progressively maturing within its length, and in which a wave of sensitivity and vulnerability passes unseen from head to tail. Early neural crest injury is unlikely to be contained by the individual segmental ganglia that emerge some days later. Injury is likely to flow into more than one presumptive segment of developing crest.

Thus several common phenomena, such as partial or incomplete sclerotome loss, and overflow onto adjacent sclerotomes, are part of the disease, and are acceptable variants of sclerotome subtraction.

The third dimension of nerve supply

Inherent in the two-dimensional sclerotome maps are neuroanatomical variables, including the interplay of different sclerotomes in the third dimension. For instance, sensory innervation of the dorsal and palmar surfaces of the skeleton of the hand do not exactly coincide (see the upper limb sclerotome maps in Figure 21.2). The thumb and index finger are supplied by the 6th and 7th cervical nerves. This provides an opportunity for dominance of one segmental nerve over the other in the formation of thumb, index and ring fingers. The interface may be oblique or even spiral. At what depth in the bone does the sclerotomal slice interface with its neighbour or competitor? Is there inherent dominance of any particular sclerotome? We do not know, but there seem to be permutations and combinations of possible sclerotomal patterns inherent in the differences between anterior and posterior surfaces of the limbs.

Left versus right in one individual

Normal variations exist between the left and right sides of the body. Few of us are strictly symmetrical. The position of the eyes and the shapes of the ears, fingers and toes are not uncommonly different in the two sides of an individual. These are normal variants.

Individual differences within a group

Normal variations exist between individuals within a group. These limited individual traits may also exist normally within the sclerotomes.

Central versus peripheral site of injury

Another source of variation is the neurological phenomenon, mapped by Kellgren,[6] that the more central (relative to the trunk) the stimulus, the more complete the zone of pain radiation. The more peripheral the site of stimulus, the more distal and the smaller the area of pain. Depending on the age of the embryo, and the site of the insult within its nervous system, so there may be variations in the ultimate deformities. This may be one explanation of different deformities within one sclerotome. For instance, a central insult to the 6th cervical sclerotome may cause it to fail throughout its whole extent, with hypoplastic scapula and humerus, and absent radius and thumb. A peripheral insult to C6 might result in absent or triphalangeal thumb. These could be examples in the embryo of that same neurological principle.

Differential vulnerability

The distribution of defects in thalidomide embryopathy may be compared and contrasted with the distribution of symptoms in thalidomide or other sensory neuropathy in adults. Both are frequently distal and symmetrical. The embryo, however, displays a segmental modification of distal distribution that is not evident in the adult.

Regulation or self-repair in the embryo

As already discussed, this inherent ability of the embryo will always tend to diminish and modify the final result. Regulation is a well-recognized fact of embryology – repair counterbalancing inflicted damage.

Conclusions

1. A spinal-segmental arrangement underlies the sensory innervation of the skeleton.
2. Sclerotome maps show the approximate sensory segmental nerve supply to skeletal structures.
3. Sclerotomes underlie their associated dermatomes and myotomes, but extend beyond them.
4. The sclerotomes obey the laws of neuroanatomy, neurophysiology, neurology and neurotoxicology.
5. They also allow expression of the laws of embryology and of neural crest anatomy and physiology.
6. Normally invisible, they can be rendered visible by disease.

References

1. Inman VT, Saunders JB de C. Referred pain from skeletal structures. *J Nerv Ment Dis* 1944; **99**: 660–7.

2. Gardner ED. The innervation of the knee joint. *Anat Rec* 1948; **101**: 109–30.

3. Skoglund S. Anatomical and physiological studies of knee joint innervation in the cat. *Acta Physiol Scand* 1956; **124**(Suppl): 36.

4. Lewis T. Suggestions relating to the study of somatic pain. *BMJ* 1938: **i**: 321–5.

5. Lewis T. *Pain*. New York: Macmillan, 1942.

6. Kellgren JH. On the distribution of pain arising from deep somatic structures with charts of segmental pain areas. *Clin Sci* 1939; **4**: 35–46.

7. Head H. *Studies in Neurology*, Vol 1. Oxford: Oxford University Press, 1920: 133–8.

8. Foerster O. The dermatomes in man. *Brain* 1933; **56**: 1–39.

CHAPTER 22

Sclerotome aplasia/subtraction

'To think is to speculate with images.'
Giordano Bruno (1548–1600)

Introduction

The sclerotome maps of Inman and Saunders are images that lend themselves to speculation. We can propose that the maps are the blueprint for limb morphogenesis. We can imagine that sclerotomes can be subtracted, divided, added or multiplied. We can speculate on what the final limbs would look like after such manipulations, which, as we have seen, can operate through the mechanism of segmental neural crest injury.[1–5]

The aim of this chapter is to explore the effect of theoretical subtraction of sclerotomes from the maps.

Theoretical sclerotome subtraction or aplasia

If one sclerotome is theoretically removed from the maps, it is like lifting one piece out of a jigsaw puzzle. If one sclerotome in the embryo fails to form, a gap is theoretically left in the skeleton. It is said that 'Nature abhors a vacuum'. This seems to be true of normal embryogenesis. The remaining sclerotomes do tend to coalesce to fill the gap. The embryo is known to have very considerable powers of self-repair, termed 'regulation'. We have already seen evidence that the neural crest is particularly efficient in repairing itself. According to Malcolm Johnston (personal communication), it is hard to inflict a permanent surgical wound upon the neural crest, because crest cells surrounding the excision tumble into the hole and tend to heal it, which is one of the many difficulties encountered when working with the neural crest in the laboratory. It is one reason why the experimenter must establish the range of damage actually achieved, as opposed to what was aimed to be achieved. These may be two very different things. It requires an extra segment of the study to harvest and examine embryos soon after the surgery. Unless the actual damage is recorded,

Chapter Summary

- Introduction
- Theoretical sclerotome subtraction or aplasia
- Theoretical sclerotome aplasia in the upper limbs
- Theoretical sclerotome aplasia in the lower limbs
- Conclusion
- References

the interpretation of results and the conclusions drawn may be completely wrong.

Because of regulation or self-healing in the embryo in general and the neural crest in particular, the sclerotomes adjacent to the absent one should theoretically tend to unite across the gap so that no cavity results in the limb skeleton. However, the total mass of skeletal tissue will be less than normal, and therefore some reduction must occur in the size of the affected bones, and the size of the limb itself. This loss of mass will be located in the area supplied by the damaged nerve.

The final reduction in size will depend upon:

(1) whether a whole sclerotome, or part of a sclerotome, or more than one sclerotome, has been eliminated; and/or
(2) modification by regulation, which means that the subtraction may not be exactly according to the maps.

Theoretical sclerotome aplasia in the upper limbs

As we have seen in Chapter 9, the commonest upper limb deficiency in thalidomide embryopathy was radial dysplasia, almost always associated with absent or deficient thumb. Because of the frequency of radial dysplasia (Chapters 7–9), and because of the possible connection between radial reduction and the 6th cervical dermatome (see Figure 7.16), the 6th cervical sclerotome was studied first.

Subtraction of the 6th cervical sclerotome (Figures 22.1 and 22.2)

Let us suppose that the C6 sensory nerve in the embryo suffers an injury, and that the 6th cervical sclerotome fails to form. The effect of this on limb morphology may be estimated by subtracting the C6 sclerotome from the map of the upper limb (see Figure 21.2 or endplates).

The *clavicle* is supplied by C4 and C5, and is therefore unaffected by loss of C6. The *scapula*, on the other hand, depends on C6 for most of the blade below the spine, except for the lateral edge, which is contributed by C7. The major portion of the *glenoid cavity* is contributed by C6. Therefore, absence of C6 should cause approximation of the C5 and C7 elements, resulting in a slender hypoplastic triangle of scapula with absent or small glenoid and a relatively large spinous process, acromion and coracoid process.

The sclerotomes C6 and C5 contribute to the *humerus* in diagonal strips. Most of the *dome* of the humeral head falls within the C6 sclerotome, so its subtraction would cause a junction of C5 and C7 elements, with loss or reduction of the humeral head epiphysis, and a smaller, more horizontal upper end. Loss of C6 from the *shaft* must diminish the bone mass of the shaft. This could be accommodated in one of three ways:

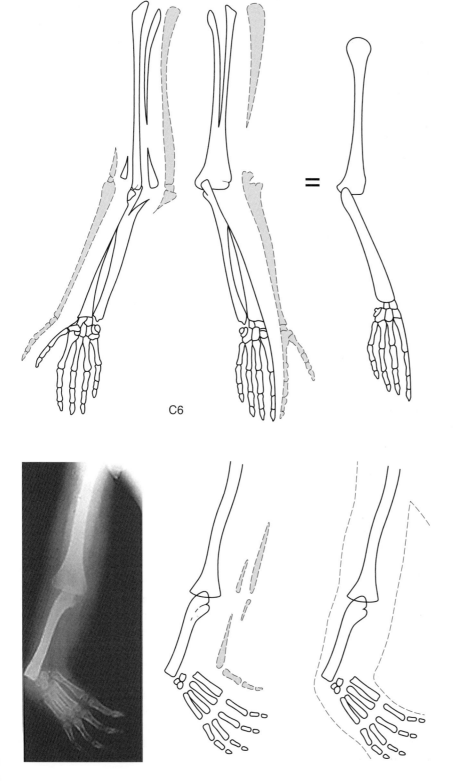

Figure 22.1 *Theoretical subtraction of C6 sclerotome reduces thumb, carpals, radius, and humerus (scapula not shown).*

C6

Figure 22.2 *Subtraction of distal part of C6 sclerotome explains radial aplasia and absent thumb.*

- as a reduction in length, resulting in a shorter bone of normal width
- as a reduction in width, leaving a slender bone of normal length or
- as a combination of these two possibilities

At the *distal end* of the humerus, the trochlea and capitulum should be absent. But the epicondyles (supplied by C7) and the posterior surface bearing the olecranon fossa (supplied by C8) would remain, causing a flat, flared distal end to the slender or short shaft, with lack of modelling of the elbow joint surface.

The C6 component of the *ulna* is the coronoid process and the radial side of the upper third posteriorly. Otherwise the ulna is a C7,8 derivative. Thus, the only effect of C6 subtraction on the ulna itself would be hypoplasia or absence of the coronoid process and the radial side of the olecranon. The trochlear notch of the elbow joint would be shallower than normal.

The shaft of the *radius* is largely within the C6 sclerotome proximally, and is shared with the C7 sclerotome distally. Loss of the C6 sclerotome would result in loss of more than half of the mass of the radius, especially at its proximal end. This would result in one or more of the following:

- shortened length and/or
- narrowed width
- absence of the proximal end with a free fragment at the distal end
- fusion of the distal radius to the distal ulna

The *thumb and index finger* are partly in the C6 sclerotome and partly in the C7 sclerotome, depending upon whether the maps are read from the front or the back of the hand. Loss of C6 could cause either absent or vestigial *thumb*, any residual part being a slender longitudinal fraction supplied by C7. Reading the sclerotomes of the hand from the dorsal side, loss of C6 might also subtract a small, longitudinal component from the *index finger*, rendering it slender and hypoplastic, but leaving a longitudinal fraction of each bone. The variants of the C6/C7 sclerotomes thus allow a longitudinal bisection of thumb or index finger. The *other fingers* should be unaffected.

In the hand, a number of variants are acceptable as part of a C6 sclerotome disorder. These include triphalangeal thumb, vestigial thumb, absent thumb, duplication of the thumb or its parts, hypoplasia or hemiplasia of the index finger, and duplication or absence of the index finger. All these indicate a disorganization of growth within C6 sclerotome, be it aplasia, hypoplasia, dysplasia or hyperplasia, and will be discussed in Chapter 27.

Subtraction of the 5th cervical sclerotome

The 5th cervical sclerotome includes a significant amount of the upper humerus, including the greater tuberosity and a band throughout the length of the humeral shaft.

The humerus can be construed as a simple rectangle, bisected diagonally by the junction of the 6th and 7th cervical sclerotomes. The 5th and 6th cervical sclerotomes comprise the upper triangle of the humeral shaft: an inverted triangle of bone with its base at the shoulder joint and its apex just distal to the elbow joint, where it supplies the anterior surface of the elbow, including a small portion of the proximal radius and ulna. Loss of the *apex* of the 5th cervical sclerotome results in proximal radio-ulnar synostosis, or failure of normal embryonic separation of radius and ulna (Figure 22.3). Loss of the *whole* of C5 subtracts the upper triangular C5 portion of the humerus and leaves a distal oblique triangle. By removing the C5 and C6 components, what remains of the humerus is composed of C7 and C8 sclerotomes. Figures 22.4 and 22.5 show progressive reduction of bones, because of increasing sclerotome subtraction.

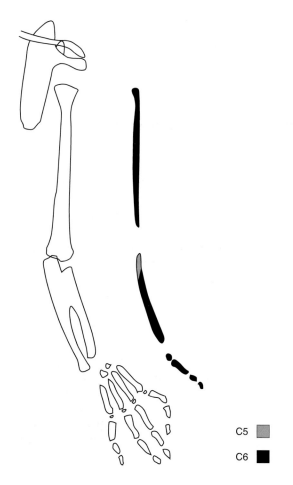

C5 ▢

C6 ■

Figure 22.3 *Proximal radio-ulnar synostosis indicates subtraction of the distal tip of C5 as well as C6.*

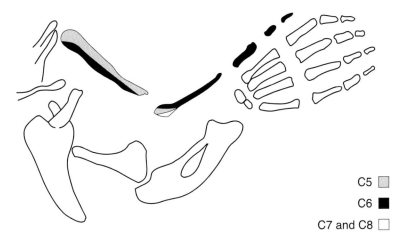

Figure 22.4 *Humeral C7/8 triangle based at the elbow after subtraction of C5 and 6. Radio-ulnar synostosis again. More of C5 is subtracted than in Figure 22.3. Residual skeleton is C7 and C8.*

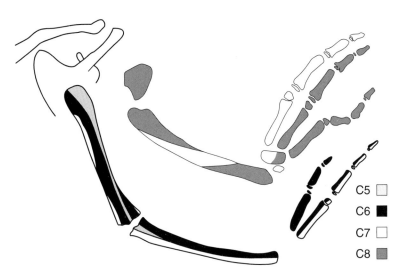

Figure 22.5 *Subtraction of all of C5 and C6, and part of C7. Moderately severe phocomelia is due to loss of all but C8 sclerotome in the distal humerus.*

Thus upper limb phocomelia is aplasia of the C5 and C6 sclerotomes as a result of C5/6 neural crest injury.

Subtraction of the 5th cervical sclerotome is a powerful way of producing upper limb phocomelia. Its disappearance always comes after, not before, loss of the 6th cervical sclerotome in thalidomide embryopathy, which means that both C5 and C6 are subtracted. From then on, in the sequence of skeletal loss, the upper limb is phocomelic in increasing degree (Figure 22.6).

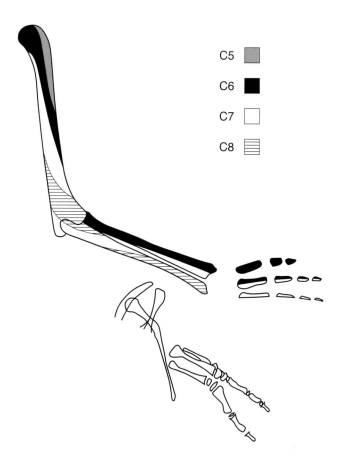

C5 ▣

C6 ■

C7 ☐

C8 ☰

Figure 22.6 *Gross phocomelia: subtraction of almost all of cervical sclerotomes 5, 6, and 7. Residual skeleton is the distal C8 sclerotome.*

Subtraction of the 7th and 8th cervical sclerotomes

Loss of part, or all, of the 7th cervical sclerotome reduces the arm still more, leaving the 8th cervical components of the humerus, ulna and ulnar digits attached to the hypoplastic shoulder girdle. Finally the 8th cervical sclerotome fails as well, and amelia results.

Theoretical sclerotome aplasia in the lower limbs

From the lower limb sclerotome maps (Figure 21.3), it can be seen that the lumbar and sacral sclerotomes curve forward in concentric bands across the pelvis, and then descend more or less vertically down the femur. During their course down the tibia and fibula towards the foot, there is evidence of a medial twist to the L3, L4 and L5 sclerotomes. As a result, sclerotomes that commenced on the lateral aspect of the hip and femur finish up on the medial side of the ankle and foot, rather like the twisted stripes on a bar of candy. This reflects the normal rotation of the lower limb in the embryo, whereby the hallux at first lies uppermost, above the other toes, but rotates medially as the leg lengthens. It follows that the sensory nerves supplying the sclerotomes exist before the lower limb elongates and rotates.

The 2nd lumbar sclerotome (L2) includes part of the sacro-iliac and iliac crest region and symphysis pubis, plus a small strip of bone on the upper medial femoral shaft. There it peters out.

Subtraction of 4th and 5th lumbar sclerotomes from the femur

Let us suppose that the 4th lumbar sclerotome is absent from the pelvis and upper femur, as shown in Figure 22.7. This would reduce the mass of the ilium, the lower margin of the pubis and the descending pubic ramus. It would reduce the depth of the acetabulum. In the thigh, L4 is the major contributor to the femoral head and neck and the upper third of the femoral shaft. L4 is a minor contributor to the femoral condyles at the knee. Aplasia of the L4 sclerotome would result in severe hypoplasia of the hip joint and the head, neck and upper shaft of the femur.

The 3rd lumbar sclerotome (L3) is very important. It comprises a continuous band of bone in the pelvis, one quadrant of femoral head, a narrow isthmus of femoral neck, a long triangular fragment of

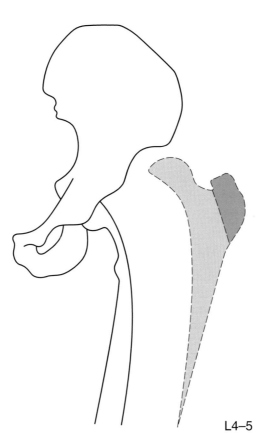

Figure 22.7 *Proximal femoral focal dysplasia (PFFD): residual femur is L3 sclerotome, plus the sacral sclerotomes, after subtraction of L4 and L5 from the head, neck and upper shaft.*

L4–5

anterior femoral shaft plus knee joint and patella, and a short tri-angular section of proximal tibia. The L3 sclerotome ends on the medial side of the upper tibia, and the muscles attached to it are mainly those of the anterior aspect of the thigh, i.e. the quadriceps, including the patellar ligament. The residual triangle of proximal tibia signals that the 3rd lumbar sclerotome is still present.

Subtraction of 4th lumbar sclerotome from tibia

The 4th lumbar sclerotome (L4) is a major contributor to the ilium, pubis and ischium, and to the acetabulum. L4 is also the major component of the femoral head and neck, whence it continues down the lateral side of the femoral shaft, including the lateral ligament of the knee joint. The L4 sclerotome then swings across the anterior aspect of the mid-tibia to the medial side of the ankle joint, thus including most of the tibial shaft. It ends on the talus and navicula.

Subtraction of L4 removes the band of skeletal elements supplied by L4 (Figures 22.8 and 22.9).

The 5th lumbar sclerotome (L5) is more posterolateral than L4. It comprises the greater trochanter, two bands of posterior femoral shaft, and sections of posterior and anterior tibial and fibular shafts. It incorporates most of the tibial mortise of the ankle joint. L5 extends on to the medial side of the foot to include the medial tarsal bones, the first metatarsal, and the hallux dorsally. Reading from the plantar surface, the bones of the 1st ray are shared with S1.

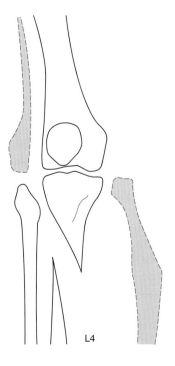

L4

Figure 22.8 *Tibial aplasia: theoretical injury to 4th lumbar nerve with loss of L4 sclerotome.*

Figure 22.9 *Another case of absent tibia after loss of distal L4 sclerotome. Note that the foot is intact, as it is supplied by L5 and the sacral sclerotomes.*

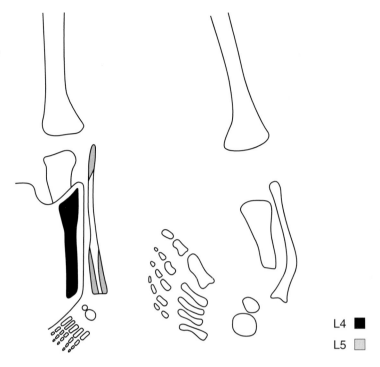

L4 ■
L5 ▨

Subtraction of 5th lumbar sclerotome in the foot

The only sclerotomes to reach the foot are L5, and sacral 1 and sacral 2 (S1 and S2). Figure 22.10 illustrates subtraction of the L5 sclerotome from the foot.

The sacral sclerotomes are best read on the posterior view. They are thin bands of bone on the femur posteriorly. L5 supplies the femoral condyles, and S1 supplies the intercondylar notch. L5, S1 and S2 between them supply the fibula. Distally, the sacral sclerotomes twist anteromedially to include the distal tibia and foot.

S1 supplies the posterior surface of the tibia, including the ankle joint, and encompasses the talus, calcaneum and associated central tarsals. The same segment includes the central rays of the foot: digits 2 and 3. S1 shares the hallux with L5, and the 4th ray with S2.

The 2nd sacral nerve (S2) supplies the lateral malleolus and the 5th ray of the foot. It shares the 4th ray with S1.

Aplasia of the L4 sclerotome may involve loss of part or all of the great toe, indicating subtraction of the distal part of L5. Involvement of more than one sclerotome was not uncommon: for example L4 plus the distal part of L5; or C6 plus the distal part of C5. It has to be remembered that in the embryo at that stage, the adjacent spinal ganglia and their segmental nerves are evolving in serial sequence from head to foot in rapid succession, and it is to be expected that adjacent levels might be clipped by the same toxic assault.

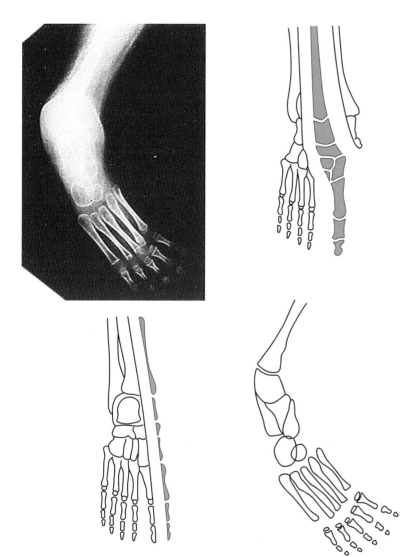

Figure 22.10 *Reduction in L5 sclerotome in the foot reduces the tibia and hallux but leaves the sacral sclerotomes intact.*
Top left: Radiograph of a thalidomide-affected foot with longitudinal reduction of the first ray.
Bottom left: Plantar aspect of L5, bisecting the first ray.
Bottom right: Subtraction of L5 from the foot. The theory explains the radiograph.
Top right: Sclerotome map of foot, with L5 shaded on the dorsal aspect. Another variant of L5 loss is a foot of four rays.

Just as pain distribution within a dermatome reveals disease involving that particular segmental sensory nerve, so a sclerotomal distribution of disease logically indicates a disease process involving the segmental sensory nerve belonging to that sclerotome. Intervertebral disc compression of a dorsal root ganglion is one example. Herpes zoster is another, where pain and the red vesicular skin eruption are located in the dermatome belonging to the infected ganglion.

Sclerotome aplasia or subtraction is a similar expression of sensory neuropathy in a segmental nerve distribution.

Conclusion

1. Correlation exists between theoretical sclerotome subtractions and the dysmorphology of the limbs in thalidomide embryopathy.
2. Sclerotome subtraction/aplasia is the only method available for interpretation of this dysmorphology.
3. It follows that the underlying pathology is situated within the sensory peripheral nervous system.

References

1. McCredie J. Segmental embryonic peripheral neuropathy. *Pediatr Radiol* 1975; **3**: 162–8.

2. McCredie J. Mechanism of the teratogenic effect of thalidomide. *Med Hypotheses* 1976; **2**: 63–9.

3. McCredie J. Sclerotome subtraction: a radiological interpretation of reduction deformities of the limbs. *Birth Defects: Original Article Series* 1977; **13** (3D): 65–77.

4. McCredie J. Thalidomide and the neural crest. In: Merker HJ, Nau H, Neubert D, eds. *Teratology of the Limbs. 4th symposium on prenatal development.* Berlin: W de Gruyter, 1980: 431–448.

5. McCredie J, Loewenthal J. Pathogenesis of congenital malformations: an hypothesis. *Am J Surg* 1978; **135**: 293–7.

CHAPTER 23

Sclerotome aplasia/subtraction in 203 cases

'One can only show how one came to hold whatever opinion one does hold.'
Virginia Woolf, in *A Room of One's Own*

Background

Twenty cases was an insufficient number for adequate evaluation of the method of sclerotome subtraction. Even within the first five Australian cases, it was apparent that the sclerotomes fitted some deformities like the proverbial glove, but an occasional case was difficult, or did not fit neatly.

The thalidomide disaster had struck West Germany hardest, and several large collections of cases there had been analysed from different viewpoints. Only one study examined the anatomy in search of a logical explanation of the pattern of the malformations. In 1969, two orthopaedic surgeons, Drs Hans-Lothar Henkel and Hans-Georg Willert,[1] published a study of 287 cases of thalidomide origin, in which they sought to define the pattern of the disease. When arranged in order of severity, the deformities formed 'a teratological sequence, linked by a common morphological pattern'. They recognized a longitudinal axis of malformation in each limb, but they were unable at that time to suggest what the basis for such longitudinal bands of tissue might be.

This was the only paper in the world literature that treated the anatomical defects in the skeleton as a continuous process rather than as a number of different and unrelated malformations. It is a landmark paper in the field of birth defects, equal in significance to the work of Lenz[2] and Nowack[3] in establishing the aetiology and the sensitive period. The Henkel and Willert[1] paper established the facts of exactly what thalidomide did to the human skeleton, i.e. the anatomical pattern of the malformations.

Their paper was adopted by the International Committee for Prosthetics and Orthotics in 1975 as the basis for a new system of classification and terminology for longitudinal reduction deformities.[4,5]

Chapter Summary
- Background
- Introduction
- Patients and methods
- Results
- Discussion
- References

On the other hand, examination of the Science Citation Index[6] since 1969 reveals the curious fact that no-one working in teratology except my group has cited or attempted to explain the pattern that Henkel and Willert[1] revealed, despite the sobriquet of 'limb patterning experts' adopted by some who claim to be investigating thalidomide's mode of action. Yet it is essential to understand the pattern of disease before one attempts to explain its pathology or pathogenesis. Perhaps this indicates how far experimental teratology has drifted away from clinical medicine and the malformed baby.

By great good fortune, thanks to Professor Sir Howard Middlemiss and Dr Ronald Murray in the UK, both Professor Willert and I had been made members of the International Skeletal Society, where we met in 1985. Professor Willert was then Professor and Head of the Department of Orthopaedic Surgery in Göttingen. He still had in his possession the X-ray films of the large series of thalidomide children on which he and Henkel had established the pattern of dysmelia in 1969. The collaborative study[7] reported here was done in the course of several short trips to Göttingen, testing my method of sclerotome subtraction in his material – a large collection of radiographs of German thalidomide children.

This chapter and the next are based upon our paper, published as the leading article in the *Journal of Bone and Joint Surgery, British Issue* of January 1999,[7] and illustrated with diagrams from his book, with permission. This study, together with the paper of 1969, explains the skeletal dysmorphology of thalidomide embryopathy.

Introduction

Most human limb deficiencies, whether sporadic or hereditary, have a wide range of dysmorphism. Because they are rare, individual cases of these malformations have been regarded as curiosities rather than as part of a biological spectrum. It was not until the thalidomide disaster that the underlying patterns were recognized.[8,9] Even so, the great variety of dysmorphology in early thalidomide children led to the belief that the distribution of these malformations was random.[10]

The large number of cases collected at that time has provided valuable material for analysis of the pattern underlying the malformations, and for determining how thalidomide worked. In a study of the nature, aetiology and pathology of what was named 'dysmelia', Willert and Henkel[1,8,9] arranged a series of 287 thalidomide cases in order of increasing severity of limb reduction.

Figures 23.1 and 23.2 summarize the pattern of malformations and the teratological sequences from the study by Henkel and Willert.[1] The defects were longitudinal, not transverse. They ranged from isolated peripheral hypoplasia to complete absence of the limb (amelia).

The sequential longitudinal reduction of the limb skeleton obeyed certain principles:

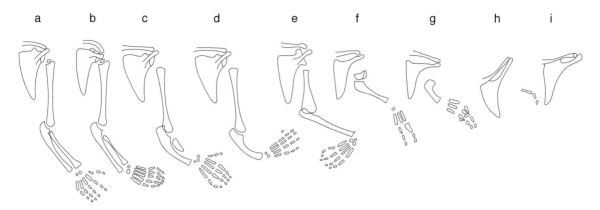

Figure 23.1 *Sequence of skeletal loss (a–i) in upper limb thalidomide defects. (From Henkel H-L, Willert H-G. J Bone Joint Surg Br 1969; **51B**: 399–414.[1])*

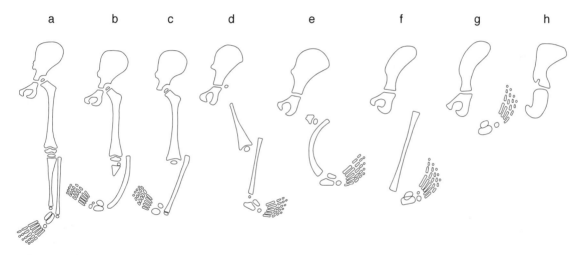

Figure 23.2 *Sequence of skeletal loss (a–h) in lower limb thalidomide defects. (From Henkel H-L, Willert H-G. J Bone Joint Surg Br 1969; **51B**: 399–414.[1])*

- Some bones as a whole, as well as defined areas within one bone, were more vulnerable than others.
- In each limb, the deficiencies occurred in a longitudinal axis of reduction.
- There was a clear interdependence between proximal and distal parts of the limb.

In thalidomide-induced dysmelia, the deficiencies were characteristically on the radial side of the upper limb and the tibial side of the lower. In the upper limb, there was progressive reduction in, and loss of, the bones of the thumb, radius and humerus, which preceded the reduction of the ulna or ulnar digits. In the lower limb, reduction began in the distal tibia or proximal femur, and affected the fibula and fibular digits last. Henkel and Willert[1] stressed that there was a common entity – an underlying pattern that had many different but related manifestations. Since the old method of classification tended to mask this, a simpler system was proposed and is now widely accepted as an international standard.[4,5]

The morphological pattern of longitudinal skeletal reduction requires explanation. The peripheral skeleton may be divided longitudinally based on the segmental sensory nerve supply of the bones and joints. This pattern of innervation has been the subject of much research since the end of the 19th century, culminating in the publication of the sclerotome maps by Inman and Saunders[11] in 1944 (see Chapter 21: Figures 21.2 and 21.3).

The sclerotomes are the counterparts of dermatomes and myotomes, and underlie but extend beyond the latter. Each sclerotome starts at the neuraxis and extends towards the periphery. Only the 6th, 7th and 8th cervical sclerotomes reach the hand; the 5th terminates in the forearm near the elbow. In the leg, only the 5th lumbar and the 1st and 2nd sacral sclerotomes reach the toes, while the 4th lumbar ends on the medial aspect of the tarsus, and the 3rd lumbar ends at the tibia below the medial side of the knee. Because of their longitudinal orientation, the sclerotomes cross joints and subdivide bones, including the pectoral and pelvic girdles, thus reorientating customary concepts of anatomy.

The sclerotomes are, like the dermatomes, normally invisible, but their presence should not be ignored. The vesicular eruption in herpes zoster, a viral infection of a segmental sensory nerve, renders an affected dermatome visible. Similarly, a sclerotome may be revealed by a disease of its nerve supply. I have suggested the concept of sclerotome subtraction for the radiological interpretation of reduction deformities of the limbs.[12,13]

We have compared the sclerotome maps with the pattern of dysmelia in a large series of cases of thalidomide-induced limb defects.[7] The skeletal deficiency in each limb was compared with the sclerotome map to determine whether or not the missing areas coincided with the sclerotomes. An attempt was made to judge if, or to what extent, these reduction defects could be interpreted by sclerotome subtraction.

We do not wish to discuss classification. The requirements for recording and labelling an individual case in a clinic differ from those needed to analyse a large series in search of a pattern of disease and a mechanism of pathogenesis.

Patients and methods

We analysed the records of 378 limbs from 203 children with thalidomide embryopathy, collected by Henkel and Willert.[1,8,9] All the infants were born between 1958 and 1962 and all had the typical signs of thalidomide embryopathy. There were cases from several centres in

Germany, and some from Oxford, UK. Radiographs, or tracings of radiographs, had been filed with the essential clinical data, including the name, date and place of birth, and the hospital attended.

We knew both the forenames and the surnames for 180 infants, but in 23 only the initials were available and their sex was unknown. In 9, the side of the malformation had not been recorded or marked on the radiograph or tracing.

In the 180 children in whom the sex was known, there were almost equal numbers of males and females (91:89).

Isolated defects of the upper limbs predominated, being present in 85% of children. Combinations of defects of the upper and lower limbs were seen in 12%, and isolated defects of the lower limb in 3%. The ratios of involvement of upper to lower to both upper and lower were 172:5:26.

Bilateral limb deficiencies were present in 90%, with a high degree of symmetry and within a limited range of morphology. Equal sex incidence, preponderance in the upper limb, and bilateral symmetry are features that have been noted in other series of thalidomide embryopathy.[2,14–21]

Henkel and Willert[1,10] used simple outline diagrams of the skeleton of the limb to record and analyse the anatomical features. Those bones or parts of bones that were missing from the radiographs were left out of the diagram. A working group of the International Society for Prosthetics and Orthotics[4,5] agreed on a system of classification based on the principles outlined by Henkel and Willert, and they advocated that the deficiencies should be named after the skeletal elements that were absent.[5] Swanson et al[22] had used a similar system, recording a condition on a silhouette drawing of the limb skeleton, with shading out of the absent parts after which the defect was named.

In our series of 203 cases, there were satisfactory radiographic records of 378 limbs. A line diagram of the skeleton was assigned to each of these and the missing parts were shaded out. The deficiencies in skeletal structure were compared with the sclerotome maps to determine whether the morphology of the malformations and the sclerotomes coincided.

We attempted to grade the quality of fit between the sclerotomes and the malformations using three grades:

Grade 1: The longitudinal defect clearly coincided with the sclerotome map.
Grade 2: The longitudinal defect had a less obvious or ambivalent match with the sclerotomes.
Grade 3: The longitudinal defect coincided poorly or not at all.

Results

There was congruence of the missing bones with all or part of the sclerotomes (grade 1) in over 73% of cases (Table 23.1). The match was less obvious in 15% (grade 2) and difficult in about 11% (grade 3). All had some evidence of sclerotome loss, even those with amelia.

A continuous pattern of deletion was seen in all malformations, which was termed the reduction tendency by Henkel and Willert.[1] Within a large series, this continuous, gradual process of reduction is a slope rather than a series of steps, illustrating a smooth progression from a minimal distal reduction to total absence of the limb. The process is a continuous gradient of skeletal reduction.

Figures 23.1 and 23.2 show that the greater part of the skeleton is still present from stages a to f, with sufficient bony landmarks to identify readily the affected sclerotome or sclerotomes. It becomes more difficult to discern particular sclerotomes after stage f, because the bony landmarks progressively disappear.

Sclerotomes are easily identified distally, where parallel digital rays and the paired bones of the forearm and lower leg provide obvious landmarks for establishing the identity of particular bones and bony remnants. Thus the sclerotome maps are easier to apply to the extremities than to the long bones in many cases. The paired forearm and lower leg bones follow the sclerotome disorders of the hand and foot, with minor variations. But difficulties arise in the humerus and femur posteriorly. Here the sclerotomes run in narrow parallel bands along the diaphyses, where anatomical landmarks are normally minimal. These facts make it difficult or sometimes impossible to distinguish which part of the humerus or femur is missing.

Absence of all or part of a single sclerotome reduces the mass and shortens the shaft of an affected long bone, presenting as hypoplasia or partial aplasia. Absence of more than one sclerotome causes further loss of bone mass, progressive shortening of long bones and increasingly severe reduction of the limb. A reduction in mass of the humerus or femur brings the hand or foot closer to the trunk (phocomelia).

Gradually, the amount of skeleton remaining and the loss of normal landmarks are such that the identity of the residual sclerotomes becomes uncertain. Amelia is the most difficult subgroup to classify. At

Table 23.1 Results of sclerotome subtraction in 378 limbs with thalidomide-induced dysmelia. The 27 amelic limbs appear transverse (grade 3), but have been classified by experts as the final stage of longitudinal deficiency (grades 1 or 2). Therefore they are placed in each grade in turn, which shows that their classification makes no significant difference to the final result of the study: that the pattern of dysmelia is closely matched by the sclerotomes in 73.5–80.8% of the limbs.

	Number of limbs (% of total)		
Grade 1	**306** (80.8%)	**279** (73.5%)	**279** (73.5%)
Grade 2	**56** (15%)	**83** (22.3%)	**56** (15%)
Grade 3	**16** (4.2%)	**16** (4.2%)	**43** (11.5%)

first sight, it appears to be a transverse rather than a longitudinal deficiency, which would not fit into any classification of longitudinal defects. In the 27 amelic limbs in our series, however, the pectoral and pelvic girdles were always abnormal, with different degrees of hypoplasia, partial aplasia or dislocation. Hypoplasia of the scapula was commonly associated with absence or hypoplasia of the glenoid process and clavicle. Absence of the acetabulum and incomplete formation of the pelvic bones were always seen in hypoplasia of the pelvis. These girdle reductions indicated deficiencies in the proximal parts of the sclerotomes, yet they were disproportionately mild compared with the gross peripheral loss.

This apparent ambivalence of amelia has been discussed previously, and all authors have concluded that amelia represents the ultimate stage of longitudinal limb deficiency. According to the Working Group of the International Society for Prosthetics and Orthotics:[4]

> '...the concept of progressive longitudinal reduction can be carried to a point where only a single digital remnant of a limb remains, and ultimately to the situation in which even this vestigial element failed to form – the true amelia. This, therefore, might be considered to be a maximum longitudinal deficiency, although presenting as a transverse type of defect.'

In order to accommodate the ambivalent appearance of amelia, we recorded our results as grades 1, 2 or 3 with three options (Table 23.1 and Figure 23.3). In spite of this ambiguity, the congruence of the

(a)

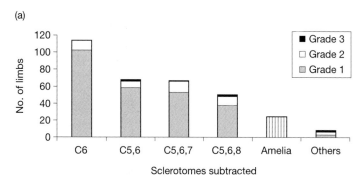

(b)

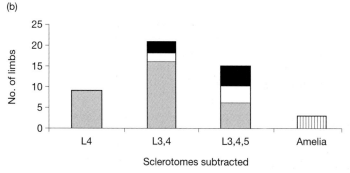

Figure 23.3 *Summary of the distribution and grades of fit of sclerotomes in 378 limbs with thalidomide-induced dysmelia: (a) upper limbs; (b) lower limbs. Note that the scale of the diagram for upper limbs is reduced to accommodate the large number of cases. The 27 amelic limbs have not been committed to any one grade, but are treated as a separate entity.*

sclerotomes with the pattern of dysmelia is still strong, between 73 and 80%. There were no cases which were not explained by the sclerotomes.

The analysis of typical cases is in the next chapter.

Discussion

The patterns of dysmelia matched the sclerotomes exactly in approximately 75% of our cases. There was evidence of sclerotome subtraction in the remainder, but the congruence of the patterns was less exact (Table 23.1). Our findings show that the absence of certain bones or areas within a bone can be explained by the sclerotomes. Some sclerotomes appeared to be more vulnerable than others, but within each subgroup of defects there was a high correlation with the anatomy.

The longitudinal axis of reduction in each limb is very clearly explained by the sclerotomes. In the upper limb, the 6th cervical sclerotome was involved in 98% (324 of 330) of limbs, either alone or in combination with adjacent levels, and is the axis of reduction in the arm. Thus the 6th cervical sclerotome is obviously most sensitive to thalidomide, while the 7th sclerotome is the most resistant.

All malformations of the lower limb showed subtraction of the 4th lumbar sclerotome. It was always the first to disappear – sometimes alone, but more often in combination with reduction in the adjacent 3rd and 5th lumbar sclerotomes. L4 is the most sensitive to thalidomide, and forms the axis of reduction in the leg. The sacral sclerotomes are the most resistant.

We do not know why the structures supplied by the 6th cervical and 4th lumbar nerves, or indeed the nerves themselves, should be more sensitive to damage or reduction by thalidomide than other segments. We have previously noted parallels in experimental teratology and phylogenesis that suggest that younger phylogenetic acquisitions are more vulnerable.[9,23] Thumb–finger opposition depends upon the 6th cervical nerve, and standing erect by knee extension involves musculoskeletal structures supplied by the 3rd and 4th lumbar nerves. Both functions have been acquired relatively recently in evolution. Bretscher and Tschumi[24] have suggested that in the competition for expression between different structures in morphogenesis, success goes to those that have been established longest in evolution.

Interdependence between the proximal and distal parts of the limb in dysmelia can be explained as progression within a sclerotome. It is possible to have proximal, distal or total lesions within one band of nerve supply, simulating the neurological distribution of adult segmental sensory neuropathies.

Since the pattern of dysmelia coincides so well with the sclerotomes, both appear to be expressions of the underlying sensory segmental innervation of the skeleton. The action of thalidomide in the embryo reveals the existence of the sclerotomes, which are otherwise invisible, and indicates the involvement of the sensory nervous system in morphogenesis and teratogenesis.

The preservation of the whole foot until the end of the reduction sequence warrants further comment. We are not convinced that the apical ectodermal ridge of the limb bud[25,26] plays a significant role in thalidomide embryopathy,[27] since if it did, the structures of the foot should be damaged from the early stages of the sequence. The resistance of the sacral nerves and sclerotomes to thalidomide explains the preservation of the foot. Interference with the function of the apical ectodermal ridge could not induce precise focal reduction of the radial digits and duplication of the great toe in radial and tibial dysmelia without damage to the other digits.

Many animal experiments have involved mechanical or surgical manipulation of limb buds, especially in the chick, but none has been able to model thalidomide embryopathy. The limb buds of the victims of thalidomide embryopathy did not suffer surgical damage. Their maldevelopment was due to a toxic effect on a normal embryo, often inflicted at a stage before the appearance of the limb.

Malformation in the arm was seen after ingestion of thalidomide from the 24th day of gestation,[3,15] but in humans the upper limb bud first arises from the trunk on the 28th day.[29] Therefore the pattern of morphogenesis of the limb is determined before the limb bud emerges from the trunk. This correlates with experimental findings, which suggest that the positional specification of neural crest cells occurs before they leave the neuroepithelium;[29] this has been established for the cranial neural crest, but not for the trunk or limbs. It is not known whether neuronal derivatives of the crest, such as sensory neurons, are similarly specified, nor is the role of *HOX* genes yet defined in the positional specification of neural crest cells.[29] Trunk neural crest cells, however, have been shown to be highly sensitive to environmental changes, which can restrict their ability to complete their differentiation into neurons, and influence the development of nerve-dependent derivatives such as skeletal structures.[30]

Genetic research has defined gene (homeobox) complexes related to particular segments of the central and peripheral nervous system, common to several phyla and including mammals.[31] The mechanism whereby homeobox genes pass morphogenetic messages to undifferentiated mesenchymal cells in the limb bud is not known. One hypothesis proposes that undifferentiated cells in the embryonic limb buds communicate positional information to one another. Even the proponents of this concept admit that 'there is not a single case in all of vertebrate development where an intercellular signal has been unequivocally identified'.[32] The hypothesis of positional information has been coupled with that of a possible diffusible morphogen emitted from the zone of polarizing activity (ZPA) of the ectodermal ridge of the limb bud. It is proposed that the genes in the mesoderm are switched on by a gradient of diminishing concentration of this morphogen as the cells are displaced proximally away from the ZPA by cell division. Evidence for the diffusible morphogen is 'indirect',[33] and evidence for the ZPA as its source is 'putative'.[34] 'Little is known about the signalling mechanisms involved in such morphogenetic events'.[34]

The sensory nervous system is constructed, in both structure and function, to transmit information in both directions between the central nervous system and the periphery. Proprioception is a sensory modality – a property of ectoderm, not of mesoderm. In the human embryo, the neural crest is present from the 18th day, 10 days before the first appearance of the upper limb bud, but during the sensitive period for thalidomide (days 21–42). Thus a mechanism that is known to be sensitive to thalidomide is present at an appropriate stage in morphogenesis for transmitting signals between the homeobox genes in the nervous system and the periphery. There is clear evidence that the neural crest plays an important role in limb morphogenesis.

The question arises as to why the possible role of nerves or sclerotomes in dysmelia was not considered at the time of the thalidomide disaster and its aftermath. There are at least two historical reasons for this.

First, sclerotome maps had been included in some anatomy textbooks for only 10 years and had been edited out by the time of the thalidomide tragedy.

Secondly, after the work of Bardeen and Lewis[35] and Lewis,[36] there was widespread belief that the limb bud of the embryo did not contain nerves and hence that the nervous system played no part in limb morphogenesis or teratogenesis. These authors reported that they did not observe axons in the limb buds of formalin-fixed embryos that had been embedded in paraffin and examined by light microscopy (standard methods in 1900). Such techniques are now known to destroy non-myelinated axons. These authors did not say that no nerves were present, although they are quoted as so doing.[37] This critical misquotation has been repeated in textbooks of embryology and in review articles,[38–40] and has diverted attention from the peripheral nervous system in embryogenesis. The presence of nerves in the limb buds has subsequently been demonstrated using modern neurohistological techniques.[41,42] Unmyelinated axons have been shown by electron microscopy to ramify into the undifferentiated limb bud before any condensation of mesenchyme.

The sclerotome pattern is not confined to thalidomide-induced dysmelia. Other reduction deformities of the upper and lower limbs also illustrate sclerotome hypoplasia and aplasia. These are dealt with in subsequent chapters.

References

1. Henkel H-L, Willert H-G. Dysmelia: a classification and a pattern of malformation in a group of congenital defects of the limbs. *J Bone Joint Surg Br* 1969; **51B**: 399–414.

2. Lenz W. Das thalidomid syndrom. *Fortschr Med* 1963; **81**: 148–155.

3. Nowack E. The sensitive phase for thalidomide embryopathy. *Humangenetik* 1965; **1**: 516–36.

4. Kay HW. The proposed international terminology for the classification of congenital limb deficiencies. *Dev Med Child Neurol Suppl* 1975; **34**: 1–12.

5. Henkel H-L, Willert H-G, Gressmann C. An international terminology for the classification of congenital limb deficiencies. *Arch Orthop Trauma Surg* 1978; **93**: 1–19.

6. Science Citation Index 1969–1999.

7. McCredie J, Willert H-G. Longitudinal limb deficiencies and the sclerotomes: an analysis of 378 dysmelic malformations induced by thalidomide. *J Bone Joint Surg Br* 1999; **81B**: 9–23.

8. Willert H-G, Henkel H-L. Die Dysmelie an den oberen Extremitäten. In: *Pathologie und Klinik in Einzeldarstellungen*. Berlin: Springer-Verlag, 1968.

9. Willert H-G, Henkel H-L. *Klinik und Pathologie der Dysmelie Die Fehlbildungen an den oberen Extremitäten bei der Thalidomid-Embryopathie*. Berlin: Springer-Verlag, 1969.

10. Wiedemann HR. Current knowledge on embryopathies with exogenous malformations in man. *Med Welt* 1962; **1**: 1343–9.

11. Inman V, Saunders JB de C. Referred pain from skeletal structures. *J Nerv Ment Dis* 1944; **99**: 660–7.

12. McCredie J. Segmental embryonic peripheral neuropathy. *Pediatr Radiol* 1975; **3**: 162–8.

13. McCredie J. Sclerotome subtraction: a radiological interpretation of reduction deformities of the limbs. *Birth Defects: Original Article Series* 1977; **13** (3D): 65–77.

14. Lenz W. Thalidomide and congenital abnormalities. *Lancet* 1962; **i**: 45.

15. Lenz W. Epidemiology of congenital malformations. *Ann NY Acad Sci* 1965; **123**: 228–36.

16. Pfeiffer RA, Kosenow W. Thalidomide and congenital malformations. *Lancet* 1962; **i**: 45–6.

17. Spiers AL. Thalidomide and congenital abnormalities. *Lancet* 1962; **i**: 303–5.

18. Cuthbert R, Spiers AL. Thalidomide-induced malformations: a radiological survey. *Clin Radiol* 1963; **14**: 163–9.

19. Ministry of Health Reports on Public Health and Medical Subjects No. 112. *Deformities Caused by Thalidomide*. London: HMSO, 1964.

20. Quibell EP. The thalidomide embryopathy: an analysis from the UK. *Practitioner* 1981; **225**: 721–6.

21. Smithells RW, Newman CG. Recognition of thalidomide defects. *J Med Genet* 1992; **29**: 716–23.

22. Swanson AB, Swanson GD, Tada K. A classification for congenital limb malformation. *J Hand Surg Am* 1983; **8**: 603–702.

23. McCredie J. Embryonic neuropathy: a hypothesis of neural crest injury as the pathogenesis of congenital malformations. *Med J Aust* 1974; **1**: 159–63.

24. Bretscher A, Tschumi P. Gestufte Reduktion von chemisch behandelen Xenopus-Beinen. *Rev Suisse Zool* 1951; **58**: 11.

25. Saunders JW. The proximo-distal sequence of origin of the chick wing and the role of the ectoderm. *J Exp Zool* 1948; **108**: 363–403.

26. Tschumi PA. The growth of the hindlimb bud of *Xenopus laevis* and its dependence upon the epidermis. *J Anat* 1957; **91**: 149–73.

27. Tabin CJ. A developmental model for thalidomide defects. *Nature* 1998; **396**: 322–3.

28. *Langman's Medical Embryology*, 10th edn. Philadelphia: Lippincott Williams & Wilkins, 2006.

29. Noden DM. Spatial integration among cells forming the cranial peripheral nervous system. *J Neurobiol* 1993; **24**: 248–61.

30. Vogel KS, Marusich MF, Weston JA. Restriction of neurogenic ability during neural crest differentiation. *J Neurobiol* 1993; **24**: 162–71.

31. Gehring WJ. Homeoboxes in the study of development. *Science* 1987; **236**: 1245–52.

32. Wolpert L. Do we understand development? *Science* 1994; **266**: 571–2.

33. Tickle C, Alberts B. Wolpert L, Lee J. Local application of retinoic acid to the hindlimb mimics the action of the polarising region. *Nature* 1982; **296**: 546

34. Dollé P, Izpisua-Belmonte JC, Falkenstein H, Renucci A, Duboule D. Coordinate expression of the murine *HOX-5* complex homeobox-containing genes during limb pattern formation. *Nature* 1989; **342**: 767–72.

35. Bardeen CR, Lewis WH. The development of the limbs, body wall and back in man. *Am J Anat* 1901; **1**: 1–36.

36. Lewis WH. The development of the arm in man. *Am J Anat* 1902; **1**: 145–83.

37. Gardner E, O'Rahilly R. Neural crest, limb development and thalidomide embryopathy. *Lancet* 1976; **i**: 635–7.

38. O'Rahilly R, Gardner E. The timing and sequence of events in the development of the limbs in the human embryo. *Anat Embryol* 1975; **148**: 1–23.

39. Poswillo D. Mechanisms and pathogenesis of malformations. *Br Med Bull* 1976; **32**: 59–64.

40. Wolpert L. Mechanisms of limb development and malformation. *Br Med Bull* 1976; **32**: 65–70.

41. Cameron J, McCredie J. Innervation of the undifferentiated limb bud in rabbit embryo. *J Anat* 1982; **134**: 795–808.

42. McCredie J, Cameron J, Shoobridge R. Congenital malformations and the neural crest. *Lancet* 1978; **ii**: 761–3.

CHAPTER 24

Radial/tibial dysmelia: Limb reductions typical of thalidomide

Introduction

Longitudinal reduction defects in the radial and tibial aspects of the limbs were typical of thalidomide embryopathy, but are not exclusive to thalidomide. Chapter 23 showed how the sclerotome maps explain radial and tibial defects as segmental sensory nerve lesions through failure of formation of their developmental fields. The aim of this chapter is to explain the morphogenesis of phocomelia. It incorporates results from Chapter 23 in its original published form,[1] amplified by extra material. Some additional cases are Australian thalidomide children, others are German children. Line diagrams and all pathological specimens are from the monograph by Willert and Henkel, *Klinik und Pathologie der Dysmelie: Die Fehlbildungen an den oberen Extremitäten bei der Thalidomid-Embryopathie.*[2] This valuable book is now out of print, but, with permission from Professor Willert and the publisher (Springer-Verlag), some of their illustrations are reproduced here with captions in English, lest valuable first-hand information be lost forever.

Upper limb

6th cervical sclerotome

Stages a–d in Figure 23.1 in the previous chapter show deletion within the 6th cervical sclerotome, including three types:

- distal – deleting the thumb and/or radius
- proximal – deleting the upper humerus; or
- central – involving all parts of the sclerotome

Associated thumb defects include absence, hypoplasia, triphalangism and occasional polydactyly; and progressive defects in the index and other fingers, all of which will be detailed in Chapter 27.

Chapter Summary
- Introduction
- Upper limb
- Lower limb
- Conclusion
- References

Figure 24.1 *Stages of radial aplasia: (a) hypoplasia; (b) mild partial aplasia; (c) severe partial aplasia; (d) subtotal aplasia; (e) total aplasia. Dotted lines show cartilaginous masses. (From Willert HG, Henkel HL. Klinik und Pathologie der Dysmelie: Die fehlbildungen an der oberen Extremitäten bei der Thalidomid-Embryopathie. Berlin: Springer-Verlag, 1969,[2] with permission.)*

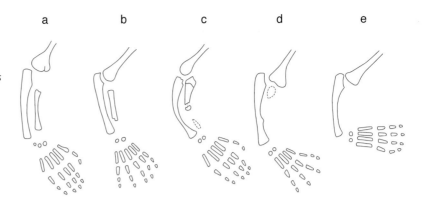

Phocomelia was due to reduction in the major long bones, particularly the humerus, but also the radius and ulna.

The radius was almost always reduced in some way (Figure 24.1). First, the styloid process was absent, with narrowing of the distal end of the radius. This progressed to reduction in width and then in length of the radius, with increasing curvature of the ulna. Further reduction led to a short residual radial fragment beside or fused to the ulnar shaft. Finally, the radius disappeared as an entity. At surgery, a fibrous band was sometimes found in its place, and was thought to increase the curvature of the ulna as a fixed string bends a flexible bow. In other cases, the ulna was increased in width by side-to-side synostosis with the residual radius. Sometimes, the outlines of two bones were evident, although they were fused side-to-side. In other cases, the distal radius had disappeared, but the head and proximal end could be discerned, and three cortical surfaces indicated fusion with the proximal ulna, which was of greater than normal width near the elbow (see Figure 11.2 in Chapter 11). The radius was commonly absent altogether, leaving the ulna to carry a hand of three or four rays, tilted to the radial side of the forearm in the typical 'radial club-hand' deformity.

The humerus could be normal, but was often slightly reduced in size and sometimes in shape (see Figures 22.2 and 22.3 in Chapter 22). The initial reduction seemed to be in width rather than length, but both could occur together.

The scapula tended to be narrow and hypoplastic. The clavicle was usually normal, but sometimes its outer end was depressed.

In our German thalidomide series, the largest single group of 34.5% (114 of 330 malformations of the upper limb) involved *only* the 6th cervical sclerotome. Grade 1 changes were seen in 102 limbs (89%) and grade 2 changes in 12 (11%), and grade 3 changes were not present.

5th and 6th cervical sclerotomes

The 5th cervical sclerotome terminates just distal to the elbow and does not reach the hand. Therefore reduction of C5 does not affect the anatomy of the hand. But failure of cell division at the tip of the C5 sclerotome would reduce the final mesenchymal mass to less than the minimum required to form separate bone ends for proximal radius and ulna.

Proximal radio-ulnar synostosis is the first sign of involvement of the 5th cervical sclerotome (Figure 24.2). It can occur with radial aplasia before the humeral shaft loses its shape. The fact that the most distal extent of the 5th cervical sclerotome is the first area to be damaged is consistent with the neurological principle that the longest nerves are most vulnerable to injury. Even the potentially longest nerves appear to comply.

The next stage shortens the upper 3rd of the arm, and phocomelia commences. In addition to the features of radial aplasia, the upper end of the humerus now fails to form and its length is reduced (Figure 24.3: stages b–d). Change in shape and reduction in size of the humerus was the characteristic feature of this group. It was seen in 68 out of 330 (20.6%) of all our malformations of the upper limb. Grade 1 changes were present in 58 limbs (85%), grade 2 in 7 (10%) and grade 3 in 3(5%).

The sclerotome maps (see Chapter 21: Figure 21.2) show that this is deletion of both 5th and 6th cervical sclerotomes. Much of the upper humerus lies in the 5th cervical sclerotome; thus the humerus is profoundly reduced by failure to form C5. Geometrically, the humerus approximates a rectangle in shape, especially in the

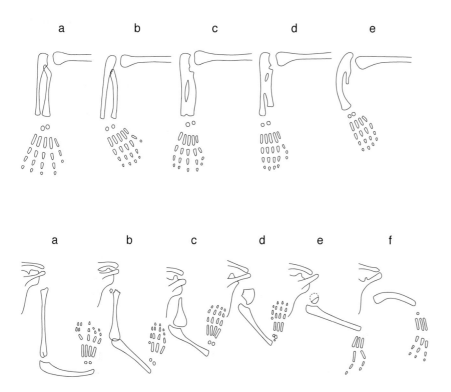

Figure 24.2 *Radio-ulnar synostosis: (a,b) hypoplasia of radial head (C5); (c,d) radio-ulnar synostosis with hypoplasia of radius (C5,6); (e) partial radial aplasia with proximal radio-ulnar synostosis and absent thumb. (From Willert HG, Henkel HL. Klinik und Pathologie der Dysmelie: Die Fehlbildungen an der oberen Extremitäten bei der Thalidomid-Embryopathie. Berlin: Springer-Verlag, 1969,[2] with permission.)*

Figure 24.3 *Radial aplasia with progressive reduction of humerus: (a,b) hypoplasia of humerus due to loss of C6; (c–e) partial humeral aplasia due to progressive subtraction of C5 and C6, encroaching on C7; (f) aplasia of ossified humerus with subtraction of C5–7. (From Willert HG, Henkel HL. Klinik und Pathologie der Dysmelie: Die Fehlbildungen an der oberen Extremitäten bei der Thalidomid-Embryopathie. Berlin: Springer-Verlag, 1969,[2] with permission.)*

posterior view, where it is divided diagonally by the border between the 6th and 7th cervical sclerotomes. Thus it is composed of two triangles: C5/6 proximo-anteriorly and C7/8 posterodistally. Adding the third dimension, the two triangles are in fact wedge-shaped pieces of bone. The wedge of C5/6 is inverted, with its base at the shoulder, while that of C7/8 is based at the elbow. If the C5/6 wedge drops out, C7/8 remains. The elbow joint is usually present but hypoplastic.

Subtraction of the 5th as well as the 6th cervical sclerotome is thus a powerful means of accelerating the transition to phocomelia without further affecting the morphology of the hand beyond basic radial aplasia.

No abnormal cells could be seen in cartilage or bone in the case in Figure 24.4(b) on light microscopy. The abundant cartilage in the

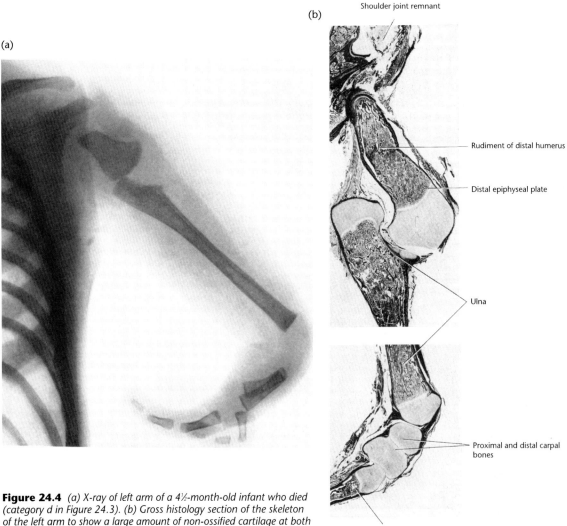

Figure 24.4 *(a) X-ray of left arm of a 4½-month-old infant who died (category d in Figure 24.3). (b) Gross histology section of the skeleton of the left arm to show a large amount of non-ossified cartilage at both ends of the radius, but only at the distal end of the humerus.*

gross longitudinal section is invisible on the radiograph. Comparisons of the gross sections with the radiographs are instructive in the facts of the situation: radiographs show more than visual inspection, but they do not reveal all the facts by any means. Cartilage cannot be seen on X-rays before it calcifies or ossifies, and a large proportion of the immature skeleton is composed of cartilage. It could be shown by ultrasound. Its presence needs to be understood. In very young fetuses in utero, the rudiment of the humerus is totally cartilaginous.

5th, 6th and 7th cervical sclerotomes (Figures 24.5 and 24.6)

In 66 (20%) malformations of the upper limb the bone loss was more severe (see Figure 22.5 in Chapter 22). This illustrates deletion of the 5th, 6th and 7th cervical sclerotomes, with some reduction of the 8th in the most severe examples. We saw no evidence of deletion of the 7th cervical sclerotome in isolation – only in combination with the 5th and 6th, and only when these were grossly involved. The remaining limb appears to be a combination of the 8th and part of the 7th sclerotome. It could also be interpreted as the 7th with part of the 8th, since insufficient limb remains to be certain which sclerotome forms the major part, but the elbow joint is derived from the 8th. Digits in the C7 sclerotome are reduced from the radial side. Grade 1 changes were seen in 52 limbs (79%), grade 2 in 13 (19%) and grade 3 in 1 limb (2%).

Note on the term 'intercalary':

The fact that the cartilaginous component of immature bones is radiologically invisible has led some to believe that no humerus is present – a so-called 'intercalary defect'.

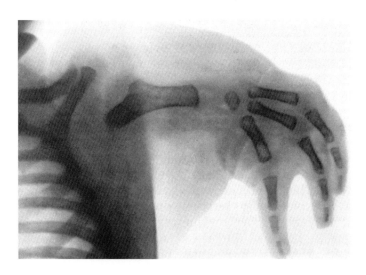

Figure 24.5 *X-ray of subtotal aplasia of humerus. Three residual digits of C7 and 8. The gap between fused forearm bones and shoulder girdle contains non-ossified cartilage, as shown in a similar case in Figure 24.6 (category f in Figure 24.3).*

Figure 24.6 *Gross histological section of upper arm of a 2-year-old girl with phocomelia. A small kernel of bone is present in the distal humeral epiphysis, posteriorly in the C8 sclerotome area. But at least three-quarters of the humeral remnant is cartilage, invisible to X-ray.*
(From Willert HG, Henkel HL. Klinik und Pathologie des Dysmelie: Die Fehlbildungen an der oberen Extremitäten bei der Thalidomid-Embryopathie. *Berlin: Springer-Verlag, 1969,[2] with permission.)*

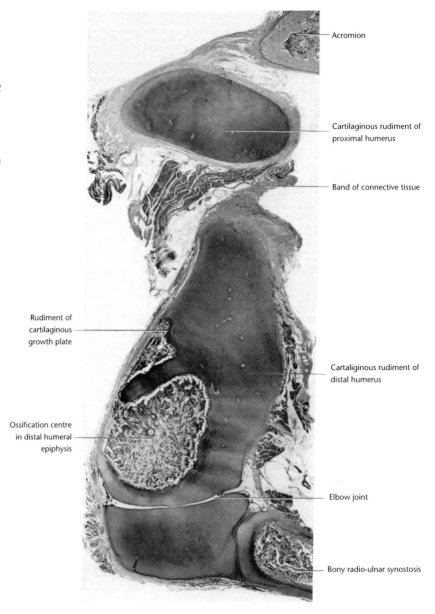

Acromion

Cartilaginous rudiment of proximal humerus

Band of connective tissue

Rudiment of cartilaginous growth plate

Cartaliginous rudiment of distal humerus

Ossification centre in distal humeral epiphysis

Elbow joint

Bony radio-ulnar synostosis

Intercalary deficiency is defined as 'absence of proximal or middle segments of a limb with all or part of the distal segment present'. It is based on the old concept of transverse segments of the limb that might allow the humerus or femur to vanish and leave a theoretical 'intercalary defect'. The anatomy is easily misconstrued in any study where no X-rays are obtained to ascertain the bony disorders within the limb, and may be further misinterpreted if the presence of invisible cartilage is not read into the image to incorporate histological and surgical observations. Early radiographs taken before ossification may show no bony humerus, although an invisible cartilage model exists.

Some authors still argue that phocomelia represents an 'intercalary' loss of limb tissue, using an outdated system of classification.[3,4]

This claim has been contradicted by numerous authors[5–10] since 1969. None found any evidence of 'intercalary malformations' in their collections. Goldfarb et al[9] propose that phocomelia is simply a severe longitudinal dysplasia:

> 'None of the 60 extremities that we studied demonstrated a true intercalary deficiency.'

Professor Willert and I found no 'intercalary' defects in over 200 German thalidomide cases. All cases of phocomelia had remnants of femur or humerus in the upper section of the limb.[1] The term 'intercalary' has been deleted from practical classification systems,[10,11] but the old term still has its adherents.

5th, 6th and 8th cervical sclerotomes (Figure 24.7)

There were 50 limbs (15%) in categories of g and h of Figure 23.1. The elbow is absent and the morphology of humero-ulnar fusion may represent the residual 7th cervical sclerotome, although it could also be residual C8 with part of C7. At this stage of reduction, there are insufficient bony landmarks and diagnosis must remain ambivalent.

Further reduction leads to more gross phocomelia, including the single-digit form (Figure 24.8).

Here the residual row of phalanges clearly belongs to a distal sclerotome that has disappeared proximally, together with the 5th, 6th, and 7th or 8th, respectively. This digit may belong to the 7th or 8th cervical sclerotome, but there are insufficient data for positive identi-

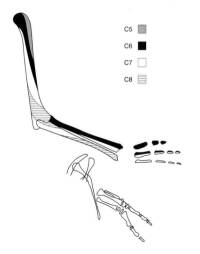

C5
C6
C7
C8

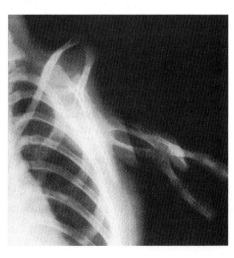

Figure 24.7 *No long bones are visible, but three digits at the shoulder are evidence of residual distal C7 or C8 sclerotomes, shown in the lower sketch. The upper sketch shows absent sclerotomes. The scapula is hypoplastic. This case is category g in Figure 23.1, tending towards category h.*

Figure 24.8 *(a) Single-digit phocomelia in a German thalidomide child. Facial bruises and abrasions are from falls. (b) Radiograph shows no ossified long bones, but cartilage residua must be assumed within the gap. Category h of Figure 23.1.*

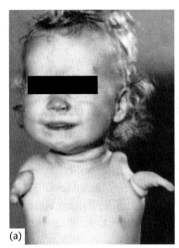

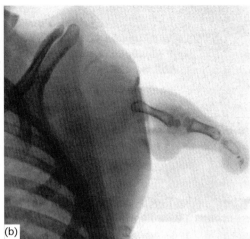

(a)   (b)

fication. Grade 1 changes were seen in 37 limbs (74%), grade 2 in 10 limbs (20%) and grade 3 in 3 limbs (6%).

5th, 6th, 7th and 8th cervical sclerotomes

Amelia was seen in 24 (7%) of our upper limbs (Figure 23.1: stage i; Figure 24.9).

Note on classification of amelia

Amelia is the only apparently transverse deficiency in the typically longitudinal defects of thalidomide origin. Henkel and Willert,[5,10] Smithells and Newman[12] and Swanson et al[13] have all drawn attention to this apparent oddity, pointing out that amelia should only be classified as transverse if the pectoral or pelvic girdle is intact. If any other parts of the limb girdles are deficient or hypoplastic, amelia should be considered a longitudinal deficiency of the most major degree. All cases of amelia in our study were associated with reduction in the limb girdles. In upper amelia, the scapula was uniformly hypoplastic, and the glenoid process was absent or hypoplastic (Figure 24.9b,c). The changes in the pectoral girdle had been emerging at early stages in the reduction, as can be seen in Figure 23.1, especially after stage e. The 24 limbs with upper amelia were interpreted as showing reduction in all sclerotomes, although identification was less obvious than in malformations where there was more skeletal residue.

Other sclerotome combinations

The remaining eight upper limbs (2%) had malformations in which sclerotomes were difficult to identify. Four showed possible subtraction of only the 5th cervical sclerotome; two retained the 5th but

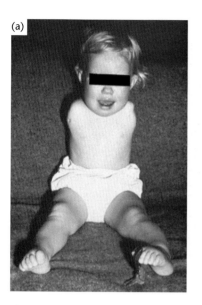 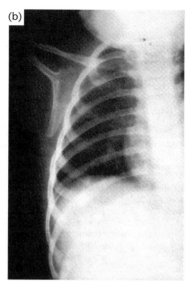 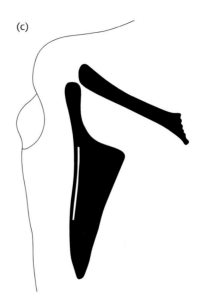

Figure 24.9 *(a) Photograph of child with bilateral upper amelia. (b) Radiograph of right upper amelia. (c) Sketch of shoulder girdle in amelia. Hypoplastic scapula is characteristic, so this is not a transverse defect.*

with subtraction of the 6th, 7th and 8th; one appeared to have subtraction of the 5th and 8th; and in one case, the 8th cervical sclerotome appeared to be missing. Two had grade 1 changes, three had grade 2 and three grade 3.

Lower limb

There were 48 defects of the lower limb, all of which exemplified the pattern of dysmelia. Figure 23.2 for the lower limb can be compared with the sclerotome map of the lower limb (Figure 21.3), working from left to right (a–h).

4th lumbar sclerotome

Figure 24.10 illustrates *distal* reduction in the 4th lumbar sclerotome. The correspondence with stages a–c of dysmelia in Figure 23.1 is obvious.

The residual triangular fragment of the proximal tibia was a characteristic finding in all published thalidomide series, and has hitherto been unexplained.

Figure 24.11 describes progressive reduction of the tibia without affecting the femur, which Willert and Henkel[2] classified as the *distal form* of leg reduction in thalidomide embryopathy.

The sclerotome maps reveal that this is the distal end of the 3rd lumbar sclerotome made visible by disappearance of the 4th lumbar. Nine limbs (18%) had this appearance, all classified as grade 1.

Figure 24.10 *Aplasia of distal tibia in three Australian thalidomide cases.*
The extraordinary triangular remnant of the proximal tibia represents the tibial component of the 3rd lumbar sclerotome, revealed by subtraction of the 4th lumbar sclerotome, which removes the medial, distal tibia.

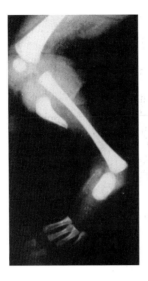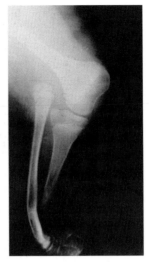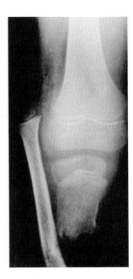

Figure 24.11 *Distal type of lower limb reduction with partial to total tibial aplasia, but virtually normal femur: (a) distal tibial hypoplasia; (b) partial tibial aplasia; (c) subtotal tibial aplasia; (d) total tibial aplasia. (From Willert HG, Henkel HL.* Klinik und Pathologie der Dysmelie: Die Fehlbildungen an der oberen Extremitäten bei Thalidomid-Embryopathie. *Berlin: Springer-Verlag, 1969,[2] with permission.)*

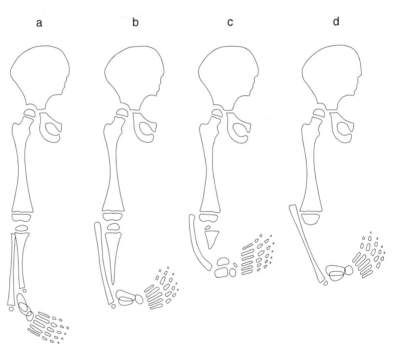

Another variant that was uncommon was the *proximal form* of lower limb reduction, in which the femur was more markedly affected than the tibia. Proximal focal femoral dysplasia resulted (Figure 24.12).

3rd and 4th lumbar sclerotomes

Increasing degrees of reduction of the 3rd and 4th lumbar sclerotomes are shown next. The distal part of the 4th lumbar sclerotome has

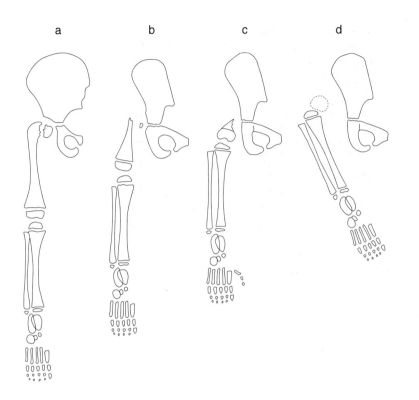

Figure 24.12 *Proximal type of leg reduction after Willert and Henkel:[2] (a) coxa vara; (b) partial femoral aplasia, hypoplastic acetabulum and vestigial femoral capital epiphysis; (c) severe partial femoral aplasia with residual distal condyles; (d) subtotal femoral aplasia. A vestige of cartilaginous distal femoral epiphysis will ossify later. The femur is reduced (PFFD), but the tibia is virtually untouched.*

disappeared, together with the lower end of the 3rd – a pattern of loss equivalent to subtraction of sclerotomes C6 and distal C5 in the arm.

The proximal part of the 4th lumbar sclerotome may also fail to form, leaving a quadrant of femoral head within a hypoplastic acetabulum. A long triangular remnant of the distal femur remains (PFFD). Figure 7.10 in the Australian cases illustrates the central type of PFFD reduction in both legs, as shown in Figure 24.13.

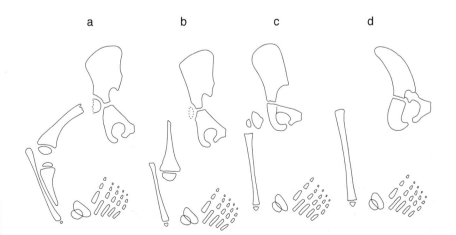

Figure 24.13 *Willert and Henkel's central type of leg reduction, in which the tibia and femur are both reduced from the start: (a) partial femoral and partial tibial aplasia; (b) partial femoral and total tibial aplasia; (c) subtotal femoral and total tibial aplasia; (d) total femoral and total tibial aplasia. Note that this also produces proximal femoral focal dysplasia (PFFD). (From Willert HG, Henkel HL. Klinik und Pathologie der Dysmelie: Die Fehlbildungen an der oberen Extremitäten bei Thalidomid-Embryopathie. Berlin: Springer-Verlag, 1969,[2] with permission.)*

Both residual femoral fragments correspond to the proximal part of the 3rd lumbar sclerotome anteriorly, or the 5th lumbar and 1st sacral sclerotomes posteriorly, or a conglomerate of all these. Loss of the patella favours reduction of the anterior sclerotomes and survival of the posterior sclerotomes.

The acetabulum and the head and neck of the femur lie in the 3rd and 4th lumbar sclerotomes. The distal triangular stump of the femur represents the 5th lumbar and 1st sacral components. The mass of the fibula is increased by incorporation of the 5th lumbar and 1st sacral sclerotomes from the posterior aspect of the tibia. The distal end of this composite bone carries a hypoplastic mortise joint for the ankle. The ambiguous identity of this bone earned it the nickname 'tibula'. In some cases, fusion of the tibia and fibula did not occur, and the two bones remained separate, despite total reduction of the femur.

This longitudinal proximal femoral focal deficiency (PFFD) can represent survival of the posterior sclerotomes, with loss of most of the anterior components. The sclerotome map of the back of the leg (Figure 21.3) shows that the 5th lumbar and 1st and 2nd sacral (posterior) sclerotomes can compose a tibia and fibula without the (anterior) 3rd and 4th lumbar sclerotomes.

The most common defect of the lower limb seen in 21 limbs (44%) of our series was deletion of the 3rd and 4th lumbar sclerotomes to varying degrees. Grade 1 changes were seen in 16 limbs (76%), grade 2 in 2 limbs (10%), and grade 3 in 3 limbs (14%).

3rd, 4th and 5th lumbar sclerotomes

In 15 limbs (32%) the 3rd, 4th and 5th lumbar sclerotomes were involved, as in Figure 24.14. There was no bone visible between the pelvis and the fibula. Involvement of the 5th lumbar sclerotome sometimes caused absence, hypoplasia, triphalangism or duplication

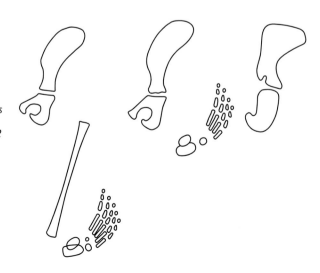

Figure 24.14 *Final sequences of lower limb reduction. Fibula and foot remain (L5, S1 and S2 sclerotomes, mainly posterior). Lumbar sclerotomes 3 and 4 have failed to form. (From Willert HG, Henkel HL.* Klinik und Pathologie der Dysmelie: Die Fehlbildungen an der oberen Extremitäten bei Thalidomid-Embryopathie. *Berlin: Springer-Verlag, 1969,[2] with permission.)*

of the hallux. Involvement of other bones within the foot was not observed. The main structure of the foot, innervated by sacral sclerotomes, was preserved until the last stage of reduction, when they became involved in the reduction process. In one case of tibial aplasia, there were three great toes.

Because the structure of the foot is little affected, difficulty in identification of individual digits does not occur in the lower limb. Lower limb reduction takes place within the major long bones and involves the deletion of the 3rd and 4th lumbar sclerotomes, which do not extend to the foot. Difficulties in interpretation can occur because of the inter-relationship of different sclerotomes on the anterior and posterior surfaces of the long bones. Six limbs (40%) had grade 1 changes, four grade 2 (26%) and five (33%) grade 3.

Note on proximal femoral focal deficiency

PFFD is seen in the middle of this reduction sequence. The residual distal femur is a triangle based where the knee should have been. This triangle comprises the posterior sclerotomes (L5, S1 and S2), the anterior sclerotomes L3 and L4 having been deleted along with the L3 and L4 elements of the tibia. The L3 triangle of upper tibia has been eliminated, and the distal femur has no tibial plateau with which to articulate. The single long bone in the lower leg is fibula (L5, S1 and S2), with the foot being intact (also L5, S1 and S2).

A *second form of PFFD* occurs with *non*-thalidomide deformities, to be discussed in Chapter 29. In this type, the residual components are anterior, the posterior sclerotomes having failed to form. A distal triangle of the femur can be read on both anterior and posterior views of the sclerotome maps, but each involves different sclerotomes.

3rd, 4th and 5th lumbar and 1st and 2nd sacral sclerotomes.

Three cases of amelia of the lower limb (6%) showed loss of all the sclerotomes in the leg (final diagram in Figure 24.14). In all cases, there were hypoplastic malformations of the bony pelvis.

Conclusion

Sclerotome subtraction explains the anatomy of the radial/tibial type of phocomelia, as seen in thalidomide embryopathy.

References

1. McCredie J, Willert HG. Longitudinal limb deficiencies and the sclerotomes: an analysis of 378 dysmelic malformations induced by thalidomide. *J Bone Joint Surg Br* 1999; **81**: 9–23.

2. Willert HG, Henkel HL. *Klinik und Pathologie der Dysmelie: Die Fehlbildungen an den oberen Extremitäten bei der Thalidomid-Embryopathie.* Berlin: Springer-Verlag, 1969.

3. Frantz CH, O'Rahilly R. Congenital skeletal limb deficiencies. *J Bone Joint Surg Am* 1961; **43**: 1202–24

4. Gardner E, O'Rahilly R. Neural crest, limb development and thalidomide embryopathy. *Lancet* 1976; **i**: 635–7.

5. Henkel HL, Willert HG. Dysmelia: a classification and a pattern of malformation in a group of congenital defects of the limbs. *J Bone Joint Surg Br* 1969; **51**: 399–414.

6. Kelikian H. *Congenital Deformities of the Hand and Forearm.* Philadelphia: WB Saunders, 1974; 891–901.

7. Swanson AB. A classification for congenital limb malformations. *J Hand Surg Am* 1976; **1**: 8–22.

8. Tytherleigh-Strong G, Hooper G. The classification of phocomelia. *J Hand Surg Br* 2003; **28**: 215–7.

9. Goldfarb CA, Manske PR, Busa R, et al. Upper extremity phocomelia re-examined: a longitudinal dysplasia. *J Bone Joint Surg* 2005; **87**: 2639–48.

10. Henkel HL, Willert HG, Gressmann C. An international terminology for the classification of congenital limb deficiencies. *Arch Orthop Trauma Surg* 1978; **93**: 1–19.

11. Kay HW. The proposed international terminology for the classification of congenital limb deficiencies. *Dev Med Child Neurol Suppl* 1975; **34**: 1–12.

12. Smithells RW, Newman CG. Recognition of thalidomide defects. *J Med Genet* 1992; **29**: 716–23.

13. Swanson AB, Swanson GD, Tada K. A classification for congenital limb malformation. *J Hand Surg Am* 1983; **8**: 479–88.

CHAPTER 25

Associated internal malformations and their embryology

'Thalidomide caused a wide variety of birth defects, not one of which was unique to that drug.'
RW Smithells and CG Newman. *Journal of Medical Genetics* 1992; **29**: 716–23

Chapter Summary
- Introduction
- The British thalidomide experience
- Cardiac malformations
- Malformations of the ear
- Malformations of the eye
- Cleft lip and palate
- Alimentary tract malformations
- Discussion
- Conclusions
- References

Introduction

In the 1960s, the British public and media, and the medical, scientific, legal and political communities were shocked by the thalidomide catastrophe in their midst. The British Government ruled that cases be notified to the Ministry of Health (MOH). From the mass of information received by 1964, the Ministry published a booklet, *Deformities Caused by Thalidomide.*[1] The simple facts of the thalidomide epidemic in UK were summarized and analysed. It was available from Her Majesty's Stationery Office for six shillings and sixpence. It is now out of print.

An essential reference used in this chapter is a paper published in the *Journal of Medical Genetics* in 1992 by Smithells and Newman,[2] two British paediatricians who devoted three decades of their professional lives to the diagnosis and clinical management of the UK group of thalidomide survivors. Their paper, 'Recognition of thalidomide defects', is a mine of information on how problems evolved over time.

It became apparent immediately that thalidomide damaged internal organs[3–11] in addition to limbs.

Many data are recorded in German and other European languages. Some German papers I have had translated into English. My colleague in Göttingen, Professor Hans-Georg Willert, to whom I am deeply indebted, often transferred information for me from German into English.

Thalidomide Embryopathy in Japan,[12] by a Japanese study group, edited by Kida and published in 1987, is a very useful reference for defects diagnosed in teenage and early adulthood. Thalidomide embryopathy continued to evolve as an entity as time passed and different defects presented. For instance, defects of the genito-urinary systems presented in the teenage and child-bearing years. Some cranial nerve lesions were diagnosed in adulthood, not childhood.

The Swedish literature is particularly good on these topics in conjunction with the Japanese data.

I have depended upon information and excellent diagrams in *Langman's Medical Embryology*, 10th edn, edited by TW Sadler.[13] I am grateful to Dr Sadler, to the illustrators Jill Leland and Susan L Sadler-Redmond, and to Lippincott Williams & Wilkins, for permission to use these excellent embryological illustrations.

The aim of this chapter is to review the internal malformations due to thalidomide, and their embryology. The question is whether internal defects, like limb defects, can be explained as neural crest injuries,[13] as hypothesized in Chapter 12.

The British thalidomide experience

Longitudinal reduction defects of the limbs became the recognized hallmark of thalidomide embryopathy from 1961. Indeed, they occurred in the majority of cases. But the drug also caused malformations in almost every internal organ.

Lenz's letter to *The Lancet*[3] in December 1961 alerted the English-speaking medical world to the breadth of the German experience. In addition to limb reductions, he listed some typical internal manifestations:

> 'absence of the auricles, haemangiomata of the nose and upper lip (wine spot variety), atresia of the oesophagus, the duodenum or the anus, cardiac anomalies and aplasia of the gallbladder and of the appendix.'

Congenital hearts, malformations of ears and of eyes were so frequently reported that the British MOH collated subgroups of these three conditions.[1]

Of 894 notified cases in the UK, 172 were dead, almost certainly from major internal defects that were life-threatening around birth, as proved in those who came to autopsy. The perinatal mortality rate was estimated to be 40%. Smithells and Newman[2] point out that serious internal defects were much less common among survivors than they were in the whole original group at birth. Stillbirths and miscarriages, misdiagnoses and failure to relate defects to the drug in the early days of the epidemic inevitably undermined statistical accuracy.

Of the 832 British birth records[1] with limb deformities, 672 infants were still alive in 1964. There were at least 323 children (about 50% of limb-deficient survivors) with deformities affecting other parts as well as the limbs, and 61 cases with malformations in other organs but no limb defects.

The occurrence of isolated non-limb defects after thalidomide exposure was first noticed by Smithells and Leck[6] in the Liverpool register of birth defects, which had been established in 1960. In 1960–61, they reported 7 cases of ear defects without limb involvement, all with proven thalidomide exposure, in a population that had seen no such cases in the previous 3 years. In the British series there were 89 of 894 children with ear defects.

There were 37 of 894 British children with deformities of the eye.[1] Although some of the eye deformities were relatively slight (e.g. ptosis or strabismus) 'the general type of deformity was of underdevelopment varying from anophthalmia to coloboma'.[1] Anophthalmia and microphthalmia with attendant blindness were often incompatable with living in a normal family, and meant life in an institution for such afflicted children.

Only 13 of 894 children were reported as having vascular naevi, typically of the nose and upper lip.[1] These wine spots faded in infancy. Although there may have been incomplete ascertainment of naevi, the British MOH concluded that at < 2% incidence, skin naevi cannot be seen as definitive of thalidomide embryopathy.[1]

Congenital heart disease, on the other hand, although it sometimes escaped diagnosis in the newborn infant, was recorded in at least 79 cases out of 894. Details of the heart condition were often not provided, yet, of those detailed, a high proportion had septal defects. Most other major cardiac malformations were also represented, but in smaller numbers.

Six children had facial palsy accompanied by eye and/or ear deformities in the early reports.[1] Strabismus was underreported in infants and children, but became increasingly recognized as a typical manifestation as they matured and could cooperate with ocular tests.

There were 12 living and 19 dead infants with intestinal atresia, all 31 with positive thalidomide exposure.[1] Three living and 18 dead infants had deformities of the kidney.

The appendix of the British MOH report[1] lists a wide variety of malformations scattered through the notified cases. Cleft palate, hare-lip, spina bifida, and atresia and stenosis of the oesophagus, duodenum and rectum are recorded more often than in the general population.

Genito-urinary malformations reflected those seen in non-thalidomide cases: absence, hypoplasia, dislocation and fusion, and cystic disease. Congenital hydronephrosis, hydroureter, stenosis, atresia, duplication, and abnormal insertion of the distal ureter were listed. Less severe malformations of kidneys and ureters presented in childhood. Malformations of the genito-urinary systems declared themselves during adolescence and the reproductive years.[2] Hypoplasia or displacement of the scrotum or labia could accompany severe lower limb deficiency. Undescended testis, duplication or atresia of the vagina and uterus, and deformities in these structures were all recorded.

Central nervous system (CNS) abnormalities such as hydrocephalus, mental retardation, epilepsy, autism, and Down's and other CNS syndromes were rarely mentioned in the British MOH series so soon after birth. But mental handicap, dyslexia, autism and epilepsy were diagnosed in childhood and adolescence more often than would be expected by chance in the normal population, and have been attributed to thalidomide.[2]

Similarly, abnormalities of the spine and knees were usually not recognized at birth, but presented in childhood or even much later. Some of these late diagnoses were never associated with thalidomide aetiology, especially in the absence of limb defects. As time passed, it became difficult to differentiate some of these conditions from normal wear and tear. Radiology has a very important part to play in sorting out differential diagnoses of spinal, renal, ear and orthopaedic problems presenting later in life in these patients. Spine X-rays of 136 Japanese thalidomide victims[12] revealed abnormal vertebrae in 104. Plain X-rays of the abdomen demonstrated defects in vertebrae and pelvic bones such as spina bifida occulta and sacral dysplasia. Later intravenous pyelography showed malrotation, crossed fused ectopia, horseshoe kidneys, pelvic kidneys and abnormalities of pelvicalyceal anatomy.[12]

Cardiac malformations (Figures 25.1 and 25.2)

In survivors, the most common malformation of the heart was septal defect: atrial septal defect (ASD), ventricular septal defect (VSD) and pulmonary stenosis. Conotruncal and other complex cardiac lesions were often recorded among the perinatal deaths.

Langman's Medical Embryology[13] illustrates the formation of the cardiac septum (Figure 25.1) as:

- union, or overlap of *two* ridges that grow forwards one another from opposite sides of the heart, or
- growth of *one* such ridge towards the opposite wall of the heart

In either case, if growth of the ridge(s) halts, the septum remains open.

The mature septum is known to contain neural elements in its conducting system: sino-atrial node, bundle of His, and atrioventricular node.

Using chick embryos, in 1966, Johnston[15] demonstrated the presence of cranial neural crest in structures beyond the face, for instance, encircling the arch of the aorta and in the cardiac septum. This was confirmed by Kirby[16] who followed labelled neural crest

Figure 25.1 *(a,b) Formation of cardiac septum by two actively growing ridges that approach one another until they fuse. (c) Septum formed by a single actively growing cell mass. (Reproduced with permission from Sadler TW, ed. Langman's Medical Embryology, 10th edn. Philadelphia: Lippincott, Williams and Wilkins, 2006.[13])*

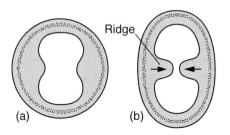 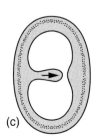

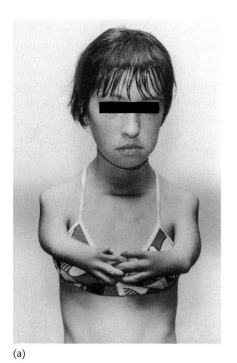

(a)

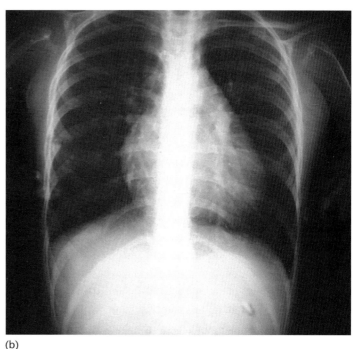

(b)

Figure 25.2 *(a) Thalidomide victim with bilateral upper phocomelia. (b) Chest X-ray of the same girl showing bilateral reduced humeri. The heart is enlarged and there is fluid overload in the pulmonary vessels, consistent with a left-to-right shunt due to an atrial septal defect.*

nuclei into the cardiac septum in chick embryo. Kirby, Gale and Stewart[16] did bilateral extirpations of chick neural crest at somites 1 and 2 and caused cardiac septal defects and transposition of the great vessels.

Interpretation by neural crest injury

Damage to autonomic innervation through the cervical sympathetic at C3–6 would damage neurotrophism and reduce the number of mitoses downstream. Reduction in cell mass of the developing ridge or ridges would mean that they fail to grow and meet as intended, and a gap in the septum would result. Hence ASD and VSD can be explained as neural crest defects.

Malformations of the ear

Of the 894 notified British cases,[2] 89 (10%) had ear deformities: anotia, microtia, accessory auricles and other external malformations, mainly bilateral and more or less symmetrical. Of 40 live children with definite thalidomide history, 16 had ear malformations alone. Others had combinations of ear with limb, or of ear with eye defects. More limb deformities were associated with eye defects than with ear defects.

Smithells and Newman[2] note that the combination of ear, eye and other associated defects is the second most common group after limb reductions; such complexes occur in a variety of permutations and combinations. Associations include external ocular palsies, facial nerve palsy, disorders of lacrimation, cleft palate, bifid uvula, hypoplasia of mandible with occlusal problems, and choanal atresia.

External ear (Figures 25.3 and 25.4)

Abnormalities of the pinna were diagnosed by inspection. Anotia is complete absence, (with the external meatus being a blind pit,) and associated profound deafness (Figure 25.4). Microtia is a less severe form, with a reduced pinna. Accessory auricles are irregular small soft skin tags at the site, sometimes associated with reduction of the pinna.

The external auditory meatus could be stenosed, tortuous, or absent altogether and replaced by a tiny pit. Accrued secretions sometimes led to cholesteatoma.

Middle ear (Figure 25.5)

D'Avignon and Barr[17] in 1964 reported 14 Swedish thalidomide infants with microtia or anotia. Of them, 11 had facial palsy, 10 had strabismus, and 8 had palatal palsy, vestibular dysfunction or were completely deaf. All 14 had some degree of impaired hearing; 8 had ossicular chain defects on X-ray. Only 6 had limb defects.

Abnormalities of the middle ear were confirmed by European clinicians in 1964,[18–19] and later in the English literature by radiologists using the then new technology of polytomography.[20–22] A British ENT surgeon, Livingstone,[23] recorded the disordered surgical

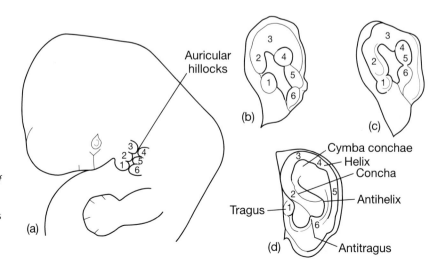

Figure 25.3 *Embryology of the pinna. (a) Lateral view of head showing six hillocks surrounding dorsal end of first pharyngeal cleft. (b–d) Fusion and progressive development of the hillocks into the auricle. (Reproduced with permission from Sadler TW, ed.* Langman's Medical Embryology, *10th edn. Philadelphia: Lippincott, Williams and Wilkins, 2006.[13])*

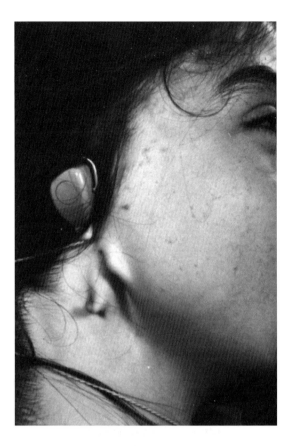

Figure 25.4 *Thalidomide child, deaf, with anotia and accessory auricles. She also had strabismus and right facial palsy.*

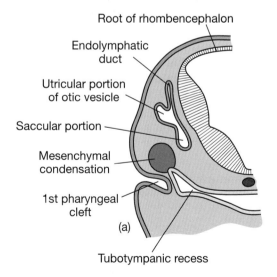

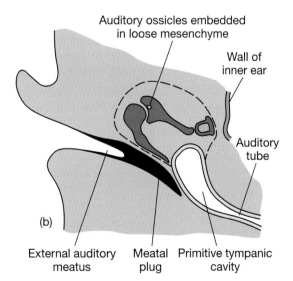

Figure 25.5 *(a) Transverse section of ear of 7-week embryo showing first pharyngeal cleft, tubotympanic recess and mesenchymal condensation in advance of development of the ossicles. (b) Middle ear showing the cartilaginous precursors of the auditory ossicles. Dashed line = future expansion of primitive tympanic cavity. (Reproduced with permission from Sadler TW, ed. Langman's Medical Embryology, 10th edn. Philadelphia: Lippincott, Williams and Wilkins, 2006.[13])*

anatomy, with later reports by Marquet,[24] among others. Over time, large contributions were made by Scandinavian, and particularly Swedish, specialists.

The middle ear cavity was sometimes full of cellular material. The three bones of the ossicular chain were abnormal in size and shape, absent totally or in part, with dislocation and/or fusion. High-definition computed tomography (CT) has now replaced poly-tomography as the investigation of choice for such lesions.

Thalidomide is the principal human teratogen recognized to affect the middle ear. A wide range of ossicular chain defects have been reported including hypoplasia, aplasia, malformation and fusion of the malleus, incus and/or stapes, fixation of the stapes to the oval window, and absence of the oval window.

Inner ear (Figure 25.6)

The inner ear was not spared by thalidomide. Polytomography and CT of the petrous temporal bone have established diagnoses that were once made only at autopsy. Polytomography or CT can show many abnormalities of the cochlea, ranging from total failure of growth of the otic vesicle to maldevelopment of the cochlea, with an incomplete number of turns.[20-21]

Vestibular system (Figure 25.7)

Malformations of the semicircular canals have been less well studied than those of the cochlea. Our knowledge of the spectrum of malformation of the vestibular apparatus is limited. With polytomography or high–resolution CT in cases with sensorineural hearing loss, abnormalities of vestibular system are found. While disorders of both are well recognized, it is difficult to establish an incidence for pure vestibular dysplasias. A large vestibular aqueduct has been described, with and without anomalies of semicircular canals or cochlea, and even without vestibular symptoms.

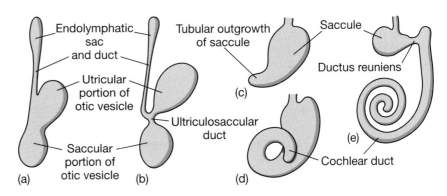

Figure 25.6 *Embryology of the inner ear. (a,b) Development of the otocyst into a dorsal utricular part that will form vestibular apparatus, and a ventral saccular portion that will develop into the cochlea. (c,d,e) Cochlear duct at 6, 7 and 8 weeks respectively. (Reproduced with permission from Sadler TW, ed. Langman's Medical Embryology, 10th edn. Philadelphia: Lippincott, Williams and Wilkins, 2006.[13])*

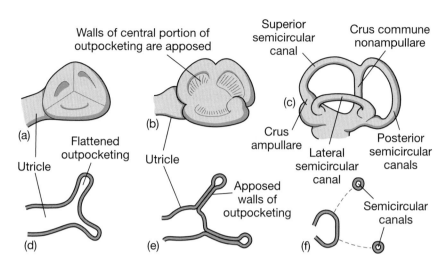

Figure 25.7 *Embryology of the vestibular system (semicircular canals). (a) 5 weeks. (b) 6 weeks. (c) 8 weeks. (d,e,f) Apposition, fusion and disappearance, respectively, of the central portions of the semicircular outpocketings. (Reproduced with permission from Sadler TW, ed. Langman's Medical Embryology, 10th ed. Philadelphia: Lippincott, Williams and Wilkins, 2006.[13])*

Interpretation by neural crest injury

Thalidomide's teratogenicity was consistently neuropathic in the cranial neural crest area, with facial palsy, external ocular palsies and other neurological lesions in association with anotia and microtia.[17–24]

According to the neural crest theory, ear defects are reduction deformities due to cranial crest injury that halts mitosis. Further development of dependant organs is arrested in mid-course. Arrest of development of the pinna before hillocks form results in anotia. Neural crest injury just after the hillocks appear leaves them as persisting accessory auricles. Later, nerve injury arrests development before the pinna has completed its growth, leaving insufficient cells to proceed. Thus, microtia and anotia can be construed as reduction deformities of the auricles due to failure of mitosis at different times. As Lenz originally observed, the timing of the thalidomide injury determines the dysmorphology.

In the middle ear, ossicles were absent, or present but deformed, smaller than normal, fused together, or dislocated. These are the same signs as in bones of the limbs (Chapters 7, 8, 10 and 11) and have already been explained as signs of embryonic neuropathy. These signs indicate that embryonic neuropathy affects the ossicular chain in exactly the same way as it affects the long bones.

In the inner ear, the cochlear canal normally achieves 2.5–2.7 spiral turns. A reduced number of turns in the cochlear spiral (usually 1–1.5) is a reduction deformity due to insufficient mesenchymal mass to complete the elongation of the cochlear duct.

The association of ear defects with cranial nerve palsies is no surprise once the primary neuropathology of physical defects is recognized, with cranial neural crest as the target organ.

Malformations of the eye

The MOH report[2] states that 'the general type of deformity was of underdevelopment varying from anophthalmia to coloboma' in its 37 cases. Some eye defects were relatively slight (e.g. ptosis or strabismus), compared with gross defects such as anophthalmia and microphthalmia.

Strabismus

Strabismus is usually due to paralysis of one of the external ocular muscles, due to abnormality of the nerve supply from the 3th, 4th or 6th cranial nerves. It was often associated with facial (7th) nerve palsy. External ocular palsy was commonly associated with eye abnormalities, and was more common in thalidomide embryopathy than in the normal population.[1]

Coloboma (Figure 25.8)

Coloboma is a slit in the iris or deeper uveal structures (see Figure 25.8c). Coloboma of the iris, with or without coloboma of the retina, was the most common eye malformation in the British series. It was

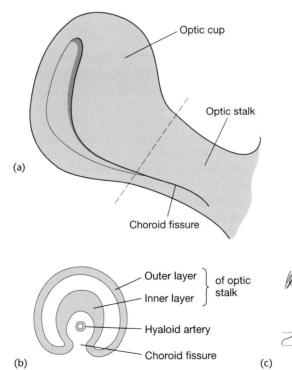

Figure 25.8 *(a) Embryology of the optic cup and stalk at 6 weeks. The choroid fissure is on the undersurface of the optic stalk. (b) Transverse section through the optic stalk. (c) Coloboma of the iris: the cleft can involve deeper structures as well. (Reproduced with permission from Sadler TW, ed. Langman's Medical Embryology, 10th edn. Philadelphia: Lippincott, Williams and Wilkins, 2006.[13])*

quite often associated with underdevelopment of the globe, presenting as anophthalmos or microphthalmos.[2]

The iris and uveal tract form by circular growth and union of the
edges of the choroid (or fetal) fissure (see Figure 25.8a–c).[13]

Anophthalmos and microphthalmos

Anophthalmos is defined as the apparent absence of the globe in
an orbit that otherwise contains normal adnexal elements.
Microphthalmos is reduction in volume of the globe (<20 mm
anteroposterior) with reduced corneal diameter.[25] Eyelids are normal
but the slit is short. Conjunctiva and lacrimal glands are present.
Rudiments of structures derived from optic vesicle, mesoderm and
neural crest are not present in primary anophthalmia. The orbit is
shallow and its volume remains small with increasing age, 'apparently
because of the absence of a trophic action of the globe on the orbit':[25]

> 'Primary anophthalmia is extremely rare and results from failure
> of the optic vesicle to bud from the cerebral vesicle; the optic
> nerves and tract are usually absent.'

Congenital paradoxical lacrimation

'Crocodile tears' or tear–saliva syndrome was occasionally associated
with ear defects and abnormal eye movements. When food is eaten,
tears rather than saliva are secreted (called after the 'sad' crocodile
who weeps rather than salivates as he devours his prey). Tears fail to
be secreted when crying. The pathology is said to be incorrect nerve
connections in the brainstem – another example of *aberrant innervation*. This odd phenomenon is not unique to thalidomide,[2] but Miller
and Strömland[26] found it in 20% of 86 Swedish thalidomiders with
ophthalmic problems in 1999. All 17 cases had strabismus (6th cranial
nerve), almost all had hearing (8th nerve) deficit, and most had facial
(7th) nerve defects and external ear malformations – adjacent cranial
nerves from adjacent cranial neural crest segments.

The neurological details of the abnormal connections in paradoxical
lacrimation are not yet established. Ramsay and Taylor[27] suggest that
there is nuclear damage or dysgenesis in or near the nucleus of the
sixth cranial nerve, and aberrant innervation of the lacrimal gland.

Dermoid cysts on the surface of the eye

These were uncommonly associated with ear defects.[2]

Duane syndrome

The review of ocular findings in 86 Swedish thalidomide cases by
Miller and Strömland[26] in 1999, because it was undertaken later in

life, is weighted towards less severe defects, with only three cases of
microphthalmia and four cases of coloboma. The association with
upper limb defects, including thumbs, is still 80%. (This suggests
exposure to more than one dose of thalidomide, to explain two
separate segmental levels.) But in their 43 cases of thalidomide-
induced strabismus, detailed ophthalmological tests revealed 26 cases
of Duane type – the largest single group (60%). Duane syndrome
occurs in only 1% of non-thalidomide cases of strabismus.

> 'Duane syndrome is felt to be due to *aberrant innervation* of the
> ocular muscles in most cases. The electromyographic data and a
> few autopsy cases support the concept that a branch of the third
> cranial nerve (which normally innervates the medial, inferior,
> and superior rectus and inferior oblique muscles)
> inappropriately innervates the lateral rectus muscle (normally
> innervated by the sixth nerve). In these patients there is usually
> little or no firing of the lateral rectus on attempted abduction,
> suggesting involvement with the 6th nerve either at the nuclear
> or peripheral site.'[26]

Miller and Strömland[26] believe that Duane syndrome has been underreported in the thalidomide literature because it is a difficult diagnosis to make in early childhood before the patient can cooperate with
electromyography.

Facial nerve palsy

This is commonly reported in thalidomide embryopathy involving
cranio-facial structures. Miller and Strömland[26] reported 17 of their
patients with facial palsy and associated strabismus in 82% and
external ear malformation and hearing deficit in 94%. These clusters
of craniofacial defects with *underlying aberrant innervation* provide
further support for the neural crest hypothesis as the pathogenesis of
thalidomide embryopathy.

Interpretation by neural crest injury

The pathogenetic mechanism of microphthalmia is said to be unclear,
according to Traboulsi,[25] who suggests that a defect in formation of
the secondary vitreous may lead to microphthalmia because of the
absence of expansive forces inside the eye.

However, there is also good evidence of neural crest injury as its
pathogenesis. Johnston's original thesis[15] on the migration of cranial
neural crest showed with the use of [³H]thymidine that the optic vesicle is surrounded by a mantle of neural crest cells. Assuming that
these crest cells stimulate mitoses, they will drive the vesicle's enlargement to form the globe of the normal eye. Figure 25.9 shows failure
of the neural crest to encircle the optic vesicle, which will result in

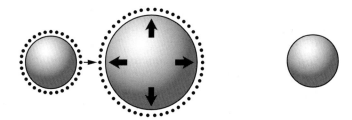

Figure 25.9 *Neural crest theory of growth of solids. Cranial neural crest cells migrate around the normal optic vesicle. Growth of the vesicle is driven by crest. If no crest cells reach the vesicle it fails to grow. This can explain anophthalmos and microphthalmos. (Reproduced with permission from McCredie J. Med J Aust 1974; 1: 159–63.[14])*

failure of neurotrophism and an eyeball that is absent (anophthalmos). Incomplete migration or reduced neurotrophism will cause a smaller than normal eye (microphthalmos).

Inadequate mitoses and reduced number of cells in the process of circular growth of the uveal tract would use up all the cells before union of the choroid fissure occurs. Insufficient cell mass to complete the full arc of growth leaves a gap: a reduction deformity of the uveal tract, presenting as incomplete growth or coloboma of the iris, choroid, or retina, or all three.

Cleft lip and palate

These occur among thalidomide victims more frequently than in the general population. However, the deformities appear to be morphologically similar to those of non-thalidomide origin.[2]

The palate normally separates the oral and nasal cavities by two shelves that grow from the lateral walls towards the midline.

Cleft palate (Figure 25.10 and 25.11) can be construed as a reduction deformity whereby the growth towards the midline halts, short of its destination, and leaves a gap between the two shelves.

The cranial neural crest is known to form at least 90% of facial structures, including the facial skeleton.[15] Neurotoxic damage during cell division would halt its progress and leave a cleft palate and/or lip. Because the cranial neural crest cells populate the facial mesenchyme in such an overwhelming proportion, their migration is comparatively easily traced by nuclear markers rather than axons. Head and neck malformations are more extensively researched than those of limbs and other organs that depend on sensory or autonomic axons.

The dental researchers Poswillo and Johnston have led work on the cranial neural crest and its relationship with congenital deformities. Although they did not work with thalidomide itself, the birth defects they examined were part of thalidomide's embryopathy. Poswillo

Figure 25.10 *(a) Frontal section through the head of a 7.5-week embryo. The horizontal palatine shelves are growing towards the midline. (b) Ventral view of palatine shelves after removal of lower jaw and tongue. The horizontal shelves are destined to unite in the midline. (Reproduced with permission from Sadler TW, ed. Langman's Medical Embryology, 10th edn. Philadelphia: Lippincott, Williams and Wilkins, 2006.[13])*

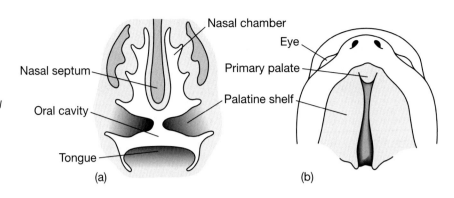

Figure 25.11 *Neural crest theory of midline growth: injury to crest halts growth towards the midline and leaves a midline gap, for example cleft palate. (Reproduced with permission from McCredie J. Med J Aust 1974; 1: 159–63.[14])*

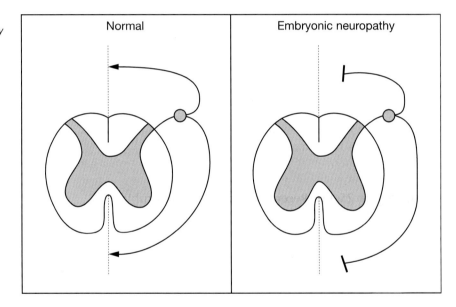

looked at the role of cranial crest in forming palate, mandible and limbs,[28] and 1st and 2nd branchial arch syndromes.[29] In experiments on the effect of excess vitamin A in pregnant rats and mice, Poswillo[30] induced Treacher–Collins syndrome in their offspring, and recorded disappearance of the anterior part of the neural crest (which relates to head structures). Poswillo attributed these malformations to deficiency of the neural crest component of facial mesenchyme.

Association between oral clefts and exposure to drugs in pregnancy was evident.[31] The cranial neural crest mechanism of malformations in the head and neck (Figure 25.11) has been firmly established in laboratory animals, using drugs other than thalidomide.[32–39]

Alimentary tract malformations

Tracheo-oesophageal complex

The trachea and oesophagus begin as one cavity, the foregut. When the embryo is about 4 weeks old, the respiratory diverticulum buds off the ventral wall of the foregut (Figure 25.12).

The upper two-thirds of the oesophagus develops a muscular wall of striated muscle, which is innervated by the vagus nerve. The lower third is smooth muscle, innervated by autonomic nerves from the splanchnic plexus.

Tracheo-oesophageal fistula (TOF) results from failure of closure of the tracheo-oesophageal septum (Figure 25.13). The cause of this failure is debated. Spontaneous deviation of the septum, or some mechanical factor pushing the dorsal wall of the foregut anteriorly, are hypothetical reasons without convincing rationale.

Oesophageal stenosis and atresia were certainly part of the British thalidomide experience,[1] although, strangely, there was no record of TOF. Many dead babies were simply labelled as multiple malformations without any details, leaving open the possibility that TOF could have been present in some. On the other hand, textbooks of birth defects treat oesophageal atresia, stenosis and TOF as one complex entity. Associated with this entity in non-thalidomide cases are cardiac, genito-urinary, anorectal, skeletal and other gastro-intestinal anomalies.[40] The embryology of TOF is therefore included here because of its integral relationship with oesophageal stenosis and atresia (Figure 25.13). Recent research in a doxorubicin rodent model of oesophageal atresia/TOF has shown inadequate mesenchyme at the site of the oesophageal lesions in the early embryo.[40]

Lungs did not escape thalidomide's attack. Abnormal lung lobation was recorded: the normal branching of the lung buds into bronchi and lobes was disordered in some cases.

The neural crest theory explains the complex of TOF as failure of innervation/mitosis of the oesophageal wall and its partition from the respiratory tract. Inadequate numbers of cells cannot complete the

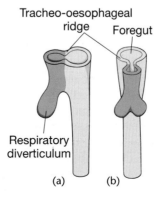

Tracheo-oesophageal ridge   Foregut

Respiratory diverticulum

(a)   (b)

Figure 25.12 *Tracheo-oesophageal separation: Embryonic growth towards midline fusion. (a) The respiratory diverticulum appears. (b) The tracheo-oesophageal septum separates it from the foregut, by union of 2 vertical ridges. (Reproduced with permission from Sadler TW, ed. Langman's Medical Embryology, 10th edn. Philadelphia: Lippincott, Williams and Wilkins, 2006.[13])*

Figure 25.13 *Variations of oesophageal atresia and/or tracheo-oesophageal fistula in order of their frequency of appearance: (a) 90%; (b) 4%; (c) 4%; (d) 1%; (e) 1%. (Reproduced with permission from Sadler TW, ed. Langman's Medical Embryology 10th edn. Philadelphia: Lippincott, Williams and Wilkins, 2006.[13])*

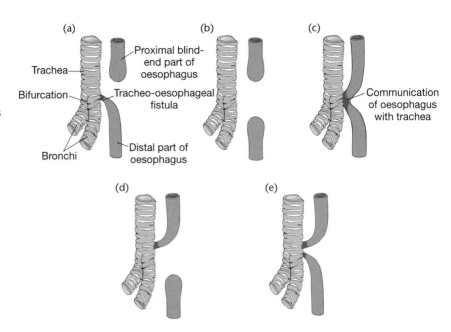

formation of the septum and/or the middle third of the oesophagus, where vagal and autonomic innervations intersect.

The first visible evidence of oesophageal atresia/stenosis/TOF in animal models is an insufficiency of mesenchyme in that region compared with normal controls. This is consistent with a failure of mitosis of undifferentiated mesenchymal cells, which in turn is consistent with embryonic autonomic neuropathy.

Duodenal atresia

The foregut becomes the midgut in the duodenum, immediately distal to the liver bud, the site of duodenal atresia or stenosis. Failure of continuity of the gut lumen here causes vomiting in the newborn baby, and is diagnosed by plain X-ray of the abdomen. The classical 'double bubble' sign is two pockets of air – one in the stomach and one in the proximal duodenum – as in Case 1 in Chapter 7 (Figure 25.14). This is a surgical emergency. The baby will perish unless the lumen is re-constituted.

Atresias and stenoses can occur anywhere in the intestine, but are most common in the duodenum. The natural incidence is 1 in 10000. Again, the pathogenesis is debated. Vascular occlusion with infarction secondary to malrotation, gastroschisis or omphalocoele may cause segmental stenosis and leave a narrowing or a fibrous cord. A less popular hypothesis is that, its lumen having theoretically been solid, the duodenum fails to recanalize in the 2nd month. There is some doubt as to whether the duodenum does have a solid stage. This has not been found in dissection of normal embryos.

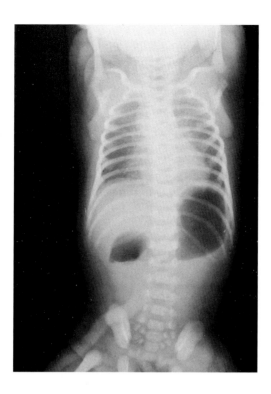

Figure 25.14 *Vertical film of newborn thalidomide baby with two fluid levels, one in the stomach and one in the duodenal cap. There is no gas beyond the duodenum. The 'double bubble' is diagnostic of duodenal atresia, a neonatal surgical emergency.*

While these hypotheses may account for some cases, they are unlikely to explain those atresias and stenoses that were part of the thalidomide syndrome, especially when associated with limb defects. Such hypotheses require a neurotoxin to change its target from nerve to blood vessel, or to whatever mechanism governs recanalization of the duodenal lumen.

Biliary malformations

The neural crest theory can explain biliary atresia and stenosis as failure of mitosis due to injury to the autonomic nerve supply at the site in the duodenum where foregut becomes midgut. Transition from one segmental nerve supply to another makes such a segment vulnerable. According to the thalidomide timetable, the insult would occur in the 4th week.

The biliary tree arises from the second part of the duodenum along with the hepatic bud. Stenosis and atresia of the bile ducts, absence and also duplication of the gallbladder were reported in thalidomide embryopathy (Figures 25.15 and 25.16). Atresia of extrahepatic bile ducts is potentially both lethal and surgically correctable, whereas the malformations of the gallbladder are usually asymptomatic unless complicated. Duplication of the gallbladder could be due to irritation rather than suppression of nerve supply, with excess mitoses allowing duplication, similar to the proposed mechanism of polydactyly.

Figure 25.15 *Malformations of the biliary tree. (a) Atresia of common bile duct, a lethal malformation. Obliteration of the common bile duct results in dilatation of gall bladder and hepatic ducts behind the blockage. (b) Duplication of gallbladder, an asymptomatic condition. (Reproduced with permission from Sadler TW, ed. Langman's Medical Embryology, 10th edn. Philadelphia: Lippincott, Williams and Wilkins, 2006.[13])*

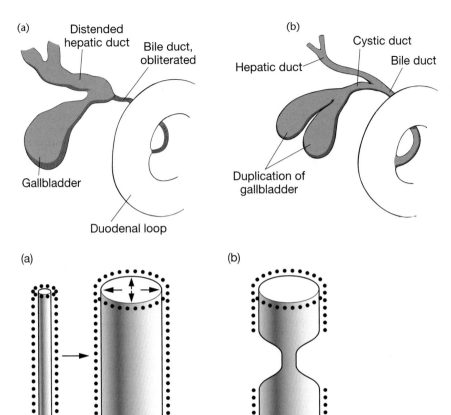

Figure 25.16 *Neural crest theory of cylindrical growth arrest based on absence of innervation. (a) Normal cylindrical growth in the presence of a mantle of neural crest cells. (b) Failure of growth in an aganglionic segment of bowel, for example Hirschprung's disease and possibly other atresias and stenoses. (Reproduced with permission from McCredie J. Med J Aust 1974; 1: 159–63.[14])*

Anorectal malformations

The cloaca of the early embryo is the common end to the urinary and gastrointestinal systems. It is divided into two cavities by the urorectal septum, which grows down to form the perineum as it reaches the skin, thus separating the genitourinary systems from the anorectal canal. At the end of the 7th week, the cloacal membrane ruptures to form the anus (Figure 25.17).

If the separation by the septum is incomplete (Figure 25.18), urorectal and rectovaginal fistulae are left at the site.

In thalidomide embryopathy, absence of the vagina and malformations of the uterus were commonly recorded in autopsies of perinatal deaths.[41] These were usually associated with lethal malformations of the cardiovascular, anorectal or urinary systems, but not necessarily with limb reduction. *Langman's Medical Embryology*[13] says:

> 'If the sinovaginal bulbs fail to fuse or do not develop at all, a double vagina, or atresia of the vagina, respectively, result.'

Survivors with absence of the genital tract were diagnosed during adolescent or reproductive years.

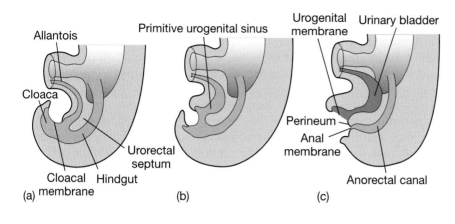

Figure 25.17 *Embryology of the perineum. (a) The hindgut enters the cloaca posteriorly and the urinary tract anteriorly. (b) The urorectal septum grows closer to the cloacal membrane. (c) The cloacal membrane breaks down to create openings for the hindgut posteriorly and the urogenital sinus anteriorly. The tip of the urorectal septum becomes the perineum. (Reproduced with permission from Sadler TW, ed. Langman's Medical Embryology, 10th edn. Philadelphia: Lippincott, Williams and Wilkins, 2006.[13])*

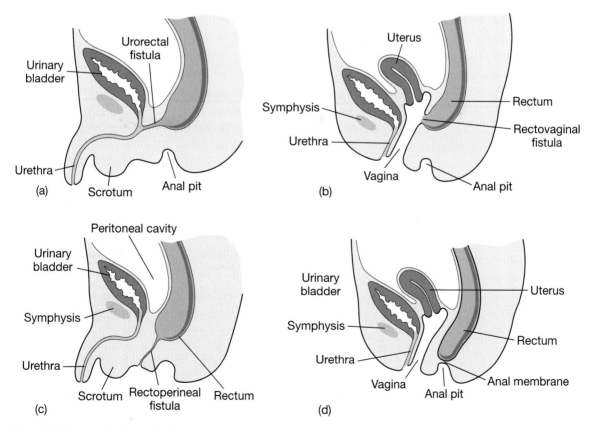

Figure 25.18 *Rectal and urogenital malformations. (a) Urorectal fistula. (b) Rectovaginal fistula. These result from incomplete separation by urorectal septum. (c) Rectoperineal fistula, which may result from vascular accident. (d) Imperforate anus due to failure of anal membrane to break down. (Reproduced with permission from Sadler TW, ed. Langman's Medical Embryology, 10th edn. Philadelphia: Lippincott, Williams and Wilkins, 2006.[13])*

Discussion

Failure of growth of the rectum to its destined length may be due to failure of the last segment of its nerve supply to generate the cell mass and length needed to complete the anus and rectum. The rectum is therefore short and does not reach the anal pit, or its distal segment is stenosed and dislocated (Figure 25.18).

In thalidomide embryopathy, anorectal and genitourinary malformations were often associated with lower limb reduction deformities. This argues in favour of both being due to sacral neural crest injury (Figure 25.16).

In general, apart from Hirschprung's disease, abnormalities of nerve supply to the gut are under-researched.[42] Tissue preparation as described by Smith[42] is recommended.

There is a dearth of research into the pathology and pathogenesis of internal organ defects in thalidomide survivors: an animal model with those internal defects induced by thalidomide is possibly too difficult to establish.

Conclusions

1. The internal malformations that featured in thalidomide embryopathy represent early or intermediate stages in normal embryogenesis of the organ concerned.
2. This developmental arrest is consistent with earlier neural crest injury, whereby the autonomic nervous system and/or cranial neural crest fail/s to stimulate cell division, and organ growth stops short of its destined endpoint.
3. Bearing in mind that no thalidomide defects were unique to thalidomide,[2] it follows that many similar, but non-thalidomide, defects share the same mechanism of pathogenesis.

References

1. Ministry of Health Reports on Public Health and Medical Subjects No. 112. *Deformities Caused by Thalidomide*. London: HMSO, 1964.
2. Smithells RW, Newman CG. Recognition of thalidomide defects. *J Med Genet* 1992; **29**: 716–23.
3. Lenz W. Thalidomide and congenital malformations. *Lancet* 1962; **i**: 45.
4. Lenz W. Das Thalidomid Syndrom. *Fortschr Med* 1963; **81**: 148–55.
5. Leck IM, Millar EL. Incidence of malformations since the introduction of thalidomide. *BMJ* 1962; **ii**: 16–20.
6. Smithells RW, Leck IM. The incidence of limb and ear defects since the withdrawal of thalidomide. *Lancet* 1963; **i**: 1095–7.
7. Kreipe U. Missbildungen innere Organs bei Thalidomid-Embryopathie. *Arch Kinderheit* 1967; **176**: 55–61.
8. Newman CGH. Teratogen Update: Clinical aspects of thalidomide embryopathy – a continuing preoccupation. *Teratology* 1985; **32**: 133–44.

9. Newman CGH. The thalidomide syndrome: risks of exposure and spectrum of malformations. *Clin Perinatol* 1986; **13**: 555–73.

10. Quibell EP. The thalidomide embryopathy: an analysis from the UK. *Practitioner* 1981; **225**: 721–6.

11. Pleiss G. Thalidomide and congenital abnormalities. *Lancet* 1962; **i**: 1128–9.

12. Kida M, ed. *Thalidomide Embryopathy in Japan*. Tokyo: Kodansha, 1987.

13. Sadler TW, ed. *Langman's Medical Embryology*, 10th edn. Philadelphia: Lippincott Williams & Wilkins, 2006.

14. McCredie J. Embryonic neuropathy: a hypothesis of neural crest injury as the pathogenesis of congenital malformations. *Med J Aust* 1974; **1**: 159–63.

15. Johnston MC. A radioautographic study of the migration and fate of cranial neural crest cells in the chick embryo. *Anat Rec* 1966; **156**: 143

16. Kirby ML, Gale TF, Stewart DE. Neural crest cells contribute to normal aorticopulmonary septation. *Science* 1983; **220**: 1059–61.

17. D'Avignon M, Barr B. Ear abnormalities and cranial nerve palsies in thalidomide children. *Arch Otolaryngol* 1964; **80**: 136–40.

18. Jørgensen MB, Kristensen HK, Buch NH. Thalidomide induced aplasia of the inner ear. *J Laryngol Otol* 1964; **78**: 1095.

19. Kittel G, Saller K. Ohrmissbildungen in Beziehung zu Thalidomid. *Z Laryngol Rhinol Otol* 1964; **43**: 469

20. Brill JF, Samuel E. Radiological and microsurgical aspects of anotia due to thalidomide. *J R Coll Surg Edin* 1965; **11**: 49

21. Rosendal T. Aplasia–hypoplasia of the otic labyrinth after thalidomide. *Acta Radiol Diagn* 1965; **3**: 225

22. Phelps PD. Congenital lesions of the inner ear, demonstrated by tomography. A retrospective study of 34 cases with special reference to the lateral semicircular canal. *Arch Otolaryngol* 1974; **100**: 11–18.

23. Livingstone G. Congenital ear abnormalities due to thalidomide. *Proc R Soc Med* 1965; **58**: 493

24. Marquet J. Congenital malformations and middle ear surgery. *J R Soc Med* 1981; **74**: 119–28.

25. Traboulsi EI. Developmental genes and ocular malformation syndromes. *Am J Opthalmol* 1993; **115**: 105–7.

26. Miller MT, Strömland K. Teratogen update: a review, with a focus on ocular findings and new potential uses. *Teratology* 1999; **60**: 306–21.

27. Ramsay J, Taylor D. Congenital crocodile tears: a key in the aetiology of Duane's syndrome. *Br J Ophthalmol* 1980; **64**: 518–22.

28. Poswillo D. Observations of fetal posture and causal mechanisms of congenital deformity of the palate, mandible and limbs. *J Dent Res* 1966; **45**: 584

29. Poswillo D. The pathogenesis of the first and second branchial arch syndrome. *Oral Surg* 1973; **35**: 302

30. Poswillo D. The pathogenesis of the Treacher–Collins syndrome (mandibulo-facial dysostosis). *Br J Oral Surg* 1975; **13**: 1.

31. Saxen I. Association between oral clefts and drugs taken in pregnancy. *Int J Epidemiol* 1975; **4**: 37

32. Johnston MC. The neural crest in abnormalities of the face and brain. *Birth Defects: Original Article Series* 1975; **11**(7): 1–18.

33. Hassell, JR, Greenberg JH, Johnston MC. Inhibition of cranial neural crest cell development by vitamin A in the cultured chick embryo. *J Embryol Exp Morphol* 1977; **39**: 267–71.

34. Johnston MC, Noden DM, Hazelton RD et al. Origins of avian ocular and periocular tissues. *Exp Eye Res* 1979; **29**: 27–43.

35. Millicovsky G, Ambrose LGH, Johnston MC. Developmental alterations associated with spontaneous cleft lip and palate in CL/Fr mice. *Am J Anat* 1982; **164**: 29–44.

36. Johnston MC, Vig KWL, Ambrose LJH. Neurocristopathy as a unifying concept: clinical correlations. *Adv Neurol* 1981; **29**: 97–104.

37. Sulik KK, Johnston MC, Webb MA. Fetal alcohol syndrome: embryogenesis in a mouse model. *Science* 1981; **214**: 936

38. Sulik KK, Johnston MC, Ambrose LJH, Dorgan DR. Phenytoin (Dilantin)-induced cleft lip: a scanning and transmission electron microscopic study. *Anat Rec* 1979; **195**: 243

39. Been W, Lieuw Kie Song, Limborgh J. Developmental anomalies of the lower face and hyoid cartilage due to partial elimination of the posterior mesencephalic and anterior rhombencephalic neural crest in chick embryos. *Acta Morphol Neerlando-Scand* 1984; **22**: 265–78.

40. Orford G. Oesophageal atresia and tracheo-oesophageal fistula: clinical and animal studies. PhD Thesis, University of Sydney, 2001.

41. Pleiss G. Thalidomide and congenital abnormalities. *Lancet* 1962; **i**: 1128–9.

42. Smith B. *Neuropathology of the Alimentary Tract*. London: Edward Arnold, 1972.

CHAPTER 26

Neurotomes and multiple malformation syndromes

Introduction

It has been proposed[1,2] that neural crest injury is not confined to thalidomide, and that it also explains other multiple malformation syndromes of longitudinal limb reduction deformities with associated internal organ defects but *without* thalidomide exposure. An association of anatomically unrelated skeletal and visceral defects may represent a single morphogenetic unit, sharing a segmental nerve supply. This chapter examines that proposal.

The neurotome concept

Whatever the unknown chemical site of action of a toxin (such as thalidomide) upon the neural crest, the result is total or partial failure of growth of tissues supplied by that segment of the neural crest (Chapters 21–25). A new term, 'neurotome', was introduced by us in 1976[1] to embrace all fields supplied by all divisions of one neural crest segment (peripheral sensory, autonomic, and other components). The concept was checked and further developed by Dr Kathryn North as part of her BSc Med project in 1982.[3]

A neurotome is a group of territories of the body supplied by one segmental level of nerve supply. It is the sum of all structures supplied by that segment, sometimes anatomically far apart. A neurotome therefore includes at least the relevant dermatome and sclerotome, plus a segmental zone of autonomic supply that we dubbed the 'viscerotome'.[2] Just as skeletal tissues in the sclerotome are absent, small or deformed by thalidomide, so the internal organs within the viscerotome may be absent, reduced in size or malformed by thalidomide or other neurotoxic agents.

The biological variants within a neurotome are similar to those within a sclerotome, as discussed in Chapters 20 and 21. Overlap onto

Chapter Summary

- Introduction
- The neurotome concept
- Concepts of neurotomes and developmental fields
- Viscerotomes and neurotomes
- Multiple malformation syndromes with upper limb defects
- Multiple craniofacial defects
- Multiple malformation syndromes with lower limb defects
- Conclusion
- References

adjacent neurotomes, modification by repair processes, etc., are operative, because a neurotome is no more rigid than a sclerotome or a dermatome.

The neurotomes could be used for classification of multiple malformation syndromes.[1,2] This approach avoids creating and naming a new syndrome to cover variations on an already-recognized group of defects.

Concepts of neurotomes and developmental fields

Opitz and Reynolds reviewed the 19th century 'developmental field' concept in an erudite historical review in a 1985 Editorial in the *American Journal of Medical Genetics*.[4] Embryologists hypothesized that there exists an intimate inter-relationship between distant parts of the embryo, and that these related parts can react together as a 'developmental field'. The developmental field concept vanished completely during the 20th century. Opitz and Reynolds saw a need for its reconsideration and noted that the 3rd edition (1982) of Moore's textbook *The Developing Human*[5] uses the word 'field' only once, referring to the 'nail field'. Small wonder that:

> 'until recently most clinical geneticists not only did not take the concept for granted, but did not know it, or, being exposed to it, were unable to connect it usefully with the observations of clinical abnormality'.[4]

Our neurotome concept revives the previous idea of the developmental field. It is the same concept really, but with a demonstrable underlying mechanism – recognizing the segmental neural crest as the underlying basis of a developmental field. Furthermore, the even older concept of developmental arrest can now be explained as damage to the neurotrophic function of the embryonic segmental nerve, with subsequent failure of mitosis within its developmental field.

Viscerotomes and neurotomes

The segmental arrangement of the autonomic nerve supply of the viscera has been depicted by Netter,[6] and is schematically modified here in Figure 26.1.

Difficult as the somatic sensory nerve fibres are to follow to their destinations, the autonomic nerve fibres are even more difficult, with more complex pathways and relays. Nevertheless, the map drawn by Netter,[6] although simplified, was based on many scientific publications.[7–17] Somite levels approximate neural crest and spinal nerve segmentation in both chick and human.[18–20]

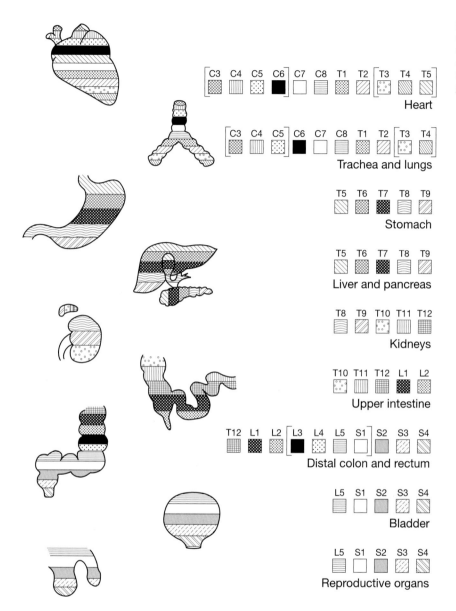

Figure 26.1 *The viscerotomes: schematic outline of segmental autonomic nerve supply to internal organs, based on Netter.[6] The stripes are purely schematic, not real.*

North[3] (1982) analysed three classical papers and compared the reviews and segmental classifications of autonomic innervation of individual organs published by Crosby et al,[21] Netter,[6] and Barr.[22] She concluded that Netter was more useful than the other two for our purpose, because only Netter made any clear differentiation between pre- and post-ganglionic sympathetic innervation. Only the post-ganglionic component is derived from the neural crest. Thus Netter's schematic segments of innervation corresponded more accurately to the embryonic neural crest origins than did either of the other two.

An approximate craniocaudal segmental order of schematic distribution in the autonomic nervous system is apparent in Figure 26.1, modified by overlap between adjacent segments (see Chapter 4: Figure 4.5). Figure 26.1 can be read in conjunction with the sclerotome maps of Inman and Saunders (see Chapter 21: Figures 21.2 and 21.3) in order to understand the associations of skeletal and visceral defects that occurred in thalidomide embryopathy and in other multiple malformation syndromes. The same spinal segmental level of nerve supply, sensory and autonomic, is identified. North designed a schematic neurotome map (Figure 26.2) for easier understanding of neural crest contributions to visceral innervation.[2,3]

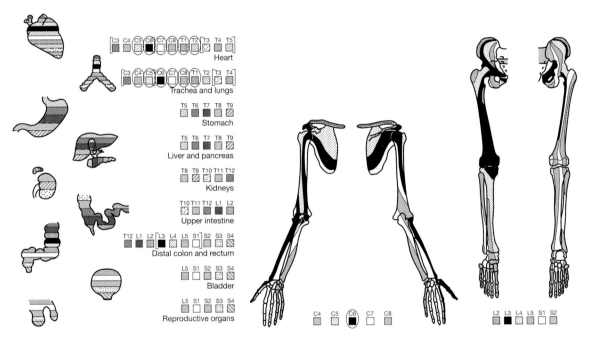

Figure 26.2 *Neurotomes: combined sclerotomes and viscerotomes, with a common key to their segments. The circled C6 sclerotome shares segmental innovation with heart, trachea, lungs and oesophagus. Thus, radial aplasia is associated with defects in these viscerotomes.*

Multiple malformation syndromes with upper limb defects

Due to thalidomide

In the British Ministry of Health (MOH) Report of 1964,[23] limb defects were recorded beside internal defects in each child. The MOH sought to record the association between limb defects and internal malformations. All cases with congenital heart disease were tabulated with their limb defects. Almost all types of congenital heart disorders were represented. Of 79 babies with mention of congenital heart disease, 69 records noted associated deficiency of upper limbs in all

Table 26.1 Number of babies alive or dead with mention of congenital heart disease. Analysis by thalidomide indication group and presence or absence of limb deformities

Thalidomide indication group	Alive		Dead		Total	
	With limb deformity	No mention of limb deformity	With limb deformity	No mention of limb deformity	With limb deformity	No mention of limb deformity
Total	28	4	41	6	69	10
I Mother certainly had thalidomide	13	1	16	1	29	2
II Mother probably had thalidomide	2	3	4	5	6	8
III No indication that mother had thalidomide	11	—	18	—	29	—
IV Mother did not have thalidomide	2	—	3	—	5	—
V Indication not clear	0	0	0	0	0	0

Reproduced from the British Ministry of Health Reports on Public Health and Medical Subjects No. 112, 1964.[23]

but one case. Ten notifications of babies with congenital heart disease did not mention limbs, and may or may not have had limb defects. A subgroup of the MOH collection headed 'Other cases' contained many reports with incomplete data. Many notifications simply stated 'multiple abnormalities', which curtailed further analysis. Many such babies would not have come to autopsy. The MOH's final figures on the association between limb and non-limb defects therefore understate the true situation. But this is the best data set available in the English language.

Table 26.1 shows that 90% of thalidomide-exposed infants with congenital heart disease had defects of the limbs. Almost all were upper limb, and the majority were of major degree. Only four were without limb deformity. Virtually all British thalidomide babies with congenital heart disease had upper limb defects of greater severity than thalidomide babies without congenital heart disease. This is an index of the severity of nerve injury – in neurology, involvement of autonomic nerves in sensory peripheral neuropathy indicates a major degree of nerve damage (Chapter 4).

The heart is innervated from the cervical sympathetic ganglia as well as from the vagus nerve (Table 26.2). Thalidomide damage to the cervical neural crest would reduce the whole neurotome related to the injured level or levels. This would include the post-ganglionic autonomic nerve supply to the heart, oesophagus, trachea and lungs.

Smithells and Newman[24] reviewed 30 years of clinical experience with 148 thalidomide victims, and summarized the main cardiac defects associated with thalidomide as:

> 'patent ductus arteriosus, VSD [ventricular septal defect], ASD [atrial septal defect], and pulmonary stenosis in survivors. Complex (especially conotruncal) lesions were seen among early deaths.'

They did not look at the correlation of limb and visceral abnormalities. But 30 years previously, Smithells[25] proved that thalidomide could cause major ear malformations in the absence of limb defects. It follows that individuals may exist with solely internal organ defects that have never been recognized as thalidomide-induced because longitudinal limb deficiencies became accepted as the drug's hallmark.

Not due to thalidomide

The dysmorphology of the hereditary Holt–Oram syndrome is very similar to that induced by thalidomide, featuring congenital heart disease and radial dysplasia. But Holt–Oram syndrome is a familial autosomal dominant condition.[26,27] Similarly, Roberts syndrome, SC syndrome and thrombocytopenia–absent radius (TAR) syndrome are autosomal recessive diseases that include similar upper limb defects.[24]

Table 26.2 Autonomic innervation of individual organs as defined by Crosby et al,[21] Netter[6] and Barr[22]

Organ	Crosby et al[21]		Netter[6]		Barr[22]	
	Parasympathetic	Sympathetic	Parasympathetic	Sympathetic	Parasympathetic	Sympathetic
Larynx and trachea	Vagus N	C4–T1	Vagus N	C1–C4	Vagus N	—
Bronchi and lungs	Vagus N	T3–T5	Vagus N	C5–T4	Vagus N	T3–T5
Heart	Vagus N	C3–T5, 6	Vagus N	C7–T5	Vagus N	T1–T6
Stomach	Vagus N	T5–T9	Vagus N	T5–T9	Vagus N	T5–T12
Liver and pancreas	Vagus N	T5–T9	Vagus N	T5–T9	—	—
Kidney	Vagus N	T10–L2	Vagus N	T10–T12	Vagus N	T11–L1
Suprarenal	Nil	T10–T12	Nil	T10–T12	Nil	T8–T11
Small intestine and caecum	Vagus N	T10–L1	Vagus N	T10–L1	Vagus N	T5–T12
Descending colon	S2–S4	T12–L2	S2–S4	L1–S2	S2–S4	T12–L2 or 3
Anus	S2–S4	T12–L2	S2–S4	L1–S4	S2–S4	T12–L2 or 3
Bladder	S2–S4	L12–L2	S2–S4	L3–S4	S2–S4	T12–L2 or 3
Penis and testes	S2–S4	T12–L2	S2–S4	L3–S4	S2–S4	T12–L2 or 3

Note that only Netter[6] makes any clear differentiation between pre- and postganglionic sympathetic innervation. Crosby et al[21] and Barr[22] refer primarily to the preganglionic sympathetic supply of the viscera.

Reproduced with permission from North K. BSc Med Thesis, University of Sydney, 1982.[3]

This suggests that a faulty gene in nuclei of crest cells can express itself through disordered segmental neurotome/s.

By reading the sclerotome maps (see Chapter 21: Figures 21.2 and 21.3) in conjunction with those of the autonomic nervous system (Figures 26.1 and 26.2), segment by segment, the possibility of neural crest syndromes predicted in Chapter 12 is reinforced. It was predicted that multiple malformation syndromes *not* due to thalidomide would fit similar patterns of reduction.

In retrospect, many multiple malformation syndromes not due to thalidomide do express reduction patterns similar to those we have seen in thalidomide embryopathy. Elimination of sclerotomes and neurotomes can explain many recorded syndromes of seemingly dissociated abnormalities.[28–33]

Two Australian studies examined associations of upper limb defects: with homolateral diaphragmatic hernia in four newborns[34] and with homolateral rib and vertebral defects and homolateral pulmonary agenesis in six cases.[35] None was due to thalidomide. All were consistent with neural crest injuries.

A third Australian study by North[2,3] examined consecutive perinatal autopsy reports in Sydney teaching hospitals over the previous 20 years (Table 26.3). She found 27 newborns or stillbirths with multiple congenital malformations that included longitudinal limb reduction defects. None had been exposed to thalidomide. Ninety-five percent of cases with upper limb dysmelia had associated cervicothoracic visceral anomalies (cardiac and respiratory) consistent with neurotome loss. Seventy-eight percent of babies with lower limb dysmelia had visceral defects in the associated lumbosacral neurotomes.

North found that:

- Multiple malformations can be categorized according to the segmental nerve supply (neurotomes) of the different organs involved.
- There is a strong association between visceral and longitudinal skeletal defects based on regional nerve supply.
- The study supports the possibility of a pathogenetic relationship between congenital defects and disruption of their nerve supply.

Table 26.3 Summary of results: relationship between skeletal and visceral anomalies on the basis of the neural crest contribution to the segmental innervation

Visceral defects	Related skeletal defects			
	Total in sample	**Cervicothoracic**	**Lumbrosacral**	**Nil**
Congenital heart defects	17	17	—	0
Upper respiratory tract (i.e. trachea, larynx, lungs, including tracheo-oesophageal fistula)	15	15	—	0
Lower intestine	11	—	7	4
Genitourinary	5	—	2	3

- Previously unexplained associations are neural crest defects whose pathology lies within the neural crest rather than in the defective organs themselves.

Neurotomes provide a logical explanation for the recurrent association of congenital defects within histologically different organs and anatomically distant sites, through a single site of insult in a particular zone of the neural crest.

Multiple craniofacial defects

Due to thalidomide

As discussed in Chapter 25, congenital defects of the eye such as anophthalmia, microphthalmia, coloboma and external ocular palsies were part of the thalidomide syndrome,[23] as were ear defects such as anotia, microtia, incomplete formation of the cochlea, and malformation, fusion and dislocation of the ossicles.[23,36] Associated with these major handicaps were cleft palate, bifid uvula, choanal atresia, cranial nerve palsies, transient midline haemangiomas, and hypertelorism.[23,24]

The MOH[23] reported that of 89 babies with ear deformities, 46 recorded associated limb deformity, all in the upper limbs, a few in both upper and lower limbs, but none in lower limbs only. Of a total of 37 babies with eye deformities, 35 reports recorded associated limb defects, 100% involving upper limbs or all four limbs. No cases were recorded where ophthalmic defects were associated with lower limb defects. In both ear and eye groups, a proportion of case records received by the MOH contained no comment on the limbs.

A review by Miller and Strömland[37] of 86 Swedish thalidomiders with ocular problems found high incidences of Duane syndrome, 'crocodile tears' and aberrant nerve connections to external ocular muscles. These are thought to be due to abnormalities of innervation (Chapter 25). Eighty percent had associated upper limb defects, illustrating injury in at least two different neurotomes, consistent with multiple doses of the drug.

Not due to thalidomide

All these birth defects occur without known cause – either alone or in conjunction with deformities in other systems of the body.[29,38]

Cranial neural crest injury explains associations of ear, eye and other craniofacial defects – suspicion that neural crest pathology was responsible in the head is not new. Hövels[39] and Stark[40] thought that Treacher Collins syndrome (which includes microtia, microphthalmia and coloboma) was a neural crest disorder (Chapter 25).

Head and neck research forged ahead of the rest of the body thanks to a dental researcher. Johnston[14] traced ^{3}H-labelled cranial neural crest nuclei into the developing facial structures, and showed that 90% of facial mesenchyme is derived from the cranial neural crest (Chapter 13). Subsequently, a number of clinical and experimental papers endorsed abnormal cranial neural crest as the underling pathology of many craniofacial syndromes of multiple malformations.[41–43] The following are examples.

In 1983, Kirby et al[44] showed neural crest cells in the septum of the heart. Kirby and Bockman[45] projected their experimental findings on cranial crest migration to include several clinical syndromes modelled by their chick experiments. They had excised segments of cranial and upper cervical neural crest and caused multiple malformations in chick embryos: clusters of developmental defects of the heart and great vessels plus thymus, parathyroids and other derivatives of the embryonic pharyngeal apparatus.

> 'The connective tissue derivatives of neural crest are necessary for normal development of these structures, and there is new experimental evidence that depletion of neural crest causes defects similar to these clinical syndromes. Therefore it is proposed that many of these syndromes are due to inappropriate development of neural crest.'[45]

They noted that, in addition to clinical entities such as Pierre Robin and DiGeorge syndromes, many teratogenic agents (dextroamphetamine, several azo dyes, X-rays, vitamin A deficiency and excess, and trypan blue) mimic neural crest extirpation.

Siebert et al[46] studied the CHARGE syndrome (a constellation of choanal atresia, coloboma, heart defects, physical or mental retardation, and genital and ear anomalies), and concluded that:

> 'many of these defects seem to result from abnormalities in the development, migration or interaction of cells of the cephalic neural crest.'

Lammer et al[47] studied 21 malformed infants from 154 pregnancies in teenage girls who had taken retinoic acid derivatives for recalcitrant acne. Ten infants had combined central nervous system, cardiac and ear defects. They concluded that:

> 'It is possible that a common teratogenic mechanism is responsible for much of the pattern – e.g., an inhibitory effect on the normal activity and interactive influence of cephalic neural crest cells.'

In 1984, Been et al[48] published a study of micro-laser excisions of particular sections of cranial neural crest in chick embryos. They induced hypoplastic mandibular structures (lower beak), some with midline cleft and absence of the tongue. They concluded that the malformations must be attributed to a lack of sufficient neural crest cells in these areas. In addition to confirming by laser injury that the cranial neural crest contributes to Meckel's and hyoid cartilages, they stressed the quantitative factors: the local deficiency was only seen in some of their chicks, probably due to insufficient damage to neural crest cells in all operated embryos.

> 'Our observations seem to indicate, in addition, that normal differentiation and growth of the cartilages at least requires the availability of a minimum number of neural crest cells.'[48]

The neural crest theory probably applies to rare diseases that affect only one side of the body or one side of the face. Hemifacial hyperplasia is a rare condition where one half of the face is larger than the other. The pathogenesis is believed to be hyperplasia of the neural crest on the affected side.[49] The opposite is another rare condition – hemifacial hemiatrophy and microsomia – where one side of the face is smaller than the other. Beals[50] investigated skeletal asymmetry involving one half of the body in overgrowth or reduced growth, with different associated conditions. Any deformities that involve one side of the face or body are almost certainly mediated through the neural crest and peripheral nervous system. No other system can divide the body into right and left sides by virtue of its normal anatomic distribution.

A 1991 textbook of perinatal pathology[51] states:

> 'As most of the cranio-facial skeleton is derived from and/or specified by neural crest cells, it is hardly surprising that disturbances in the latter cause a variety of disorders.'

Multiple malformation syndromes with lower limb defects

Due to thalidomide

Lower limb defects and visceral associations were less frequent than upper limb complexes in thalidomide embryopathy. Nevertheless, reduction deformities of the legs were sometimes associated with atresia or stenosis of the colon, rectum and anus, and abnormalities of the bladder, all representing lumbosacral neurotome deletions.

The MOH report[23] confirmed these associations. The autonomic nerve supply of the bladder, genitalia, rectum and anus is L5–S4. The neural crest injury in such cases would be lower lumbar and sacral segments of the crest, and the common factor linking the limbs (L2–S2) with the internal organs is their nerve supply. That is, the damaged structures would all lie in the L2–S2 neurotomes.

Smithells and Newman[24] summarized abdominal and pelvic abnormalities associated with thalidomide as any of the following:

- Urinary tract abnormalities:
  'absent, horseshoe, ectopic, hypoplastic, rotated kidney; hydronephrosis, megaureter, ectopic ureter, vesicoureteric reflux, inert bladder'.
- Abnormalities of the genital tract:
  'undescended, small or absent testis, hypospadius, cyst of hydatid of Morgagni; vaginal atresia, interruption of the Fallopian tube, bicornuate uterus'.
- Alimentary tract abnormalities:
  'duodenal atresia, pyloric stenosis, inguinal hernia, imperforate anus with fistula, anorectal stenosis, anterior displaced anus. Congenital absence of appendix and gall bladder have been noted at necropsy'.

Smithells and Newman[24] stress that:

> 'thalidomide caused a wide variety of birth defects, not one of which was unique to that drug. Thirty years later, subjects are still coming forward (albeit in small numbers) with claims that they have birth defects which have (or may have) been caused by thalidomide taken by their mothers during early pregnancy.'

Not due to thalidomide

Lower limb defects can be predicted from the maps (see Chapters 21: Figures 21.2 and 21.3) in association with malformations of rectum, anus, bladder and external genitalia (lumbosacral neurotomes in Figures 26.1 and 26.2).

Clusters of visceral and lower limb defects unrelated to thalidomide are well recognized in the literature.[29,32,33,52–54] The caudal regression syndrome of diabetic embryopathy is an example[52] where 'pseudo-thalidomide' deformities[55] of the lower limbs are accompanied by sacral agenesis and various anorectal and vesico-urinary malformations. The multiple malformation syndromes simply tell us that thalidomide and diabetes cause sensory and autonomic neuropathy in the embryo.

Conclusion

Neural crest injury offers a logical explanation for the distribution and pathogenesis of multiple malformation syndromes that include dysmelic limb defects.

The concept is simple. It avoids both ancient terminology and modern eponym. It requires only anatomical knowledge of the segmental nerve supply to affected parts. The defect can then be named after the missing neurotome.

It unifies a number of previously unrelated conditions under the common title of 'neural crest defects'.

These comprise a natural category adjacent to the well-recognized 'neural tube defects'.

References

1. McCredie J. Neural crest defects: a neuroanatomic basis for classification of multiple malformation syndromes. *J Neurol Sci* 1976; **28**: 373–87.

2. North K, McCredie J. Neurotomes and birth defects: a neuroanatomic method of interpretation of multiple congenital malformations. *Am J Med Genet* 1987; **Suppl 3**: 29–42.

3. North K. A study of teratogenic mechanisms in the embryo. BSc Med Thesis, University of Sydney, 1982.

4. Opitz J, Reynolds JF. Editorial Comment: The developmental field concept. *Am J Med Genet* 1985; **21**: 1–11.

5. Moore KL. *The Developing Human: Clinically Oriented Embryology*, 3rd edn. Philadelphia: WB Saunders, 1982.

6. Netter FH. *The Ciba Collection of Medical Illustrations*. Volume 1: *The Nervous System*. New York: Case-Hoyt, 1975.

7. Kuntz A, Bateson OV. Experimental observations on the histogenesis of the sympathetic trunks in the chick. *J Comp Neurol* 1920; **32**: 335–45.

8. Kuntz A. Experimental studies on the histogenesis of the sympathetic nervous system. *J Comp Neurol* 1922; **34**: 1–36.

9. Kuntz A. *The Autonomic Nervous System*. Philadelphia: Lea & Febiger, 1953.

10. Jones DS. The origin of the sympathetic trunks in the chick embryo. *Anat Rec* 1937; **70**: 45–66.

11. Jones DS. Further studies on the origin of sympathetic ganglia in the chick embryo. *Anat Rec* 1941; **79**: 7–16.

12. Yntema CL, Hammond WS. Depletions and abnormalities in the cervical sympathetic system of the chick following extirpation of neural crest. *J Exp Zool* 1945; **100**: 237–63.

13. Horstadius S. *The Neural Crest*. Oxford: Oxford University Press, 1950.

14. Johnston MC. A radioautographic study of the migration and fate of cranial neural crest cells in the chick embryo. *Anat Rec* 1966; **156**: 143–56.

15. Weston JA. A radioautographic analysis of the migration and localisation of trunk neural crest cells in the chick. *Dev Biol* 1963; **6**: 279–310.

16. Weston JA. The migration and differentiation of neural crest cells. *Adv Morphogen* 1970; **8**: 41–114.

17. Le Douarin N. A biological cell labelling system and its use in experimental embryology. *Dev Biol* 1973; **20**: 217–22.

18. Romanoff AL. *The Avian Embryo – Structural and Functional Development*. New York: Macmillan, 1960.

19. Hamilton WJ, Mossman HW. *Human Embryology*. Cambridge: Heffer/ Baltimore: Williams and Wilkins,1972.

20. King AS, McLelland J. *Outlines of Avian Anatomy*. London: Baillière Tindall, 1975.

21. Crosby EC, Humphrey T, Laver EW. *Correlative Anatomy of the Nervous System*. New York: Macmillan, 1962.

22. Barr ML. *The Human Nervous System – An Anatomical Viewpoint*. Hagerstown, MD: Harper & Row, 1979.

23. Ministry of Health Reports on Public Health and Medical Subjects No. 112. *Deformities Caused by Thalidomide*. London: HMSO, 1964.

24. Smithells RW, Newman CG. Recognition of thalidomide defects. *J Med Genet* 1992; **29**: 716–23.

25. Smithells RW. Thalidomide and malformations in Liverpool. *Lancet* 1962; **i**: 1270–3.

26. Holt M, Oram S. Familial heart disease with skeletal malformations. *Br Heart J* 1960; **22**: 236

27. Kaufman RL, Rimoin D, McAlister W, Hartmann A. Variable expression of the Holt–Oram syndrome. *Am J Dis Child* 1974; **127**: 21.

28. D'Avignon M, Barr B. Ear abnormalities and cranial nerve palsies in thalidomide children. *Arch Otolaryngol* 1964; **80**: 136.

29. Rubin A. *Handbook of Congenital Malformations*. Philadelphia: WB Saunders, 1967.

30. Stoll C, Levy J-M, Francfort J-J, Roos R, Rohmer A. L'association phocomélie–ectrodactylie – malformations des oreilles avec surdité, arythmie sinusale, constitue-t-elle un nouveau syndrome héréditaire? *Arch Franc Pediatr* 1974; **31**: 669.

31. Landing H. Syndromes of congenital heart disease with tracheo-bronchial anomalies. *AJR Am J Roentgenol* 1975; **123**: 679.

32. Pinsky L. A community of human malformation syndromes involving the Mullerian ducts, distal extremities, urinary tracts and ears. *Teratology* 1974; **9**: 65–79.

33. Pinsky L. A community of human malformation syndromes that shares ectodermal dysplasia and deformities of the hands and feet. *Teratology* 1975; **11**: 227.

34. McCredie J, Reid IS. Congenital diaphragmatic hernia associated with homolateral upper limb malformation: a study of possible pathogenesis in four cases. *J Pediatr* 1978; **92**: 762–5.

35. Osborne J, Masel J, McCredie J. A spectrum of skeletal anomalies associated with pulmonary agenesis: possible neural crest injuries. *Pediatr Radiol* 1989; **19**: 125–32.

36. Brill JF, Samuel E. Radiological and microsurgical aspects of anotia due to thalidomide. *J R Coll Surg Edin* 1965; **11**: 49

37. Miller MT, Stömland K. Teratogen Update: A review with a focus on ocular findings and new potential uses. *Teratology* 1999; **60**: 306–21.

38. Norman AP. *Congenital Abnormalities in Infancy*. Oxford: Blackwell, 1971.

39. Hövels O. Zur systematik der missbildungen des I. viscaeralbogens unter desonderer berücksichtigung der dysostosis mandibulofacialis. *Z Kinderheilkd* 1953; **73**: 532–67.

40. Stark RB. The pathogenesis of harelip and cleft palate. *Plast Reconstr Surg* 1954; **13**: 20

41. Poswillo D. The pathogenesis of the Treacher Collins syndrome (mandibulofacial dysostosis). *Br J Oral Surg* 1975; **13**: 1–26.

42. Strömland K, Miller M, Cook C. Ocular teratology. *Surg Ophthalmol* 1991; 35: 429–46.

43. Johnston MC, Vig KWL, Ambrose LJH. Neurocristopathy as a unifying concept: clinical correlations. *Adv Neurol* 1981; **29**: 97–104.

44. Kirby ML, Gale TF, Stewart DE. Neural crest cells contribute to normal aorticopulmonary septation. *Science* 1983; **220**: 1059–61.

45. Kirby ML, Bockman DE. Neural crest and normal development: a new perspective. *Anat Rec* 1984; **209**: 1–6.

46. Siebert JR, Graham JM, MacDonald C. Pathologic features of the CHARGE association: support for involvement of the neural crest. *Teratology* 1985; **31**: 331–6.

47. Lammer EJ, Chen DT, Hoar RM et al. Retinoic acid embryopathy. *N Engl J Med* 1985; **313**: 837–41.

48. Been W, Song LK, Limborgh J. Developmental anomalies of the lower face and hyoid cartilage due to partial elimination of the posterior mesencephalic and anterior rhombencephatic neural crest in chick embryos. *Acta Morphol Neerl Scand* 1984; **22**: 265–78.

49. Pollock RA, Newman MH, Burdi AR, Condit DP. Congenital hemifacial hyperplasia: an embryologic hypothesis and a case report. *Cleft Palate J* 1985; **22**: 173–84.

50. Beals RK. Hemihypertrophy and hemihypotrophy. *Clin Orthop Rel Res* 1982; **166**: 199–203.

51. Wigglesworth JS, Singer DB. *Textbook of Fetal and Perinatal Pathology.* Boston: Blackwells, 1991.

52. Blumel J, Evans EB, Eggers GWN. Partial and complete agenesis or malformation of the sacrum with associated anomalies. *J Bone Joint Surg* 1959; **41A**: 497

53. Thompson W, Grossman H. The association of spinal and genito-urinary abnormalities with low ano-rectal anomalies (imperforate anus) in female infants. *Radiology* 1974; **113**: 693.

54. Obeid M, Corkery J. Importance of the urinary tract in imperforate anus. *Proc R Soc Med* 1974; **67**: 203.

55. Lenz W. Bone defects of the limbs – an overview. *Birth Defects: Original Article Series* 1969; **5**(3): 1.

CHAPTER 27

Hands and feet in thalidomide embryopathy: Histology and sclerotomes in the digits

Having defined the pattern of thalidomide dysmelia in the long bones of the limbs in German in 1968–69[1,2] and in English in 1969,[3] Willert and Henkel published the pattern of dysmelia in the hand and feet[4] in 1970, based on about 300 cases in Germany and Switzerland, with all radiographs and some anatomical specimens including histopathology. They found the same fundamental underlying process as in the long bones of the limbs.

'Dysmorphogenesis of longitudinal reduction deformities: anatomical and histological principles expressed in the digits'[4] was never published in the English language literature on thalidomide, and has been bypassed as a reference by subsequent researchers. Yet it is a seminal paper for understanding the principles behind polydactyly, syndactyly, brachydactyly (short digits) and other defects that are still being debated to this day.[5–7]

This paper was translated from German to English by my Australian friends Mrs Gertrude Muldoon and Professor Ernest Finck (retired Director of Sydney's largest Institute of Pathology). Professor Willert and I revised the discussion in 2004, in order to incorporate three decades of biological research that we thought shed light on the pathogenesis of these birth defects. Further revision was suspended by his failing health. The paper is published here for the first time in English and dedicated to the memory of Professor Willert, who died on 25 September 2006. The contributions of Professors Willert and Henkel to international research into thalidomide embryopathy rank with those of the great Professor Lenz.

Introduction

Of the five anatomical subgroups of longitudinal reduction deformities of the hands and feet (radial, tibial, ulnar, fibular and central), radial and tibial reduction defects were the hallmark of thalidomide

Chapter Summary

- Introduction
- Materials and methods
- Radiology of reduction in the radial digits
- Histology of reduction in the radial digits
- Supernumerary skeletal elements of radial and tibial rays
- Histology of supernumerary skeletal elements
- Discussion
- Sclerotomes and the distribution of defects
- Embryology of the digits
- The cell cycle and neurotrophism: apoptosis and interdigital spaces
- Conclusion
- References

embryopathy. The radial rays of the hand were most commonly affected, then the radius itself, followed by the humerus. In the leg, the tibia, tibial ray of the foot and the femur were affected in that order.

Central, ulnar and fibular reduction defects did not occur in thalidomide embryopathy.

Single cases of malformations in all five anatomical subgroups were recorded both before and after the thalidomide era of 1958–62. During that short period there was a steep rise in the incidence of radial and tibial reductions, but not of the other three groups.[4]

Materials and methods

In the Willert and Henkel thalidomide cases, developmental changes in the radial fingers or tibial toes appeared alone, or combined with reductions in the radius or tibia respectively. The changes were of two main types: reductions or additions.

In the hand, reductions were characteristic. Additions such as triphalangeal thumb or polydactyly were relatively rare, and occurred mainly with less severe reductions of the radius.

The facts were different in the foot. Digital reductions were rare. As a rule, the toes were unaffected, even in cases of severe reduction in tibia or femur.[8] Additions sometimes occurred on the tibial aspect of the foot in the form of triphalangeal hallux or polydactyly.[9,10] Reductions in the hallux similar to those in the thumb are on record, but are exceptional.

Radiology of reduction in the radial digits

Thumb (Figure 27.1)

Reduction begins in the thumb and proceeds from the radial to the ulnar side of the hand, with increasing severity. There is a gradual reduction in mass, with narrowing in the shape and size of the 1st metacarpal, which is affected early and disappears progressively from its proximal end until this bone vanishes completely. The phalanges

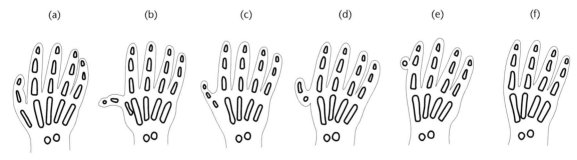

(a)   (b)   (c)   (d)   (e)   (f)

Figure 27.1 *Thumb reduction in thalidomide embryopathy. As severity of damage increases, the thumb and 1st metacarpal are reduced from normal to total absence, through hypoplastic and triphalangeal morphology to pedunculated remnants, and then no thumb at all. (Reproduced with permission from Willert HG, Henkel HL. Z Orthop Ihre Grenzgeb 1970; **107**: 663–75.[4])*

follow this proximodistal progress. In the most advanced stage of thumb reduction, a minute phalangeal vestige is attached to the radial side of the index finger.

In thalidomide infants, such a flail or pedunculated digit was non-functional (except for sucking, which encouraged oedema and infection). It was usually surgically removed.

Index finger (Figure 27.2)

After disappearance of the thumb, reduction progresses to the index finger, where there is underdevelopment of the 2nd metacarpal and its phalanges. The middle phalanx is the first to be reduced, producing brachymesophalangy or a short middle phalanx of a digit.

The middle phalanx then vanishes, so the index finger has only two out of three phalanges. Thereafter, reduction follows the same pattern as the thumb – a proximodistal progression from the base of the 2nd metacarpal. Finally, vestigial phalanges were attached to the 3rd digit as they in turn receded.

The morphology of the index finger varied from normal to complete absence. Between these two extremes, the 2nd metacarpal and phalanges were often hypoplastic. A common morphology was longitudinal bisection to create a hemisected digit, or 'hemi-digit' (see Chapter 7: Figure 7.3).

Occasionally, polydactyly of another digit (usually the middle finger) accompanied absence of the thumb and/or index finger (see Chapter 7: Figure 7.3).

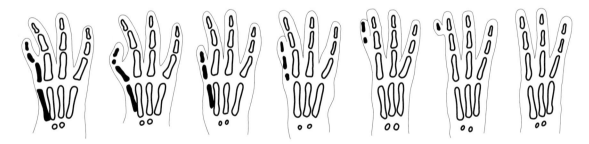

Figure 27.2 *Index finger reduction from normal to nil. The 2nd metacarpal disappears before the phalanges. Two or three phalanges may be reduced in size and/or fused to the adjacent 3rd ray by syndactyly of soft tissues or by a narrow pedicle (flail digit). (Reproduced with permission from Willert HG, Henkel HL. Z Orthop Ihre Grenzgeb 1970;* **107***: 663–75.[4])*

Third finger

Reduction of the 3rd ray follows the same pattern. In most cases, the adjoining digit shows some signs of reduction by the time its radial neighbour has diminished to a rudiment. The metacarpal disappeared ahead of the phalanges.

Interdigital spaces

In conjunction with reduction of the bones, variable soft tissue changes appear between the affected rays, representing different stages of syndactyly. They are relics of the palette stage of the embryonic hand.

Carpal bones

The carpal bones were frequently abnormal, showing absence of scaphoid and/or trapezium, and synostosis of two or more carpals in the same row. Carpal bones were frequently synchondrosed en bloc, in two rows (see Chapter 7: Figures 7.5 and 7.6) or just to their neighbouring carpal. Carpal coalition was seldom evident in X-rays at birth, because the carpals are cartilaginous and invisible on radiographs at that age. Synchondrosis is seen in Professor Willert's pathology specimens (see Figures 27.3–27.5). Carpal coalition becomes visible radiologically at a later date, after ossification.

Histology of reduction in the radial digits

In the reduced radial digits, the microscopic appearance of the cells is normal, but the sizes and shapes of the bones are highly abnormal – an unusual discordance. The histological details are as follows.

Insufficient building material

Histopathology of longitudinal sections of brachymesophalangeal digits (Figure 27.3) shows that there is insufficient building material to form a normal middle phalanx. However, under the light microscope, the cartilage and bone of the skeletal rudiments show an absolutely normal structure with typically normal appearance of cells and matrix, despite the abnormal size and shape of the bone.

There was no evidence of haemorrhage, vascular pathology, cell death or necrosis. There were no abnormal mitotic figures.

Loss of normal shape

Along with reduction in mass due to a lack of building material (mesenchyme), we observed loss of normal shape of the affected bone. The normal organization of the phalanx into diaphysis, metaphysis and epiphysis was absent within these short plump rudiments. They ossify from only one centre of ossification, without formation of a bony perichondrial splint, which normally identifies the diaphysis. The epiphyseal growth plate was usually absent (anepiphyseal ossification).[10]

Joint deformity, fusion and notches

The interphalangeal joints of the reduced bones show slanted bone ends (clinodactyly and camptodactyly: Figures 27.3 and 27.4), which

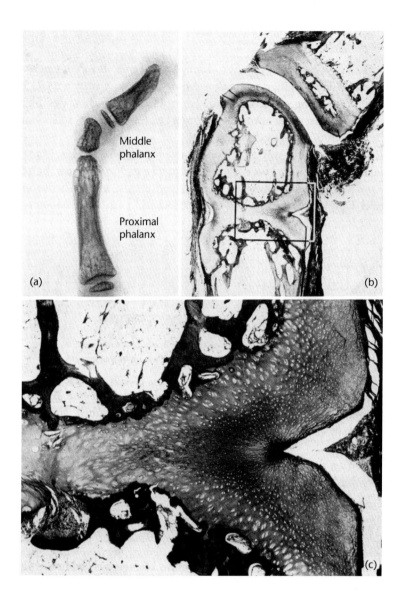

(a)

Middle
phalanx

Proximal
phalanx

(b)

(c)

Figure 27.3 *Histology of brachymesophalangy. A 5-year-old child with radial aplasia, absent thumbs, and synchondrosis of the proximal and middle phalanges of the index finger. Note the sloping bone ends at the distal interphalangeal (IP) joint. (a) X-ray showing small middle phalanx with sloping joint surface at the distal IP joint, and without epiphyses. (b) Gross histology shows no joint cleft at the proximal IP joint site. (c) Cartilaginous fusion where the proximal IP joint should be (x26). There were no abnormal cells. (Reproduced with permission from Willert HG, Henkel HL. Z Orthop Ihre Grenzgeb 1970; 107: 663–75.[4])*

frequently proved to be incorrectable. Malformations of articular surfaces are observed at neighbouring less-affected joints, for instance at the heads of the proximal phalanges and metacarpals (Figure 27.4).

Skeletal remnants are frequently attached to an adjacent, less-affected bone, to which they remain united. During infancy, this union was cartilaginous (synchondrosis), proving that the cause of the malformation predated the cartilage model (Figures 27.3 and 27.4). As enchondral ossification advances, the cartilage bridge will be replaced by a bony bridge (synostosis). At this stage, the failure of separation becomes visible on the radiograph. Sometimes the vestige of a joint cleft is seen as a lateral notch or notches at the site where the joint should have been, while in the centre the phalangeal remnants are united. Remnants of structures

Figure 27.4 *Histology of brachymesophalangy and synchondrosis of index finger. A 4-year-old boy with aplasia of the radius and thumb. The index finger shows brachymesophalangy and synchondrosis between the distal and rudimentary middle phalanges. (a) Radiograph. (b) Gross section. (c) Histology (x26). There is no evidence of any past or present joint space. There is continuous solid cartilage across the joint site. (Reproduced with permission from Willert HG, Henkel HL. Z Orthop Ihre Grenzgeb 1970; 107: 663–75.[4])*

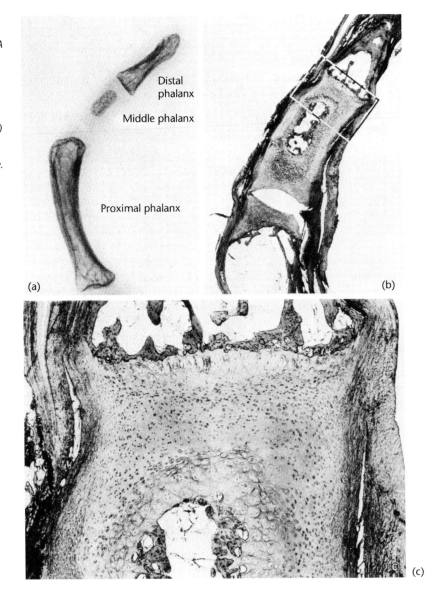

belonging to the joint capsule and ligaments are also found nearby. The cells and fibres of hyaline cartilage fanned out radially from the bottom of such clefts (Figure 27.3c). However, the cartilaginous connection to the normal phalanx could be seamless, without any trace of a joint cleft, and after ossification this appeared to be identical with assimilation–hypophalangism as in Figure 27.4.[11]

Delayed ossification

The commencement of enchondral ossification is delayed. In infancy, the various damaged skeletal elements are present as hyaline cartilage.

The middle phalanx of a malformed index finger often contains only a small ossification centre at a stage when enchondral ossification should normally have been complete (Figure 27.4).

Normal histology but disturbed maturation

Lack of ossification of hyaline cartilage is also evident in malformed thumbs (Figure 27.5). With light microscopy, no structural change could be found in the cartilage to explain this phenomenon, but the delayed ossification suggested a disturbance in maturation of the cartilage resulting in deformity.

Because of the delay in ossification, radiographs in early childhood reveal only part of the picture, with hidden malformations in unossified cartilage. Ossification may not have commenced when the infant was first X-rayed. When ossification occurs, this is not new bony material, but delayed ossification of existing cartilage. If the radiographs show 'empty spaces' between the bony parts of the rudiment and the neighbouring bones, one can assume that these empty spaces contain cartilage tissue.

Brachymesophalangy

Characteristic underdevelopment of the middle phalanx during the reduction process in the radial rays expresses three morphological characteristics:

- reduction in mass and loss of normal shape of the middle phalanx and its cartilaginous growth plate

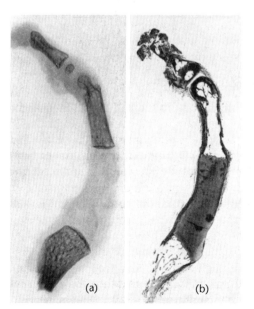

(a)   (b)

Figure 27.5 *Hypoplastic thumb fused to the index finger. A 6-year-old boy with hypoplastic thumb partially fused to the index finger. (a) Radiograph of excised hypoplastic thumb and 1st metacarpal, without a metacarpophalangeal joint. (b) Gross histology of a section showing no joint space, but a very long cartilage segment. There is a distal pseudoepiphysis on the proximal phalanx. (Reproduced with permission from Willert HG, Henkel HL. Z Orthop Ihre Grenzgeb 1970; 107: 663–75.[4])*

- impairment of joint development in less severe cases and absence of joint development in more severe cases, including absence of joint cleavage, and fusion of a rudimentary phalanx to its neighbour (synchondrosis or synostosis)
- delay in ossification of hyaline cartilage

Each of these findings is always combined with one or both of the other two. The final presentation is a matter of the degree of reduction, varying with the severity of the malformation.

Supernumerary skeletal elements of radial and tibial rays

Excess rather than insufficient building material is the main characteristic of supernumerary skeletal elements. Triphalangism of the thumb or great toe can be associated with duplication and syndactyly of the first ray, especially in the foot. As in the reduction defects, there were various stages (Figure 27.6) in the formation of the supernumerary skeletal elements.

Figure 27.6 *Teratological sequence of stages in triphalangeal thumb, with all epiphyses present in final stage. (Reproduced with permission from Willert HG, Henkel HL. Z Orthop Ihre Grenzgeb 1970; 107: 663–75.[4])*

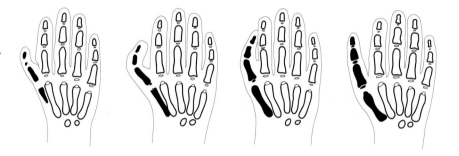

Triphalangeal thumb or hallux

For triphalangeal thumb (Figure 27.7), there are also serial degrees of malformation, the final stage being a fully developed but often weak triphalangeal digit. The additional bone is like a normal phalanx, with epiphysis, diaphysis, cartilaginous growth plate and ossification centre. The first metacarpal sometimes shows a rudimentary distal epiphysis (Figure 27.7).

In a less well-developed middle phalanx, the basal epiphysis disappears first. The additional phalanx is smaller than normal, varying in size right down to a mere bony rudiment. The corresponding first metacarpal tends to be hypoplastic. The hypoplastic form of triphalangeal thumb appears at the beginning of the teratological series and provides a link to a normal biphalangeal thumb. It seems plausible that the presence of a distal pseudo-epiphysis in a rudi-

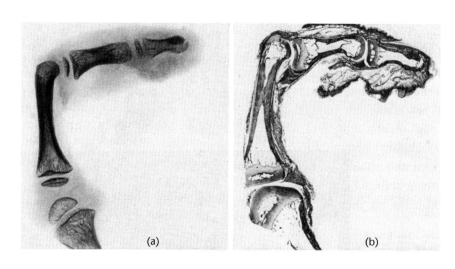

(a)   (b)

Figure 27.7 *Functionless triphalangeal thumb with epiphysis on the head of 1st metacarpal. (a) Radiograph. (b) Gross histological specimen (x16). Three phalanges are present, with an eccentric proximal interphalangeal joint surface with fixed subluxation. (Reproduced with permission from Willert HG, Henkel HL. Z Orthop Ihre Grenzgeb 1970; 107: 663–75.[4])*

mentary phalanx of a normal thumb indicates a tendency to triphalangism (see Figure 27.5).

A thumb with brachymesophalangeal triphalangism is automatically similar to a hypoplastic finger. In general, there appears to be a great similarity between the different stages of triphalangeal thumb and the reduction of the index finger.

Supernumerary toes: polydactyly

Because abnormalities of the toes were much rarer than those of the thumb and fingers in thalidomide embryopathy, the original case material is insufficient to determine whether there are corresponding variations of triphalangism between the great toe and the thumb. However, the characteristics of triphalangeal thumbs were observed in supernumerary toes on the tibial side of the foot, as long as they were triphalangeal. Underdeveloped middle phalanges in supernumerary toes mimicked brachymesophalangism (Figure 27.8).

Like reductions, duplications and supernumerary skeletal elements have been discussed in the literature, particularly the progressive stages of triphalangeal thumb, tracing every step from a barely recognized rudiment up to a normally formed middle phalanx.[11–16]

Comparing the two processes (reduction versus addition of digits), the same principles and processes are operating. The only difference between the two is the reverse direction of the deviation from the norm (minus or plus).

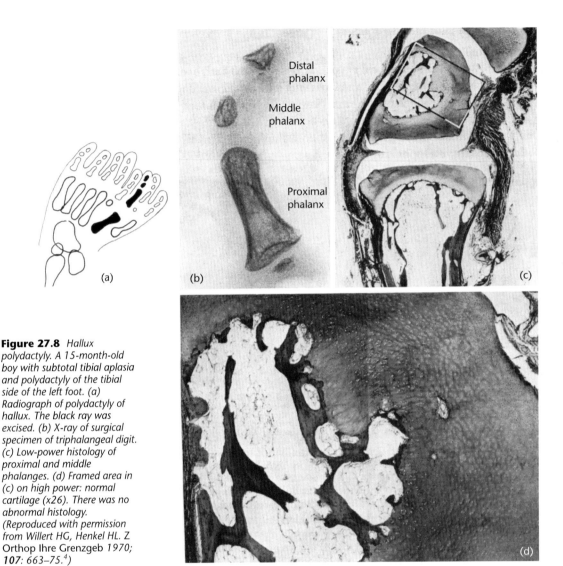

Figure 27.8 *Hallux polydactyly. A 15-month-old boy with subtotal tibial aplasia and polydactyly of the tibial side of the left foot. (a) Radiograph of polydactyly of hallux. The black ray was excised. (b) X-ray of surgical specimen of triphalangeal digit. (c) Low-power histology of proximal and middle phalanges. (d) Framed area in (c) on high power: normal cartilage (x26). There was no abnormal histology. (Reproduced with permission from Willert HG, Henkel HL. Z Orthop Ihre Grenzgeb 1970; 107: 663–75.[4])*

Histology of supernumerary skeletal elements

Normal middle phalanx

Macroscopically and microscopically, the middle phalanx of a triphalangeal thumb, having developed exactly like that of an index finger, is structurally indistinguishable from a normal phalanx (see Figure 27.7). Sometimes, the kernel of a distal epiphysis (pseudo-epiphysis) could be recognized in middle phalanges of normal size. This applies also to triphalangeal toes.

Reduced middle phalanx

If the middle phalanx is small, the proximal epiphysis disappears, but the proximal cartilaginous joint surface is still present. The changes in very small middle phalanges and triphalangeal thumbs and toes, including supernumerary toes, are the same as in the similarly reduced index fingers (brachymesophalangeal reduction): loss of normal shape, disappearance of epiphysis and diaphysis, loss of bony cortex and growth plate in the smaller rudiments, and ossification of a residual phalanx starting at the central core.

Joint deformity

Slanting joint surfaces (Figures 27.3 and 27.6) cause angulation and consequent deformities of the digit (campto- or clinodactyly), yet the histology of the cartilage and bone tissues of these supernumerary rudiments is completely normal.

Finally, slanting joint surfaces are observed at the heads of the proximal phalanges, metatarsals and metacarpals respectively, similar to reduction deformities of the radial digits. These slanting surfaces mainly point in the direction of the bend, causing an uncorrectable angulation at the affected joint (Figure 27.7). In some cases, there is fusion of the rudimentary middle phalanx to a neighbouring phalanx in the thumb or great toe.

Discussion

The outstanding feature of malformed digits was too much or too little building material (plus or minus). The quantity of undifferentiated mesenchyme in the human limb bud has rarely been addressed in the medical literature, yet it is pivotal to these digital deformities.

As discussed in previous chapters, normal growth depends upon normal neurotrophism to generate a normal number of mitoses from which the mass of mesenchymal 'building material' is composed. Neurotrophism is driven by sensory nerves, but it can be accelerated, slowed or halted by interference with the nerves or neural crest.

Segmental neural crest injury provides a mechanism for both addition and reduction in numbers of basic mesenchymal cells in peripheral developmental fields.

There is supportive evidence from animal experiments.

The first sign of polydactyly is excess mesenchyme

From his study of hundreds of thalidomide-exposed rabbits, Vickers[17–18] established that a circumscribed proliferation of mesenchyme in the preaxial edge of developing hindpaws of embryonic rabbits was the first visible sign of an accessory digit (Figure 27.9).

Figure 27.9 *Polydactyly of hallux in a black rabbit fetus exposed to thalidomide in utero. This is equivalent to polydactyly in the L5 human sclerotome.*

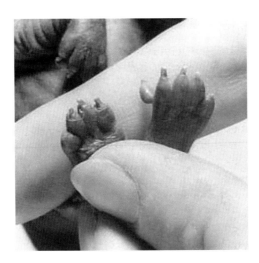

Dose specificity governs polydactyly, hypo/aplasia

Using 6-aminonicotinamide in mice, Neubert and Dillmann,[19] toxicologists and pharmacologists in Berlin, established that a 'dose specificity' exists in the embryo, whereby polydactyly results from low dose, phocomelia follows a medium dose, and amelia results from high dosage.

This can now be interpreted as a low dose irritating the nerve and causing extra mitoses, hence an extra digit; higher doses suppress nerve function in a dose-related fashion. Neurotrophic control of mesenchymal mass is biphasic, and exceeds or fails in proportion to dose. The response to dose levels exhibits the classical biphasic response of nerves to injury (Chapter 4).

Timing of dosage influences polydactyly

Skalko[20,21] has shown that limb buds in culture (excised from the trunk) do not increase in cell number, but progress to differentiation. Skalko reported that when such limb bud cultures are dosed with a polydactyly-inducing drug, no polydactyly occurs.

However, if the dam is given the drug 24 hours before the embryo is harvested, polydactyly follows in the limb bud culture.

In that 24 hours after dosage and before excision, the peripheral nerves to the embryonic limb bud are intact, still function, and neurotrophism operates. The nerves receive the stimulus for overgrowth *before* the limb bud is excised. In the first experiment, excision of limb buds for culture severs the peripheral nerves from their cell bodies in the spinal ganglia; *subsequent* stimulation of these *denervated* limb buds fails. There is no neurotrophic response, because of denervation *before* stimulation.

Sclerotomes and the distribution of defects

Another compelling piece of evidence emerges by comparing the anatomy/distribution of digital defects with the sclerotomes of the hand and foot (Figures 27.10 and 27.11).[22,23]

The morphology of radial aplasia and its associated bones is visible in the sclerotome maps of the forearm and hand. Clearly, the thumb or the index finger can be divided longitudinally by the border between sclerotomes 6 and 7, depending on whether the maps are read from the front or the back of the hand. Depending on the variables inherent in the sclerotomes, a range of reduction is to be expected between the thumb and index fingers.

The biphasic response to nerve injury is difficult to read in long bones, where the sclerotomes are thin parallel longitudinal bands, locked together without borderline markers. Nature has teased out three of the segments in the hands (C6–8) and feet (L5, S1 and S2). This separation facilitates a clear reading of the sclerotomes.

Where a digit is supplied by a single segmental nerve, and that nerve is damaged, the finger or toe fails to form. Similarly, if several digits are supplied by one segmental nerve, they will tend to react together as a unit, with excess or reduced growth of all.

In the thumb, index finger and great toe, the nerve supply is divided between two segmental nerves, each with its own area. Injury to the outer, marginal nerve causes dysplasia in the area it supplies: excess or deficiency of digits. Elimination of one of the sclerotomes (i.e. one half of the digit) bisects the digit longitudinally. The outer half vanishes; the inner longitudinal half of the digit forms. Such digits may even have a bisected fingernail. These 'hemi-digits' match the longitudinal divisions of the thumb and index finger in the sclerotome maps of the upper limb, where the 6th and 7th cervical nerves share innervation of thumb and index finger. Similarly, the great toe is innervated by L5 and S1, and a 'hemi-digit' here indicates

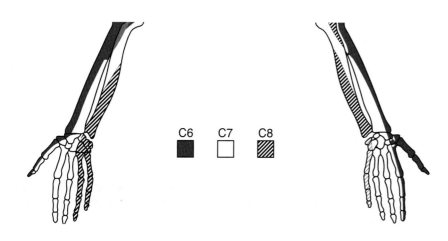

C6   C7   C8

Figure 27.10 *Sclerotomes of the hand skeleton. Palmar aspect on left, dorsal aspect on right. Cervical nerves 6, 7 and 8 reach the fingers.*

Figure 27.11 *Sclerotomes of the foot skeleton. Dorsal view on the left, plantar view on the right. Lumbar 5 and sacral 1 and 2 reach the toes.*

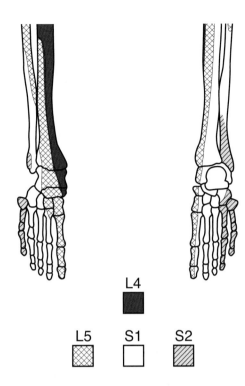

that the S1 sclerotome is present but the 5th lumbar sclerotome is absent.

Extra digits and hemidigits most often occur where a vulnerable sclerotome meets a thalidomide-resistant sclerotome. There must be a reason for this, but I do not know what it is. The phenomenon exists. Normally some modification occurs at an interface of two sclerotomes due to overlap of nerve supply from adjacent normal segments (see Chapter 4). But this regulation is unusual at the interface between vulnerable and resistant sclerotomes (C6 with C7, and L5 with S1).

Extra digits or hemidigits in the hand occur at the interface of the 6th and 7th sclerotomes, parallel or attached to the thumb or the index finger. In the foot, extra digits appear at the hallux, where the 5th lumbar sclerotome abuts the first sacral sclerotome. Extra toes may have two phalanges and appear to duplicate the hallux, or the hallux may be absent, with three phalanges in the extra digit, duplicating the second toe. There seems to be a sliding scale of possibilities for the final morphology.

Embryology of the digits

The sensitive period for triphalangeal thumb in thalidomide embryopathy was days 32–35, at the end of the 5th week of gestation, before differentiation began.

According to Sadler,[24] differentiation in the limb bud begins during the 6th week. First, condensation of mesenchyme appears at the sites for midshafts of future long bones. Then some cells in the mesenchymal condensations differentiate into chondroblasts, and thence into chondrocytes, which start to lay down the hyaline cartilage model for the future bone. Still in the 6th week, the extremity flattens into a palette, within which five ridges develop at the site of future digital rays. Joint interzones appear. The end of the 6th week, day 42, is the end of the 'thalidomide-sensitive period'.

On day 48, the web spaces begin to form, as cells of the apical ectodermal ridge between the digital rays begin to die. This initiates the phenomenon known as 'programmed cell death' or 'apoptosis', which is fundamental to digit separation (Figure 27.12).

Sadler[24] says:

'Normally, mesenchyme between prospective digits in hand and footplates is removed by cell death (apoptosis). In 1 per 2000 births this process fails and results in fusion between two or more digits.'

Death of cells in the potential web spaces between the digits causes the interdigital spaces to disappear, while the multiplying cells in the digital rays cause fingers to enlarge. Apoptosis frees the digits from the palette, allowing them independent development thereafter; their separation from one another is complete by day 56 (the end of the 8th week).

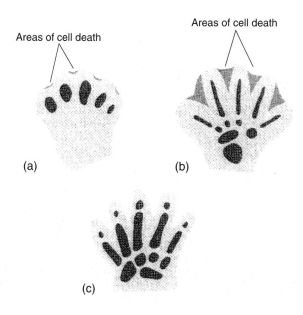

(a) (b) (c)

Figure 27.12 *Schematic of human hand formation. (a) At 48 days, cell death in the apical ectodermal ridge creates a separate ridge for each digit. (b) At 51 days, cell death in the interdigital spaces separates the digits. (c) At 56 days, digit separation is complete. (Reproduced with permission from Sadler TW, ed.* Langman's Medical Embryology, *10th edn. Philadelphia: Lippincott, Williams and Wilkins, 2006.[24])*

The cell cycle and neurotrophism: apoptosis and interdigital spaces

How cells in the web spaces know that they must die is an unresolved puzzle in biology. Could it be explained as a return to their primary cell cycle[28] in the absence of neurotrophism? Neurotrophism appears to interfere in the normal life cycle of a cell by effectively forcing it to divide, preventing it from fulfilling its natural destiny – which is to die. If nerves vacate an area, neurotrophism is removed: there is no demand for mitosis. Does this allow cells in that area to relapse into their original cell cycle, live out the remains of their lifespan, and die?

A possible mechanism that has not been considered in the search for what controls apoptosis is the fact that the digital nerves turn away from the webspaces to innervate the digits. Cells in the interdigital spaces are no longer innervated, and are free to resume their original fatal course. Absence of mitosis and presence of cell death in the non-innervated interdigital spaces contrasts with normal mitosis in the growing, innervated digits. Positive growth in digits and negative growth in web spaces allows the digits to grow as the interdigital spaces shrink. Thus digits separate from one another.

Absence of the neurotrophic imperative to divide must allow cells in the web spaces to resume their original program, complete their lifespan, and die. This is indeed programmed cell death.

Conclusion

- The same principles apply to digits as to the long bones of the limbs.
- Polydactyly and hypoplasia/aplasia of digits in thalidomide embryopathy is an expression of the biphasic response of nerves to injury.
- The sclerotomes explain the distribution and dysmorphology of dysmelic digits.
- Embryogenesis, absent neurotrophism, and the normal cell cycle provide a new explanation for programmed cell death and the formation of interdigital spaces.

References

1. Willert HG, Henkel HL. Die Dysmelie an den oberen Extremitäten. In: *Pathologie und Klinik in Einzeldarstellungen*. Berlin: Springer-Verlag, 1968.

2. Willert HG, Henkel HL. *Klinik und Pathologie der Dysmelie*. Berlin: Springer Verlag, 1969.

3. Henkel HL, Willert HG. Dysmelia: a classification and a pattern of malformation in a group of congenital defects of the limbs. *J Bone Joint Surg Br* 1969; **51**: 399–414.

4. Willert HG, Henkel HL. Pathologisch–anatomische Principien bei Extremitätenfehlbildungen, dargestellt am Beispiel der Finger. *Z Orthop Ihre Grenzgeb* 1970; **107**: 663–75.

5. Talamillo A, Bastida MF, Fernandez-Teran M, Ros MA. The developing limb and the control of the number of digits. *Clin Genet* 2005; **67**: 143–53.

6. Galois L, Mainard D, Delagoutte JP. Polydactyly of the foot: literature review and case presentations. *Acta Orthop Belg* 2002; **68**: 376–80.

7. Biesecker LG. Polydactyly: How many disorders and how many genes? *Am J Med Genet* 2002; **112**: 279–83.

8. Blauth W, Willert HG. Klinik und Therapie ektromeler Missbildungen der unteren Extremität. *Arch Orthop Unfall-Chir* 1963; **55**: 521.

9. Refior HJ. Die Triphalangie der Grosszehe – ein Beitrag zu den metrischen Variationen des Fusses. *Z Orthop* 1967; **103**: 498.

10. Schinz HR, Baensch WE, Friedl E, Uehlinger E. *Lehrbuch der Röntgendiagnostik*. Stuttgart: Thieme-Verlag, 1952.

11. Pol R. Brachydactylie, Klinodactylie, Hyperphalangie und ihre Grundlagen. *Virchows Arch* 1921; **229**: 388.

12. Cotta H, Jäger M. Die familiare Triphalangie des Daumens und ihre operative Behandlung. *Arch Orthop Unfall-Chir* 1965; **58**: 282.

13. Hilgenreiner H. Neues zur Hyperphalangie des Daumens. *Beitr Klin Chir* 1910; **67**: 196–221.

14. Müller W. *Die angeborenen Fehlbildungen der Hand*. Leipzig: Thieme-Verlag, 1937.

15. Witt AN, Cotta H, Jäger M. *Die angeborenen Fehlbildungen der Hand und ihre operative Behandlung*. Stuttgart: Thieme-Verlag, 1965.

16. Blauth W, Olason AT. Classification of polydactyly of the hands and feet. *Arch Orthop Trauma Surg* 1988; **107**: 334–44.

17. Vickers TH. Concerning the morphogenesis of thalidomide dysmelia in rabbits. *Br J Exp Pathol* 1967; **48**: 579–91.

18. Vickers TH, Wrba H. Further observations on the thalidomide embryopathy in rabbits. *Exp Pathol* 1970; **4**: 81.

19. Neubert D, Dillmann I. On the problem of phase specificity in limb teratogenesis. In: Merker HJ, Nau H, Neubert D, eds. *Teratology of the Limbs. 4th Symposium on Prenatal Development* Berlin, New York: Walter de Gruyter, 1980: 243–52.

20. Skalko RG. Pharmacological concepts and developmental biology. *Ann NY Acad Sci.* 1989; **562**: 21–30.

21. Kwasigroch TE, Vannoy JF, Church JK, Skalko RG. Retinoic acid enhances and depresses in vitro development of cartilaginous bone anlagen in embryonic mouse limbs. *In Vitro Cell Dev Biol* 1986; **22**: 150–6.

22. McCredie J, Willert H-G. Longitudinal limb deficiencies and the sclerotomes: an analysis of 378 malformations induced by thalidomide. *J Bone Joint Surg Br* 1999; **81**: 9–23.

23. Inman VT, Saunders JB de C. Referred pain from skeletal structures. *J Nerv Ment Dis* 1944; **99**: 660–7.

24. Sadler TW *Langman's Medical Embryology*, 10th edn. Philadelphia: Lippincott Williams and Wilkins, 2006.

25. Flatt AE. *The Care of Congenital Hand Anomalies*. St Louis: Mosby, 1977.

26. Temtamy S, McKusick VA. Polydactyly as an isolated malformation. In: Temtamy S, McKusick VA, eds. *The Genetics of Hand Malformations. Birth Defects*. New York: Alan Liss, 1978.

27. McKusick VA. *Mendelian Inheritance in Man*, 10th edn. Baltimore: Johns Hopkins University Press, 1992.

28. Mitchison JM. *The Biology of the Cell Cycle*. Cambridge: Cambridge University Press, 1971.

CHAPTER 28

Other disorders of similar sclerotomes

This chapter outlines some disorders other than thalidomide embryopathy in which sclerotomes can explain the segmental distribution of skeletal lesions.

The following conditions can be interpreted as skeletal expressions of sensory neuropathy:

- 'thalidomide look-alikes'
- polydactyly; triphalangeal thumb
- diabetic embryopathy
- melorheostosis
- macrodactyly of congenital neurofibromatosis

'Thalidomide look-alikes': non-thalidomide sclerotome subtractions of C5, 6 and L3, 4 – longitudinal limb reductions of unknown cause but thalidomide type

This is a large group of longitudinal reduction deformities of the limbs, some of which are similar to thalidomide dysmelia in their anatomy, but with no history of thalidomide exposure. Radiologically, there is often evidence of subtraction within the same sclerotomes as thalidomide: C6 and L4 (Figure 28.1). They were dubbed 'thalidomide look-alikes' during the thalidomide era, and were a cause of concern during compensation assessments of thalidomide children.

This group was referred to in Chapter 24. Thalidomide attacked the neural crest at certain levels to induce its wide range of malformations, as we have seen. Characteristic defects in radius and tibia have been explained as the axes of malformation being the 6th cervical sclerotome in the arm and the 4th lumbar sclerotome in the leg. The

Chapter Summary

- 'Thalidomide look-alikes': non-thalidomide sclerotome subtractions of C5, 6 and L3, 4 – longitudinal limb reductions of unknown cause but thalidomide type

- Polydactyly; triphalangeal thumb

- Diabetic embropathy

- Melorheostosis

- Macrodactyly in neurofibromatosis

- References

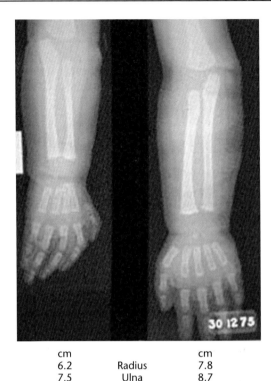

Figure 28.1 *Unilateral hypoplasia of the radius and thumb compared with the normal arm. Similar to thalidomide but born many years later.*

cm		cm
6.2	Radius	7.8
7.5	Ulna	8.7

reasons for the selection of these segmental levels of crest by that drug are unknown and speculative. The same distribution of defects is found in these cases of unknown aetiology and in other cases of genetic origin.

Autosomal recessive disorders such as Roberts syndrome and SC syndrome include reduction deformities of the limbs. Another autosomal recessive disorder is TAR (thrombocytopenia–absent radius) syndrome, where neonatal thrombocytopenia tends to improve and disappear in infancy. The absent radii are associated with normal thumbs. In Cornelia de Lange syndrome, the limb defects are bizarre and asymmetrical.

Many reductions of unknown origin either mimic or have components in common with thalidomide embryopathy. This suggests that there may be other neurotoxins in the environment, acting upon the neural crest. Injury to the neural crest then emerges as a final common pathway for expression of a number of teratogenic influences.

Aetiology and incidence

Wynne-Davies and Lamb,[1] in their study of 387 congenital malformations of the upper limb in Edinburgh, stressed the basic need to search for the cause of these defects.

'In some instances the cause is known, for example, the auto-somal dominant inheritance of the central longitudinal "absence" defects (lobster claw deformity) and the defects associated with thalidomide. Others clearly occur as only one feature of a malformation syndrome; these in turn frequently have a genetic origin. However, patients presenting with upper limb anomalies that have an unknown cause probably amount to about 85% to 90% of all cases.'

This large and common group of defects demands explanation, and will challenge future researchers.

In non-thalidomide reduction deformities of the limbs, where the cause is unknown and the pharmacokinetics of the causative agent is therefore also unknown, there is wide scope for anatomical variants to appear. There may or may not be other target tissues. The primary action may involve metabolic pathways common to two or more tissues or organs. These variables were not present with thalidomide. Such factors will cause variations in the ultimate anatomy.

But because the anatomy is often similar to that of thalidomide defects, it suggests that the target tissue is the same, i.e. the neural crest. Given that the neural crest is the target, the pharmacokinetics of suspected teratogens need to be examined.

By any parameters, the pharmacokinetics of thalidomide were exceptional. The teratogen was the intact molecule, which hydrolysed rapidly into inert by-products. The teratogenic action was uncomplicated: a short pulsed injury.

Other teratogens may have teratogenic by-products. Their pattern of attack would therefore be the sum of the activity of the parent and the active by-product(s). The teratogenic act would be more prolonged than that of thalidomide. As a longer period of embryotoxicity played across the craniocaudal development of the neural crest, a different pattern of damage would result: not single sclerotome subtractions, but a spread of damage across several sclerotomes. The anatomy of these defects would differ from the thalidomide model and would probably be more difficult to read. But the principles that have emerged from the analysis of thalidomide could still be applied, and the principles remain.

Polydactyly; triphalangeal thumb

Polydactyly

Polydactyly is not uncommon in the general population, unrelated to thalidomide. It is a feature of a number of genetic syndromes, as well as being a frequent sporadic malformation of unknown cause. Flatt[2] in a large review of congenital hand anomalies, listed 361 cases of polydactyly, 443 cases of syndactyly and 31 cases of ulnar hypoplasia. The three types of polydactyly were:

- 162 cases of radial (preaxial) polydactyly (thumb, C6)
- 130 cases of ulnar (postaxial) polydactyly (5th digit, C8)
- 69 cases of central polydactyly (2nd, 3rd, 4th digits, C7)

The incidence of polydactyly in the general population is 0.5–2 per 1000 live births, with more males, and is up to 20% familial in some series. Its aetiology is unknown. Teratogens, genes, aspirin and testosterone have been suggested. Many cases are sporadic.

A number of associations and associated syndromes are recorded. It is beyond the scope of this book to attempt to review the large literature on this topic, beyond making the general suggestion that most polydactyly represents the irritative phase of embryonic neuropathy, and is a response to a sensory neurotoxin, injury or irritant. Further discussion of cases of genetic and sporadic polydactyly can be found in Temtamy and McKusick's textbook[3] and similar publications on genetic syndromes.

Triphalangeal thumb

Rarely, three phalanges in the thumb may occur as a normal variant, as a sporadic malformation or as a familial trait. Triphalangism is also associated with other congenital defects of the thumb, such as duplication or absence of the opposite thumb in thalidomide embryopathy, Holt–Oram syndrome and Fanconi anaemia. It appears to be associated with eight other syndromes, as well as with various anomalies of other digits. Defects of pectoral muscles, ears, tibia and anus are possible associations.

Diabetic embryopathy

Pregnant women with unstable insulin-dependent diabetes are at risk of having birth defects in their infants, known as diabetic embryopathy.[4,5] Diabetic embryopathy is anatomically similar to thalidomide embryopathy in some cases. Longitudinal reduction deformities in the femur,[6] sacral agenesis and gross defects in the lumbar spine constitute the caudal regression syndrome.[7] Cardiovascular malformations were over-represented in Day and Insley's study[5] of 205 diabetic mothers. Those on insulin at the time of conception ran a 15% risk of malformation in their baby, and also bore a sixfold risk of stillbirth and neonatal death, with or without congenital malformations.

Most limb defects in diabetic embryopathy involve similar sclerotomes to thalidomide, but are not as neat a fit (Figure 28.2). One difference is that sacral agenesis is common in diabetic embryopathy but rare with thalidomide.[7–10] The associated cardiovascular, alimentary and genito-urinary malformations account for many perinatal deaths.

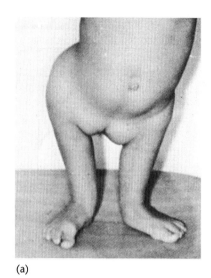

(a)

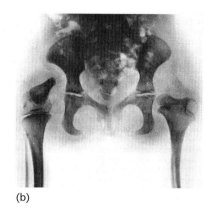

(b)

Figure 28.2 *Longitudinal reduction defects in both legs in diabetic embryopathy (a), with proximal femoral focal deficiency (PFFD) shown in the radiograph (b). (Reproduced from Saxén L, Rapola J. Congenital Defects. New York: Holt, Rinehart & Winston, 1969: 59.[9] The case is from Kucera et al.[10])*

Clinically and anatomically, the limb malformations can be identical. In their experience of assessing the compensation claims for thalidomide damage, Smithells and Newman[11] stated that:

'The differential diagnosis between thalidomide and diabetic embryopathy depends on the clinical history of unstable diabetes in the mother.'

Note on the term 'pseudo-thalidomide'

Diabetic embryopathy has been called the 'pseudo-thalidomide syndrome',[12] although the term is confusing because it has also been applied to an autosomal recessive condition of growth retardation, limb reductions and craniofacial abnormalities, now thought to be the same entity as Roberts syndrome.[13] The latter involves somatic growth and mental retardation, tetraphocomelia and midline craniofacial abnormalities.[14–17] These are genetic disorders with no diabetic aetiology.

Diabetic neuropathy

Not only do thalidomide and diabetes share a similar embryopathy, but they also share the complication of peripheral neuropathy, a fairly common side-effect in patients with diabetes mellitus.[18–24] It can afflict either young type 1 (insulin-dependent) diabetics with unstable control or elderly type 2 (non-insulin-dependent) diabetics. Once established, its progress is usually slow and irreversible. It involves sensory, motor and/or autonomic nerves, and thus differs from thalidomide neuropathy, which is virtually purely sensory. The neuropathology is axonal degeneration in both thalidomide and diabetes. Associated autonomic neuropathy in diabetes causes functional disturbances in the heart, gastrointestinal tract and other organs.

Diabetic peripheral neuropathy afflicts the longest nerves of the body, with initial sensory symptoms in the feet. Late in the course of the peripheral neuropathy, chronic 'trophic' complications of the neuropathy itself occur in the skin (trophic ulcers) or in the skeleton (diabetic osteoarthropathy, as discussed in Chapter 10), both involving weight-bearing areas such as the heel or the ball of the foot. Sometimes complicated by infection, trophic ulcers resist treatment and frequently break down. The cause of the trophic ulcers is believed to be a combination of sensory neuropathy, vascular abnormality and intercurrent infection, to all of which diabetics are prone.

Pathogenesis of diabetic embryopathy

A logical suggestion is that diabetes, like thalidomide, can cause embryonic sensory peripheral neuropathy. The common pathogenetic pathway for similar congenital malformations is the neural crest, although the causative agent acting upon that pathway is different. In the case of thalidomide, it is a chemical sensory neurotoxin; in diabetes, it is some aspect of the metabolic imbalance conveyed to the embryo from the maternal bloodstream. Acidosis, hyper- or hypoglycaemia, and hyper- or hypoinsulinaemia are just some of the fleeting disorders of unstable diabetic physiology that may trigger an injury to the embryonic neural crest.

The tetraphocomelic baby drawn by Goya in 18th century Spain (Figure 28.3) was not a thalidomide baby, although the malformations are almost identical to those of case 4 in Sydney, and to others in the German and British series. This mother may have had

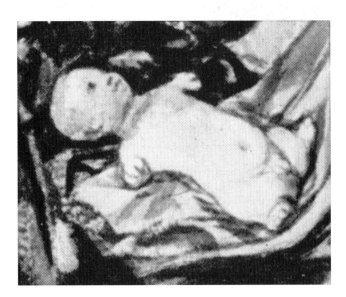

Figure 28.3 *Goya's sketch of a tetraphocomelic baby in pre-thalidomide Spain.*

type 1 diabetes, or she may have been exposed to an unknown sensory neurotoxin in early pregnancy. Thalidomide was not invented until a century later.

Melorheostosis

Melorheostosis (literally 'honey-flowing bone') is a rare condition of unknown origin in which overgrowth of thick, sclerotic cortical bone occurs in longitudinal strips down the long bones (Figures 28.4–28.7). The abnormal cortical bone is often lumpy and irregular, with an appearance like trickles of honey or candle wax flowing down the outside of the bony shaft.

The phenomenon can occur in most bones, and is associated in some cases with abnormalities in adjacent soft tissues and rarely in various internal organs. Most patients live a normal life and die of some other disease, but those with gross involvement of internal organ systems may not reach their full span. The common presenting symptom is chronic pain in the affected limb, but sometimes the condition may be totally asymptomatic, found only incidentally on radiographs taken for another reason.

At the other extreme, bony excrescences and contractures of the soft tissues may cause cosmetic deformities and orthopaedic complications of such severity that amputation is necessary. The woman in Figure 28.5 presented because she could no longer remove her rings. The surgeon excised a slice of thickened cortex from the shaft of the proximal phalanx of the ring finger. The pathologist, Dr Fiona Bonar, reported that this was histologically normal cortex, but thickened (Figure 28.6).

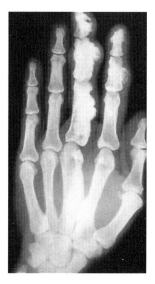

Figure 28.4 *Melorheostosis in the 7th cervical sclerotome of the hand.*

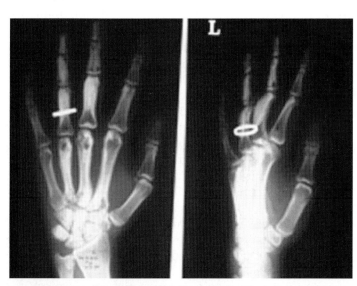

Figure 28.5 *Another case of melorheostosis of the C7 sclerotome. (Courtesy of Dr Fiona Bonar, Pathologist, Sydney.)*

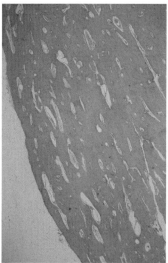

Figure 28.6 *Histopathology of the case shown in Figure 28.5, which demonstrates excess cortical bone, but normal cells. (Courtesy of Dr Fiona Bonar, Pathologist, Sydney.)*

The disease is usually limited to a single limb in which several bones may be affected (Figure 28.7). The typical sclerotic densities are clearly defined and usually affect only one longitudinal segment of the bone or series of bones, always in a linear arrangement parallel to the longitudinal axis of the limb. The lesions are often peripheral, involving the small bones of the hands and feet. Ectopic bone may be present within para-articular soft tissue masses.

The peculiarly segmental distribution does not correspond to the anatomical course of the blood vessels, nor to the mixed nerve roots in the limbs, and was thought to be a developmental error as a result of an embryonic metameric disturbance. In an extensive review of the subject in 1968, Campbell et al[25] observed that the distribution of the limb lesions resembles that of paraxial hemimelia and suggested that the disorder is congenital, postulating 'that it is initiated early in embryonic life *prior to formation of the limb buds*'.

Following republication of the sclerotome maps of Inman and Saunders,[26] and their application to the pattern of thalidomide deformities by 'sclerotome subtraction',[27] Dr Ronald Murray, Senior Radiologist at the Institute of Orthopaedics, Royal National Orthopaedic Hospital, in London, realized that the sclerotomes might also explain the linear pattern of melorheostosis. During my next visit to London, he invited me to look at the Institute's collection of 30 cases of melorheostosis. We tested them against the sclerotomes, and published our joint paper in *Skeletal Radiology* in 1975.[28]

The case histories were incomplete, and sometimes only the plain X-ray films were available to examine. Cases had been referred to the Institute over many years and from all over the world. Briefly, our results were as follows.

As far as facts were available, there was equal sex incidence, and an age range from childhood to 76 years. Bone pain was the predominant symptom, with deforming exostoses and contractures necessitating surgery in the worst affected cases. Overall, the disease was predominantly unilateral and left-sided. Two-thirds of the patients had a single sclerotome involved: 8 upper and 11 lower limbs. Another 11 patients had multiple sclerotome involvement, and these patients had correspondingly more severe clinical findings.

In the 19 patients with single-sclerotome lesions, the sclerotome distribution was particularly accurate, especially in the hand and foot, where the hyperostosis typically affected a bone in the forearm plus part of the carpus, metacarpus and contiguous phalanges. There was predeliction for involvement of the 7th cervical sclerotome (C7) in the upper limb (Figures 28.7–28.9). In the leg, the distribution was fairly equal among the major sclerotomes L3 to S1. In the 11 patients with multiple-sclerotome sclerosis, half had ossification in the soft tissues adjacent to the joints, and occasional vascular hypertrophy.

The sclerotomes explain the main features of melorheostosis:

- Involvement of one longitudinal row of several appendicular bones, including the pelvis and pectoral girdle, can only be explained by the presence of an invisible longitudinal subdivision of these bones based on their segmental spinal innervation.
- Involvement of one side of the bone, with a clear-cut line of demarcation between normal and abnormal sections, and extension of this demarcation line into the distal smaller bones of the appendages, is explained as the border between the normal and the affected sclerotomes.
- The same patterns repeat themselves in different patients, proving the presence of a common underlying mechanism in all.

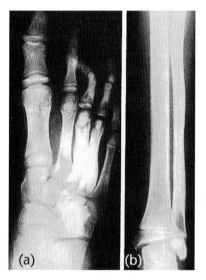

Figure 28.7 *Melorheostosis of the 1st sacral sclerotome: (a) foot; (b) mid-fibula of the same patient.*

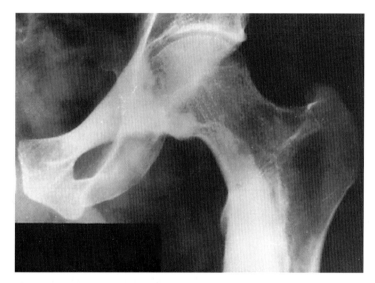

Figure 28.8 *Melorheostosis of the femur and pelvis in the L3 sclerotome.*

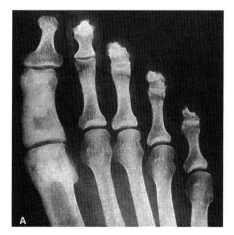

Figure 28.9 *Melorheostosis in the L5 sclerotome of the foot.*

There are differences between the application of the sclerotomes in melorheostosis and in dysmelia. In melorheostosis, there is overgrowth of the cortex of the bone. In dysmelia, there is total or partial failure to form the sclerotome, including the cortex. In melorheostosis, the lesions fit less neatly into the maps than do those of dysmelia. In melorheostosis, the sclerotome sclerosis is unilateral, asymmetrical and more random in distribution, whereas in dysmelia, the involvement is bilateral and symmetrical in the majority (80%) of cases. This raises the possibility that melorheostosis may be some form of pre- or post-natal peripheral neuropathy, affecting segmental spinal sensory nerves in a manner similar to herpes zoster, with scarring of bone rather than skin. Hyperostosis is *overgrowth*, and may represent nerve root *irritation* and excessive trophic (mitogenic and osteogenic) action. This contrasts with dysmelia, where segmental skeletal aplasia and hypoplasia reflect *suppression* of the sensorineural segment and failure of its trophic effect on mitosis in the undifferentiated embryonic mesenchyme. Excessive osteogenesis and segmental overgrowth in melorheostosis may include the soft tissues and explain the para-articular bony masses, local vascular hypertrophy and occasional linear skin lesions. The mixed tissues that can be affected by melorheostosis suggest that there is an underlying mechanism with a common origin, such as nerve.

The aetiology of melorheostosis remains unknown. But approximation of the anatomical distribution to the sclerotomes in the majority of cases suggests a major if not a primary role for the sensory nerve in the pathogenesis of this condition. Perhaps the spinal sensory ganglia are the initial sites of pathological change, reflecting some form of sensory neuropathy due to a specific insult that culminates in the development of segmental sclerotic bony lesions. The question may be asked whether other skeletal disorders, including such entities as macrodystrophia lipomatosa, neurofibromatosis and even fibrous dysplasia, might be based on these patterns of segmental innervation of the bones. Further investigation of these possibilities must await appropriate neurohistological studies.

Since our paper appeared in *Skeletal Radiology*, numerous case reports and over 50 citations have substantiated our argument that the distribution of melorheostosis is sclerotomal, consistent with a neurological disease.[29–32]

Melorheostosis is important despite its rarity. It adds a further dimension to our understanding of the interface between nerves and bones.

Macrodactyly in neurofibromatosis

Neurofibromas are tumours or swellings of the peripheral nerves.[33] They may be single or multiple, sporadic or familial, benign or malignant. They arise from the connective tissue of nerves; histologically, they are fibromas, or occasionally myxomas or lipomas. Because they are believed to originate from the perineurium or endoneurium, they can degenerate into fibrosarcoma. The nerve fibres may be spread over the surface of the tumour, which is often eccentric. Axons are not incorporated into the tumours.

Neurofibromatosis, or von Recklinghausen's disease, is an uncommon condition where many of these tumours form thickenings or beads along nerve trunks and under the skin, in the spinal canal, or in the walls of internal organs.

The presenting symptom is usually pain or deformity. There may be multiple pigmented patches in the skin, known as café-au-lait spots. Neurofibromatosis may present at birth, or may develop at puberty.

The infantile form presents at birth with a rare complication, organ gigantism,[34,35] or macrodactyly that follows the sensory distribution of a major peripheral nerve[36] (Figures 28.10 and 28.11). The nerves to involved digital rays are consistently found to be grossly thickened.[37] The digit is enlarged and continues to grow faster than the other rays of the hand or foot (Figure 28.12) – a histologically benign lesion that behaves like a malignancy.[38] The excessive growth may be so rapid and extreme that the remainder of the appendage is severely

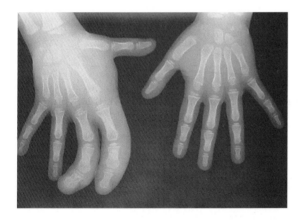

Figure 28.10 *Neurofibromatosis: macrodactyly in the 7th cervical sclerotome.*

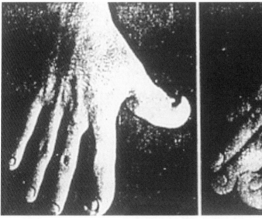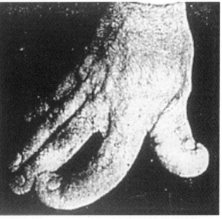

Figure 28.11
Neurofibromatosis: progressive growth of macrodactyly in the 6th cervical sclerotome over time.

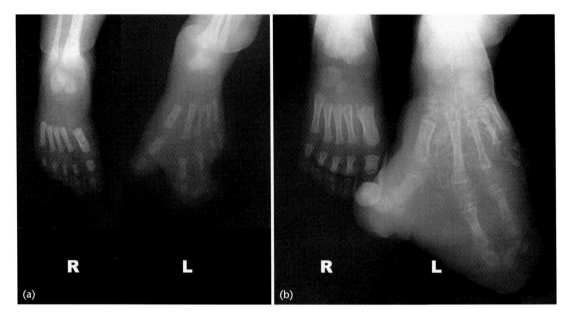

(a) (b)

Figure 28.12 *(a) Newborn baby with infantile neurofibromatosis in L5, S1 sclerotomes of left foot. (b) Some months later there is disproportionate growth in the affected area of left foot, known as macrodactyly or organ gigantism.*

distorted. Management presents exceedingly difficult problems.[38] Segmental resection of the overgrowth and its nerve is often necessary,[39] although skin flap necrosis is a common postoperative complication.[36]

Figure 28.12a shows a baby born in our hospital with enlarged first, second and third rays of one foot. Review some months later (Figure 28.12b), shows grossly accelerated enlargement of these three rays, which came to segmental resection.

The pathophysiology is uncertain. However, a neurofibroma is a tumour of neural crest-derived cells. Dell[36] noted that macrodactyly 'involves cell types that are predominately affected by neurogenic growth control' and follow a sensory nerve distribution. Turra et al[39] proposed that macrodactyly was based on the concept of 'neuro-induction', because of consistent histopathological findings in the plantar nerve and its terminal branches.

A consensus is emerging that overgrowth of the digit(s) results from increased neurotrophism emanating from an *enlarged* nerve. The enlargement of the nerve supplying the overgrowth is consistent with the principles of neurotrophism in amphibian biology (Chapter 14), and with the quantitative laws of neuropathy (Chapter 4). Increased neurotrophism increases the number of cells within the area supplied by that nerve. The result is segmental overgrowth.

References

1. Wynne-Davies R, Lamb DW. Congenital upper limb anomalies: an etiologic grouping of clinical, genetic, and epidemiologic data from 387 patients with 'absence' defects, constriction bands, polydactylies, and syndactylies. *J Hand Surg [Am]* 1985; **10**: 958–64.

2. Flatt AE. *The Care of Congenital Hand Anomalies.* St Louis: Mosby, 1977.

3. Temtamy SA, McKusick VA. *The Genetics of Hand Malformations.* New York: Alan R Liss, 1978.

4. Pedersen LM, Tygstrup I, Pedersen J. Congenital malformations in newborn infants of diabetic women. *Lancet* 1964; **i**: 1124.

5. Day RE, Insley J. Maternal diabetes mellitus and congenital malformation: study of 205 cases. *Archv Dis Child* 1976; **51**: 935–8.

6. Lenz W, Maier W. Congenital malformations and maternal diabetes. *Lancet* 1964; **ii**: 1124.

7. Passarge E, Lenz W. Syndrome of caudal regression in infants of diabetic mothers: observations of further cases. *Pediatrics* 1966; **37**: 672.

8. Blumel J, Burke Evans E, Eggers GWN. Partial and complete agenesis or malformation of the sacrum with associated anomalies. *J Bone Joint Surg Am* 1959; **41**: 497–518.

9. Saxén L, Rapola J. *Congenital Defects.* New York: Holt, Rinehart & Winston, 1969: 59.

10. Kucera J, Lenz W, Maier W. [Malformation of the legs and caudal section of the spine in infants born to diabetic mothers.] *Dtsch Med Wochenschr* 1965; **90**: 901–5 [in German].

11. Smithells RW, Newman CG. Recognition of thalidomide defects. *J Med Genet* 1992; **29**: 716–23.

12. Herrmann J, Feingold M, Tuffli GA, Opitz JM. A familial dysmorphogenetic syndrome of limb deformities, characteristic facial appearance and associated anomalies: The 'pseudo-thalidomide' or 'SC syndrome'. *Birth Defects: Original Article Series* 1969; **5**: 81–9.

13. Roberts JB. A child with double cleft of lip and palate, protrusion of the intermaxillary portion of the upper jaw and imperfect development of the bones of the four extremities. *Ann Surg* 1919; **70**: 252.

14. Tomkins D, Hunter A, Roberts M. Cytogenetic findings in Roberts–SC phocomelia syndrome(s). *Am J Med Genet* 1979; **4**: 17–26.

15. Fryns H, Goddeeris P, Moerman F, Herman F, van der Berghe H. The tetraphocomelia–cleft palate syndrome in identical twins. *Hum Genet* 1980; **53**: 279–81.

16. Holden KR, Jabs EW, Sponseller PD. Roberts/pseudothalidomide syndrome and normal intelligence: approaches to diagnosis and management. *Dev Med Child Neurol* 1992; **34**: 534–9.

17. Van Den Berg DJ, Franche U. Roberts syndrome: a review of 100 cases and a new rating system for severity. *Am J Med Genet* 1993; **47**: 1104–23.

18. Mencer Martin M. Diabetic neuropathy: a clinical study of 150 cases. *Brain* 1953; **76**: 594–624.

19. Thomas PK, Lascelles RG. The pathology of diabetic neuropathy. *Q J Med* 1966; **35**: 489–509.

20. Editorial. Diabetic autonomic neuropathy. *Lancet* 1985; **i**: 379–80.

21. Lloyd-Mostyn RH, Watkins PJ. Defective innervation of heart in diabetic autonomic neuropathy. *BMJ* 1975; **iii**: 15–7.

22. Hosking DJ, Moody F, Stewart IM, Atkinson M. Vagal impairment of gastric secretion in diabetic autonomic neuropathy. *BMJ* 1975; **ii**: 588–90.

23. Clouse ME, Gramm HF, Legg M, Flood T. Diabetic osteoarthropathy. Clinical and roentgenographic observations in 90 cases. *AJR Am J Roentgenol* 1974; **121**: 22–34.

24. Kraft E, Spyropoulos E, Finby N. Neurogenic disorders of the foot in diabetes mellitus. *AJR Am J Roentgenol* 1975; **124**: 17–24.

25. Campbell CJ, Papademetriou T, BonFigurelio M. Melorheostosis. A report of the clinical, roentgenographic and pathological findings in 14 cases. *J Bone Joint Surg Am* 1968; **50**: 1281–304.

26. Inman VT, Saunders JB de C. Referred pain from skeletal structures. *J Nerv Ment Dis* 1944; **99**: 660–7.

27. McCredie J, Segmental embryonic peripheral neuropathy. *Pediatr Radiol* 1975; **3**: 162–8.

28. Murray RO, McCredie J. Melorheostosis and the sclerotomes. *Skel Radiol* 1975; **3**: 162–8.

29. Greenspan A. Sclerosing bone dysplasias: a target-site approach. *Skel Radiol* 1991; **20**: 561–83.

30. Rhys R, Davies AM, Mangham DC. Sclerotome distribution of melorheostosis and multicentric fibromatosis. *Skel Radiol* 1998; **27**: 633–6.

31. Brown RR, Steiner GC, Lehman WB. Melorheostosis: a case report with radiologic–pathologic correlation. *Skel Radiol* 2000; **29**: 548–52.

32. Freyschmidt J. Melorheostosis: a review of 23 cases. *Eur Radiol* 2001; **11**: 474–9.

33. Dyck PJ, Thomas PK. *Peripheral Neuropathy*, 4th edn. Philadelphia: Elsevier Saunders, 2005.

34. Holt JF. Neurofibromatosis in children. *AJR Am J Roentgenol* 1978; **130**: 615–39.

35. Hoyt CS, Billson FA. Buphthalmos in neurofibromatosis: Is it an expression of regional gigantism? *J Pediatr Ophthalmol* 1977; **14**: 228–34.

36. Dell, PC. Macrodactyly. *Hand Clin* 1985; **1**: 511–24.

37. Gamstorp I. Neurological disorders and growth disturbances in infancy and childhood. *Eur Neurol* 1972; **7**: 1–25.

38. Dufresne CR, Hoopes JE. Pseudomalignancies. *Clin Plast Surg* 1987; **14**: 367–81.

39. Turra S, Santini S, Cagnoni G, Jacopetti T. Gigantism of the foot: our experience in seven cases. *J Pediatr Orthoped* 1998; **18**: 337–45.

CHAPTER 29

Segmental and truncal neuropathies in sclerotomes not affected by thalidomide

Segmental limb malformations *not* due to thalidomide

The significance of sensory neurotrophism, the segmental sensori-neural site of this embryonic pathology and the fact that longitudinal developmental fields are sclerotomes, has been the message of this book. Because thalidomide has been the model, the radial–tibial distribution (sclerotomes C6 and L4) has been explored.

But there are other sclerotomes and other malformations. Some of the other sclerotomes appear to be implicated in the pathogenesis of longitudinal limb deficiencies unrelated to thalidomide. There are four major groups:

- femur–fibula–ulna defects (C8 and S2)
- central defects: split hand or foot (C7 and S1)
- multiplication of sclerotomes
- distal limb reductions, possibly truncal neuropathies

C8 and S2 sclerotome defects: femur–fibula–ulna reductions

A different anatomical distribution of defects is seen in this group of longitudinal reduction deformities of unknown origin. The defects are in the femur, fibula and ulna, and are known as the FFU syndrome. The sclerotome maps apply to these malformations, and sclerotome subtraction is easily confirmed, but the sclerotomes are not those of thalidomide embryopathy. Whereas thalidomide deficiencies typically involve the radial (C6) and tibial (L4) aspects of the limbs, FFU defects are typically ulnar (C8) and fibular (L5, S1 and 2). These defects will be discussed in turn.

Chapter Summary

- Segmental limb malformations *not* due to thalidomide

- C8 and S2 sclerotome defects: femur–fibula–ulna reductions

- C7 and S1 sclerotome defects: central and genetic – 'split' hand or foot

- Sclerotome multiplication

- Non-segmental neuropathies

- References

Ulnar reduction

Definition

Congenital reduction or absence of the ulna (ulnar ray defect, ulnar dysmelia or ulnar deficiency) is a condition in which some or all of the following skeletal parts may be absent: ulna, ulnar carpals, ulnar metacarpals and ulnar digits. When the ulna is entirely absent, or when its distal end is deficient, the hand is deflected towards the ulnar side (manus valga). The forearm is shortened and the radius is curved towards the ulnar side, either fused to the humerus or dislocated at its head.

Classification

Ulnar defects may be total or partial, depending on whether all or only some of the bone elements are missing. Partial deficiencies are subdivided into proximal (ulna missing but fingers present) or distal (fingers missing but ulna present).

Anatomy

The anatomy has been reviewed by O'Rahilly,[1] Lausecker,[2] and Kelikian.[3] The essential features were described by Kelikian[3] as follows:

> 'The ulna serves as the main skeletal element of the forearm at the elbow. It supports the elbow in the same manner that the radius supports the wrist. In defects of the ulnar ray, the elbow bears the brunt of the distortion; deformities of the wrist are minimal. At the elbow, the proximal end of the radius is often fused with the humerus or is dislocated. The radius is short. The hand tilts in the ulnar direction and is slightly flexed. This deformity is not as conspicuous as the radiopalmar deflection of the hand in connection with defects of the radial ray. There is increasing tendency for the digital rays to fail as one passes from the ulnar to the radial aspect. The surviving digits exhibit degrees of stunting, syndactyly or symphalangism. Defects of the ulnar ray are only occasionally bilateral; they are seldom symmetrical. Absence of the ulna is more often incomplete than complete.'

In addition to complete and partial absence, the range of ulnar deficiency includes delayed appearance of the ulnar ossification centre, and a fibrocartilaginous band tethering the ulnar fragment to the carpus or distal radial epiphysis (thought to represent the vestige of the missing ulna). Carpal bones on the ulnar side are absent or fused. The 4th and 5th metacarpals and their digits are very often absent, sometimes fused (syndactyly). Thumb, index and middle fingers are usually present and relatively normal, except that the middle finger ray may be smaller than normal.[4]

Card and Strachman[5] pointed out that the radiolucent region between ossified humerus and radius in the radiograph of a newborn baby with ulnar ray defect is actually made up of cartilage, which ossifies a few months after birth with absence of the elbow joint. Warkany and Schraffenberger[6] induced humeroradial synostosis in fetal rats irradiated on the 13th day of gestation, and demonstrated a continuous cartilaginous connection between the humerus and radius, with no elbow joint.

Ogden et al[4] noted that the radius is frequently smaller than that of the normal arm. As the child grows, the radius may become progressively bowed because of the ulnar band, unless it is surgically released. There is frequently dislocation of the head of the radius.

The elbow joint may be normal, absent, hypoplastic, fused or dislocated. Radio-humeral synostosis replaces the elbow joint, and occasionally includes the proximal ulnar remnant in the union.

From these descriptions of the bones and joints, it is apparent that the pattern of malformation in ulnar dysmelia has the same component features as radial dysmelia, but involves the other side of the limb.

Associations

In contrast to radial aplasia, there are very few associations with thoracic and abdominal organs, although diaphragmatic hernia and dental, facial and renal anomalies have been reported. But there are frequent malformations elsewhere in the skeleton, such as deficiency of fibula, patella and femur, club-foot, scoliosis, and spina bifida.

Also in contrast to radial aplasia, ulnar deficiency is usually unilateral. Familial cases have been reported, but are rare. A syndrome of deficiencies in ulna, femur and fibula is recognized – the FFU syndrome. Rarely, ulnar defect has been reported in association with syndromes such as Cornelia de Lange, mesomelic dwarfism and sickle cell anaemia.

Incidence

In 1949, Birch-Jensen[7] calculated the statistical incidence of ulnar ray defect in Denmark to be 1 in 100 000 births. It is thus three to four times less frequent than radial ray defect in a pre-thalidomide population.

In a post-thalidomide population study from the Swedish Register of Congenital Malformations 1969–1979, Kallen et al[8] reported 58 reductions of the radius compared with 19 reductions of the ulna, an incidence ratio of approximately 3:1, in a total of 855 infants with 1046 limb reductions, a significant change.

Lamb et al[9] in the 1980s published a collection of upper limb anomalies in Edinburgh, analysed in terms of their causes. Of these

387 Scottish cases, 24 had longitudinal absence defects known to be due to thalidomide. Of the 72 longitudinal defects apparently not caused by thalidomide, 20 were amelia/phocomelia, 31 were absent radius, 9 were absent ulna and 12 were central defects (lobster claw). This suggests that radial–tibial defects of unknown cause are about five times as common as either ulnar or central defects in the population around Edinburgh. In view of the difficulties recorded in confirmation or denial of thalidomide exposure, the possibility remains that some of the 72 non-thalidomide reduction deformities in this particular era in Edinburgh may have had thalidomide aetiology. The experience of Spiers and Cuthbert[10] in establishing thalidomide exposure in their series of cases around Stirling in central Scotland (Chapter 1) is relevant to interpretation of the Edinburgh cases. If not thalidomide, there must be some other explanation for the high radial–ulnar ratio.

Aetiology

The majority of ulnar reductions are sporadic and of unknown cause. Rare cases have been reported with dominant inheritance[11–13] or recessive inheritance in association with micromelic dwarfism and hypoplasia of the fibula.[14] Hereditary factors overall account for less than 10% of cases.

The role of environmental factors is unknown. Animal experiments confirm that prenatal environmental factors can induce ulnar ray defects. Maternal riboflavin deficiency in rats causes shortening of both foreleg bones, although the radial defect tends to be more pronounced than the ulnar.[15] Prenatal irradiation induces frequent and severe ulnar deficiencies in rats.[6]

Weicker[16] did not observe isolated ulnar aplasia in his series of 100 thalidomide cases, although the ulna was reduced in size, deformed or absent in 85% of his cases secondary to radial defects of the upper extremity. Lenz et al[17] reported that the incidence of ulnar aplasia did not rise, as did radial ray defect, during the thalidomide epidemic in Germany, which was confirmed in Willert and Henkel's collection of thalidomide and non-thalidomide cases[18] (Chapter 27).

Concerning the differential diagnosis of thalidomide defects, Smithells and Newman[19] say:

> 'Longitudinal reduction defects of the ulnar side of the hand and forearm, or of the fibular side of the foot and lower leg, grouped as the femur–fibula–ulna (FFU) syndrome, usually unilateral, are not seen in thalidomide embryopathy and should cause no trouble.'

Radiology: sclerotome subtraction in ulnar reductions

Comparison of radiographs with the sclerotome maps (see Chapter 27: Figure 27.11) shows that absence of the ulna and ulnar digits represents subtraction of the *8th cervical* sclerotome (Figures 29.1 and 29.2).

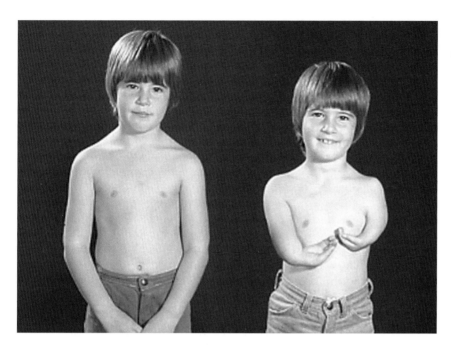

Figure 29.1 *Identical twins – one with bilateral upper phocomelia.*

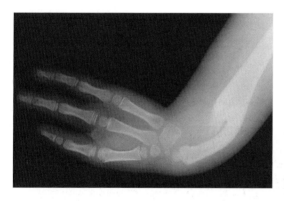

Figure 29.2 *X-ray of forearm: aplasia of 8th cervical sclerotome.*

Figure 29.2 shows C8 subtraction. The distal ulna and the ulnar carpals, metacarpals and digits have been eliminated. The thumb, index and middle fingers are present, although the latter is smaller than normal, consistent with hypoplasia adjacent to the subtraction. There is radio-ulnar synostosis. A pointed prong of bone arising from the area of the synostosis can be interpreted as the residuum of the 7th cervical sclerotome of the ulna. There is carpal coalition in the centre of the wrist.

Scoliosis is a recognized accompaniment of ulnar ray defect. It is not difficult to suppose that a neural crest injury at C8 may overflow onto C7, and also in the other direction onto the upper thoracic neural crest. Damage here can be predicted to reduce growth in the upper thoracic vertebrae. If the neural crest injury is unilateral, the future growth of the upper thoracic vertebrae will be reduced on one side compared with the other. This asymmetry will produce a slowly progressing upper thoracic scoliosis as the child grows up. Imbalance of growth between the two sides is a possible explanation for scoliosis in general, but particularly so when there is an associated ipsilateral ulnar defect. The neural crest damage in a child such as this may be read as extending from C7 down to the upper thoracic crest, maximum at C8.

Humerus and elbow joint

The C8 sclerotome incorporates the elbow joint within its territory on the posterior aspect of the distal humerus. Loss of C8 would theoretically include elbow joint deficiencies, ranging from normality through hypoplasia to total absence of the joint, with ultimate humero-radial fusion.

Deletion of both C7 and C8 leaves a forearm and hand composed of C6. One of our patients, an intelligent young woman of 18, had bilateral arm defects with cubital pterygia (Figure 29.3). Her father accompanied her to X-ray, and his hands (Figure 29.4) revealed the hereditary nature of these defects.

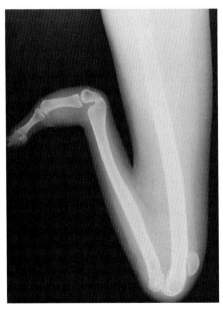

Figure 29.3 *Arm composed of the 5th and 6th cervical sclerotomes, with aplasia of C7 and C8. There is cubital pterygium.*

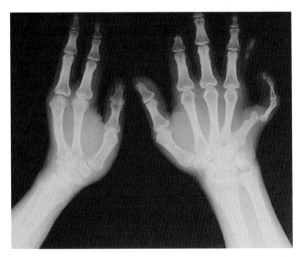

Figure 29.4 *The father of the woman in Figure 29.3 had aplasia of C8 on the left, and hypoplasia, polydactyly and dislocation within C8 on the right. There is traumatic amputation of the right index finger.*

Fibular reduction

Fibula and foot

Reference to the pattern of dysmelia[20] shows that the fibula and foot remained intact until last in the reduction sequence of thalidomide embryopathy.

Thalidomide targeted the lumbar nerves and spared the sacral nerves for some unknown reason. Absence of the fibula is not seen in thalidomide embryopathy unless all other long bones have disappeared from the leg, for example in the last stage before amelia of the lower limb in Figure 29.5. The lateral side of the lower leg, like the foot, is not vulnerable to thalidomide.

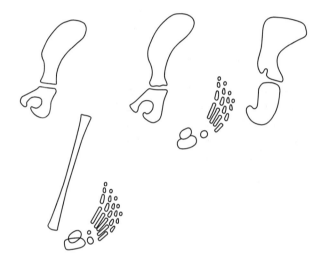

Figure 29.5 *Thalidomide preserved fibula and foot until last. There is aplasia of the tibia from injury to lumbar nerves. Survival of sacral sclerotomes was typical of thalidomide embryopathy.*

Sclerotome subtraction in fibular reductions

However, in the general population, primary absence of the fibula and the one or two lateral rays of the foot is more common than absence of the tibia. Fibular hypoplasia almost always presents with deleted lateral rays of the foot, in contrast to tibial hypoplasia, where the foot is spared. The range of fibular defects is wide.

Fibular pathology varies from hypoplasia to total absence of the fibula and one or two lateral rays (Figure 29.6). Associated with fibular defects are hypoplastic changes in the mid-foot: talocalcaneal synostosis, other tarsal coalitions, and hypoplasia of the 2nd and 3rd metatarsals and phalanges. The distal tibial epiphysis is wedge-shaped, with its base medial and its apex pointing towards the absent lateral sclerotome. Wedge-shaped epiphyses generate greater bone production on the thicker side, with bending of the tibia as growth proceeds. A fibrous band replacing the fibula and the wedge-epiphysis cause disalignment of weight-bearing as the child grows, and may necessitate amputation to fit a prosthesis for ambulation.

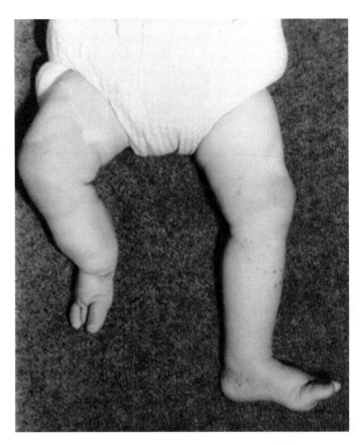

Figure 29.6 *Infant with short right leg and absent lateral two digital rays. There is aplasia of the 2nd sacral sclerotome.*

Figures 29.7 and 29.8 illustrate absence of one sclerotome and hypoplasia in the adjacent sclerotome. In terms of response to nerve damage, this amounts to total failure of growth in one segment of nerve supply, and partial growth failure or hypoplasia in the adjacent band of nerve supply. This indicates a gradient of neurotrophic failure from gross to moderate across adjacent sclerotomes.

Occasionally, both sacral sclerotomes are obliterated and the residual foot is formed of the 5th lumbar sclerotome alone (Figures 29.9 and 29.10).

As discussed in Chapter 17, ablation of the sacral neural crest in the chick embryo resulted in total absence of the foot and ankle. There was a corresponding reduction in dorsal root ganglion mass, which predated the formation of the foot. The equivalent defect in humans is longitudinal apodia, where all sclerotomes of the foot are absent.

Chapter 18 showed that reduction deformities have a moderate to severe reduction of nerve supply, and that mild reduction in nerve supply can occur without skeletal deformity.

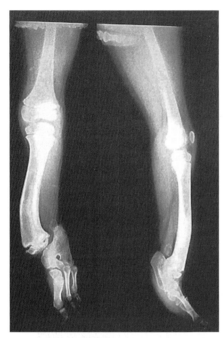

Figure 29.7 *Aplasia of S2, hypoplasia in S1. There is tibiofibular synostosis. The distal tibial epiphysis is wedge-shaped, and the tibia is curved. A calcified distal fibular epiphysis is faintly visible.*

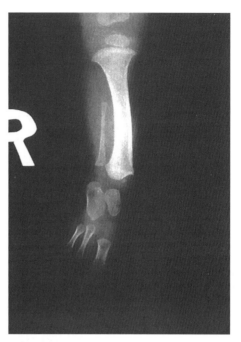

Figure 29.8 *The same sclerotomes are involved as in Figure 29.7. A fragment of the S1 component of the fibula remains. The 4th and 5th rays of the foot have not formed (S2).*

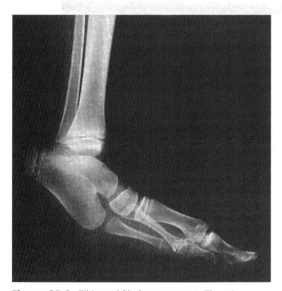

Figure 29.9 *Tibia and fibula are present. There is aplasia of S2 and hypoplasia of S1, with hypoplastic S1 digits and talocalcaneal synostosis.*

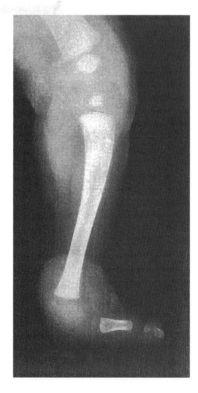

Figure 29.10 *There is total absence of S1 and S2. The residual leg is L5. The sole bone in the lower leg is the L3, 4, 5 tibial sclerotomes, bearing the 1st metatarsal and hallux. The S1 and S2 tarsals and metatarsals have not formed.*

Because that experiment in rabbits was based on thalidomide, the defects were on the tibial (medial) aspect of the foot. Were there some way of inducing fibular defects in rabbits, one would anticipate a similar quantitative neuropathology in relation to the sacral nerves supplying the fibula and fibular rays on the lateral side of the foot.

The femur in fibular and tibial defects

Femur

Reduction in mass of the femur is a common feature associated with fibular hypo/aplasia – so common that the complex is dubbed 'FFU syndrome'.

As noted in Chapter 24, a second type of proximal focal femoral dysplasia (PFFD) can accompany reduction of the fibula and loss of the lateral toe or toes of the foot. The morphology of the distal femur is superficially similar to the PFFD of thalidomide embryopathy, but there are some differences. While the presence of a distal triangular remnant of femur, based at the knee, is common to both, in FFU, the triangle has a less sharp apex, and may have more bone fragments at the proximal end, or a proximal pseudarthrosis connecting the fragments to the shaft, or even a short formed femur.

Sclerotome anatomy

Reading the reduction of the femur with the sclerotome maps (see Chapter 21: Figure 21.3), its morphology is consistent with proximal reduction in the sacral sclerotomes on the posterior surface of the femur, tending to bow or bend the femoral shaft forward. A logical explanation can be derived from the sclerotome maps. We have seen that thalidomide deleted the anterior sclerotomes: L3, L4 and L5 (Chapter 24). This left the posterior aspect of the femur, which composed the long triangle of PFFD from the residual sclerotomes: part of L5 and all of S1 and S2.

In FFU, the opposite happens. The posterior sclerotomes, S1 and S2, are deleted. In the femur, the posterior aspect loses S1, which is the longitudinal core of the limb, encompassing the intercondylar notch and its contents, including the cruciate ligaments. The anterior sclerotomes remain – L3, L4 and part of L5 – and they too form a longitudinal triangle based at the knee joint.

Thus there are two ways of generating the distal femoral triangle that typifies PFFD, *depending upon whether the anterior or posterior sclerotomes are deleted* (Figures 29.11 and 29.12).

Either of these subtractions can generate a characteristic upper femoral deficiency of PFFD – when associated with FFU, it tends to have a greater volume of residual bone, and makes a better attempt to attain the normal anatomy. However, it can also delete the intercondylar notch and its contained ligaments with bifurcation of the distal end of the femur – the most rare and bizarre of all its forms.

The distal end of the femur may be branched or bifid.[25] Van de Kamp et al[26] dissected an amputation specimen of a bifid distal femur in two cases with FFU syndrome. The cruciate ligaments and patellar ligament were absent. They appear to travel with the intercondylar notch.

Ogden[25] in 1976 published a case of bifurcation of the distal femur in a child with tibial aplasia (Figure 29.11). He noted that 'tibial hemimelia was definitely present in three and probably four of the other reported cases.' Thalidomide was not mentioned. According to the sclerotome maps and to the thalidomide records, Figure 29.11

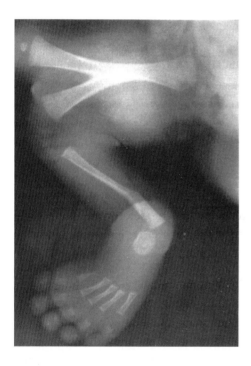

Figure 29.11 *Radiograph of femoral bifurcation associated with tibial aplasia and intact foot. (Reproduced with permission from Ogden JA, J Bone Joint Surg Am 1976; **58**: 712–13.[25])*

shows typical subtraction of L4 in the lower leg, together with subtraction of the tibial triangle of L3. Additional more proximal damage to L3 appears to have eliminated the core of the distal anterior triangle of the femur supplied by L3. This extraordinary split or bifid femur is consistent with total deletion of L3 and 4 in Ogden's case. But Van de Kamp's two cases of bifid distal femur are reported to have FFU syndrome, so that the posterior femoral triangle supplied by S1,2 may have been deleted instead. Thus similar femoral defects may have two different aetiologies, and two possible sclerotome interpretations may exist for the same defect. The presence of two sclerotomal triangles back to back on the distal femur creates this apparent ambiguity. The key to interpretation lies in the defects in the lower leg and foot.

Lewin, Opitz and Reynolds[27] reviewed fibular aplasia and hypoplasia, and recognized two distinct developmental fields in

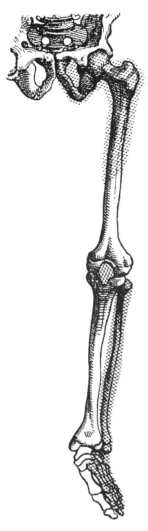

the lower leg – a tibial and a fibular field (Figure 29.12). I agree with them, but I would take their discussion further, and I would interpret their developmental fields as areas of nerve supply, or sclerotomes. Each developmental field is one sclerotome, or a group of sclerotomes, either tibial/lumbar/anterior or fibular/sacral/posterior. When they express injury from embryonic neuropathy, the field defects are very different below the knee, but superficially alike above the knee, in the distal femur, because of the similar back-to-back triangles there.

The malformations in the rays of the foot and the tarsal coalitions indicate that sacral sclerotomes are missing or disordered in the lower leg. The foot is the key to the femur. Using the sclerotome maps, one can read the foot sclerotomes first – identify the residual sclerotomes – and follow up them into the distal femur. Sacral sclerotomes in the femur are posterior. When they drop out, the anterior sclerotomes remain, and the femoral triangle is formed by lumbar 3–5 anteriorly.

This is the opposite to the PFFD in thalidomide embryopathy. Figure 29.5 is a reminder that all the sacral structures (the foot, tarsus and fibula) remain intact until last in thalidomide embryopathy, all in the posterior sclerotomes (S1 and S2). Meanwhile the proximal three-quarters of the femur has disappeared, leaving PFFD. In thalidomide, the triangle of distal femur is the remaining posterior triangle. The anterior sclerotomes (L3–5) are lost in the tibia and femur. They do not reach the foot.

Therefore one cannot say that PFFD is typically a fibular developmental field defect: *PFFD can be either a tibial or a fibular field defect.*

Histopathology of PFFD

Boden et al[28] analysed the histology of growth plates and epiphyses of a 21-week fetus with PFFD. The defect was characterized by 'altered proliferation and maturation of chondrocytes' manifested in every zone of the growth plate. The chondrocytes appeared rounded in shape, resembling embryologically primitive, less differentiated cells, which failed to organize into a growth plate with normal vertical columns of proliferating cartilage cells. Consequently, the septa of the cartilage matrix were horizontal and honeycombed rather than vertical.

The hypertrophic zone was narrow: 2–3 cells thick instead of the normal 8–10 cells at this age. The chondrocytes here were relatively immature. Vessels invaded the hypertrophic zone in a disorderly manner and created an abnormal pattern of osteoid deposition that led to later disorganized geometry for mineralization. Boden et al[28] concluded that the cause of PFFD is 'a defect affecting the regulation of proliferation and maturation of chondrocytes and collagen synthesis' before differentiation. Their observations could be explained by reduced neurotrophism, reduced mitoses, and fewer cells to construct the normal growth plate.

Figure 29.12 *The 'fibular' developmental field of the lower limb, hatched upon Vesalius' drawing of the skeleton of the human leg (Tabulae Sex, Andreas Vesalius, 1538). Reproduced from Lewin SO, Opitz JM and Reynolds JF,* Am J Med Gen *1986;* **25***(S2): 215–38.[27]*

C7 and S1 sclerotome defects: central and genetic – 'split' hand or foot

Synonyms include central hypoplasia, ectrodactyly and lobster claw (Figure 29.13).

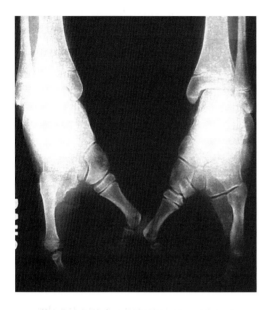

Figure 29.13 *'Lobster claw foot': deletion of the S1 sclerotomes.*

Anatomy

Absence of the central ray or rays of the hand or foot is often associated with syndactyly (fusion) of the remaining digits. The third digit is most commonly absent, then the index finger. A more extreme form is monodactyly, where only one digit remains, resembling the thumb, and the long bone of the forearm appears to be the radius. There is overlap with ulnar reduction in some families, as illustrated in Figures 29.3 and 29.4.

Incidence

According to Birch-Jensen,[7] this is 1 in 90 000 births.

Aetiology

This is genetic. Familial inheritance can be dominant or recessive, with variable penetrance. Many are autosomal dominants.

Associations

Various anomalies of face, palate, eyes, ears, nails, heart and lower limbs are recorded.[29] It can be a component of several syndromes.

Radiology

Variable bone defects underlie the cleft.

Sclerotome subtraction

In the hand, the *7th cervical* sclerotome is subtracted, and hypoplasia, synostosis, etc. are seen in the adjacent sclerotomes. The digital ray of the middle finger is nearly always absent, and sometimes the index finger as well, either bilateral or unilateral. Some cases are peripheral and do not involve the carpus; others extend proximally and reduce the metacarpal and carpal bones.

In the foot, the *1st sacral* sclerotome is subtracted, with variable hypoplastic changes in the adjacent 2nd sacral and 5th lumbar distributions. Cleft-hand and cleft-foot may occur together.

Cleft-hand and -foot indicate that a genetic abnormality can be expressed through the peripheral nerve supply, with subtraction of those sclerotomes that were most resistant to thalidomide.

This raises the question of why the central rays of the extremities were resistant to thalidomide's attack. Leaving aside any other arguments, the point can be made that the innervation of the central rays of the extremities is reinforced, as it were, from overlap of three nerves. In the hand, the central (C7) section receives nerve fibres from three segments, C6–8, obeying the neurological principle of a one-segment overlap each way. The central part of the foot (S1) is similarly supplied by three segments, L5, S1 and S2. In contrast, the edges of the extremities are only supplied by one to two segments.

Resistance to a toxic insult such as thalidomide may be directly proportional to the number of available sources of segmental innervation. Multiple segments may help to ensure resistance to an outside neurotoxin. But numerous segments will not over-rule inherent gene expression.

Sclerotome multiplication

These bizarre malformations were very rarely recorded in thalidomide embryopathy (Figure 27.6), but they are also reported sporadically as non-familial birth defects of unknown aetiology. The hand or foot has more than five digits (Figure 29.14). There is usually associated absence of the radius or tibia, and, as in thalidomide embryopathy, the missing bone may be replaced by a fibrocartilaginous band. However, there is excess mesenchymal mass at the extremity, resulting in extra digits – in contrast to a general reduction in mass in thalidomide cases. The most extreme forms have duplication of the ulna or fibula as well as distal structures, termed dimelia. Judging from reports in the literature, there is a role for sclerotomes in the morphogenesis of these cases. One could predict that such cases express intense neurological irritation, similar to polydactyly, but greater in degree and more proximal.

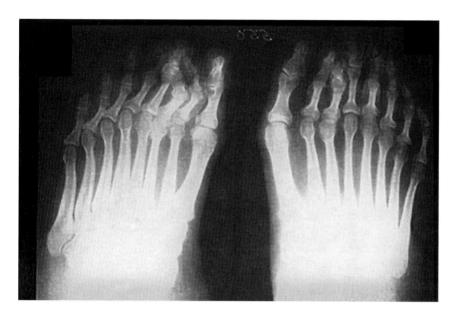

Figure 29.14 *Duplication of the S1 sclerotome in the foot.*

Non-segmental neuropathies

Transverse and distal reduction defects

This section describes a mixture of congenital malformations that are clearly not of segmental origin. They tend to be distal in the extremities and do not involve proximal structures such as major long bones. Their distribution appears to be related to the main nerve trunks rather than to the spinal segments. The presence of partly formed hand elements suggests that the injury occurred later than the thalidomide-sensitive period, during late embryonic or early fetal periods.

There can be no certainty about these predictions in the absence of maps of the truncal nerve supply to the skeleton. One has to match the photographs of defects with the maps of skin innervation, which is a comparatively crude method. Whether or not other deformities relate to non-segmental nerve supply is not known. The following are largely hypothetical notions, but they might stimulate future research.

Truncal and other neuropathies may explain the distribution of some distal reduction defects

War injuries that require surgery to damaged peripheral nerves have stimulated the publication of textbooks on the surgical anatomy of the limbs with details on the effects of sensory nerve injury:[30]

> 'The area supplied by any one nerve varies from patient to patient, and depends on the extent to which its territory is overlapped by adjacent nerves; particularly the median and ulnar nerves.'

The skin supplied by peripheral nerve trunks and their branches has been mapped in such books.[30,31] These maps can be applied to congenital malformations in the group that do not correlate with the sclerotomes.

Transverse defects are not segmental nerve lesions. Some might be explained as nerve trunk injuries, occurring later in embryonic life, at a stage when the hand has already been initiated as far as nubbins or a miniature hand shape. The hand ceases to progress beyond that size and shape, but the upper arm, which is still innervated, continues to grow normally.

Trans-humeral defects could be whole-brachial-plexus injury excluding T2, or a residual C5 arm.

Below-elbow amputation (BEA) defects could be due to later injury to radial, musculo-cutaneous and medial cutaneous nerves combined. Nubbins are common; more advanced hands are rare. The elbow joint is present. These forearm transverse defects are the most common single malformation in any series of limb deficiencies of unknown origin. They are almost always unilateral, with no other associations.

Digital defects of fingers and finger tips with preservation of thumb and little finger could be median nerve injury later in the embryo (Figures 29.15 and 29.16).

Absence of digits on the ulnar aspect of hand, but without loss of the ulna itself, could indicate a later ulnar nerve injury (Figures 29.17 and 29.18).

Defects of the toes without loss of major long bones could be injury to medial popliteal or posterior tibial nerves (Figures 29.19–29.21). The areas eliminated appear to correspond to the modality of light touch rather than pin prick on neurological testing.

The dimple in the shoulder in amelia is related to the deltoid muscle and the overlying skin supplied by the circumflex nerve (C5 and 6).

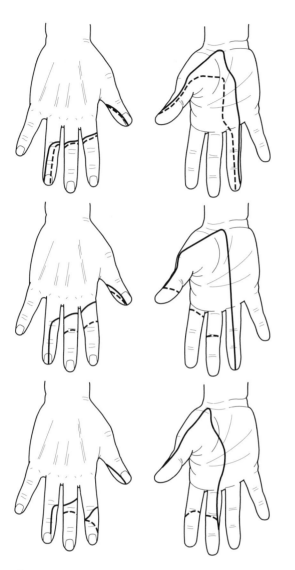

Figure 29.15 *Variants of sensory loss following median nerve injury.*

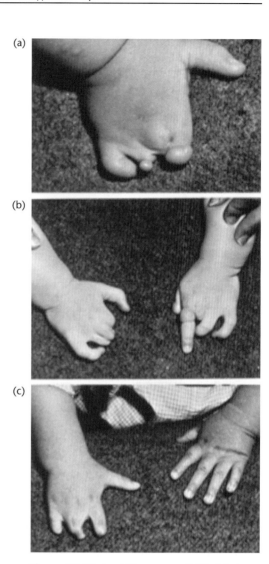

Figure 29.16 *(a–c) Three cases of birth defects suggesting prenatal median nerve damage. The cases shown in (a) and (b) are complicated by constriction bands.*

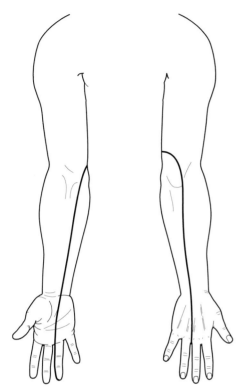

Figure 29.17 *Sensory loss in ulnar truncal neuropathy.*

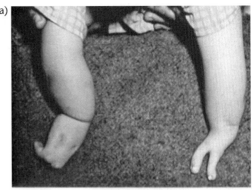

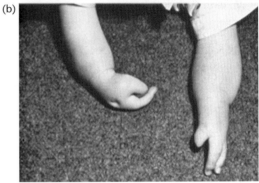

Figure 29.18 *(a,b) Two cases of distal reduction in similar areas of forearms and hands.*

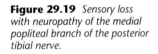

Figure 29.19 *Sensory loss with neuropathy of the medial popliteal branch of the posterior tibial nerve.*

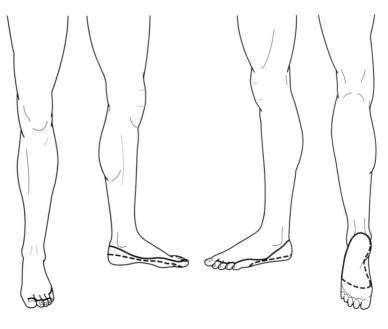

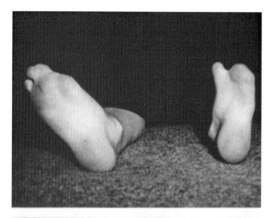

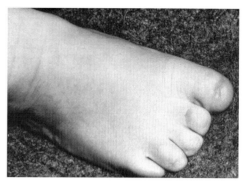

Figure 29.21 *Distal limb reduction in the area of the medial popliteal branch of the posterior tibial nerve.*

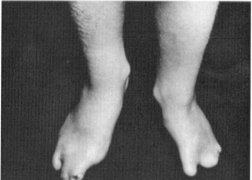

Figure 29.20 *Distal reduction in the same area.*

Glove-and-stocking distribution

Some sensory neuropathies in medicine are not segmental in distribution, but transverse. They are sometimes described as 'glove-and-stocking' neuropathies. They obviously do not lie in the distribution of segmental sensory nerves. The sensory symptoms start at the periphery and work up the limb as the disease progresses.

Could this explain transverse skeletal defects? Could congenital transverse 'amputation' defects of the limbs be the equivalent of glove-and-stocking anaesthesia in the embryo?

References

1. O'Rahilly R. Morphological patterns in limb deficiencies and duplications. *Am J. Anat* 1954; **89**: 135–94.

2. Lausecker H. Der angeborene Defect der Ulna. *Virchows Arch Path Anat* 1954; **325**: 211

3. Kelikian H. *Congenital Deformities of the Hand and Forearm*. Philadelphia: WB Saunders, 1974.

4. Ogden JA, Watson HK, Bohne W. Ulnar dysmelia. *J Bone Joint Surg Am* 1976; **58**: 467–75.

5. Card RY, Strachman J. Congenital ankylosis of the elbow. *J Pediatr.* 1955; **46**: 81–5.

6. Warkany J, Schraffenberger E. Congenital malformations induced in rats by Roentgen rays. *AJR Am J Roentgenol* 1947; **57**: 455–63.

7. Birch-Jensen A. *Congenital Deformities of the Upper Extremities.* Copenhagen: Munksgaard, 1949.

8. Kallen B, Rahmani TM, Winberg J. Infants with congenital limb reduction registered in the Swedish Register of Congenital Malformations. *Teratology* 1984; **29**: 73–85.

9. Lamb DW, Wynne-Davies R, Soto L. An estimate of the population frequency of congenital malformations of the upper limb. *J Hand Surg* 1982; **7**: 557–62.

10. Spiers AL, Cuthbert R. Thalidomide-induced malformations – a radiological survey. *Clin Radiol* 1963; **2**: 163–9.

11. Roberts AS. A case of deformity of the forearm and hands with an unusual history of congenital deficiency. *Ann Surg* 1886; **3**: 135.

12. Southwood AR. Partial absence of the ulna and associated structures *J Anat* 1927; **61**: 346–51.

13. Pfeiffer RA. Beitrag zur erblicken Verkürzung von Ulna und Fibula. In: Wiedemann HR, ed. *Dysostosen.* Stuttgart: Gustav Fischer, 1966: 130.

14. Lenz W. Anomalien des Wachstums und der Körperform. In: Becker PE, ed. *Humangenetik.* Stuttgart: Georg Thieme, 1964.

15. Warkany J. *Congenital Malformations: Notes and Comments.* Chicago: Yearbook Medical Publishers, 1971.

16. Weicker H. 100 children with thalidomide embryopathy. In: Proceedings of XIth International Congress of Pediatrics, 1965.

17. Lenz W, Zygulska M, Herst J. FFU complex: an analysis of 491 cases. *Hum Genet* 1993; **91**: 197–200.

18. Willert HG, Henkel HL. Pathologisch–anatomische Prinzipien bei Extremitätenfehlbildungen, dargestellt am Beispiel der Finger. *Z Orthop Ihre Grenzgeb* 1970; **107**: 663–75.

19. Smithells RW, Newman CG. Recognition of thalidomide defects. *J Med Genet* 1992; **29**: 716–23.

20. Henkel H-L, Willert H-G. Dysmelia. A classification and a pattern of malformation in a group of congenital defects of the limbs. *J Bone Joint Surg Br* 1969; **51**: 399–414.

21. Anton CG, Applegate KE, Kuivila TE, Wilkes DC. Proximal focal femoral deficiency (PFFD): more than an abnormal hip. *Semin Musculoskel Radiol* 1999; **3**: 215–25.

22. Fordham LA, Applegate KE, Wilkes CD, Chung CJ. Fibular hemimelia: more than just an absent bone. *Semin Musculoskel Radiol* 1999; **3**: 227–37.

23. McCredie J. Sclerotome subtraction: a radiologic interpretation of reduction deformities of the limbs. *Birth Defects Original Article Series* 1977; **13**: 65–77.

24. Dennis MG. Proximal femoral focal deficiency, 2006. http://www.emedicine.com/orthoped/topic547.htm.

25. Ogden JA. Ipsilateral femoral bifurcation and tibial hemimelia: a case report. *J Bone Joint Surg Am* 1976; **58**: 712–13.

26. Van de Kamp JM, van der Smagt JJ, Bos CFA, et al. Bifurcation of the femur with tibial agenesis and additional anomalies. *Am J Med Genet* 2005; **138A**: 45–50

27. Lewin SO, Opitz JM, Reynolds JF. Fibular a/hypoplasia: review and documentation of the fibular developmental field. *Am J Med Genet* 1986; **25**(S2): 215–38.

28. Boden SD, Fallon MD, Davidson R, et al. Proximal focal femoral deficiency. *J Bone Joint Surg Am* 1989; **71**: 1119–29.

29. Temtamy SA, McKusick VA. *The Genetics of Hand Malformations*. New York: Alan R Liss, 1978.

30. *Aids to the Investigation of Peripheral Nerve Injuries* (MRC: War Memorandum No. 7). London: HMSO, 1972.

31. Sunderland S. *Nerves and Nerve Injuries*, 2nd edn. Edinburgh: Churchill Livingstone, 1978.

CHAPTER 30

Review of actions of thalidomide

'A new scientific truth does not triumph by convincing its opponents and making them see the light, but rather because its opponents eventually die, and a new generation grows up that is familiar with it.'

Max Planck in *A Scientific Biography* (1949)

Actions of thalidomide

Thalidomide is believed to have the following actions:

Proven:
1. Teratogenic
2. Hypnosedative
3. Neurotoxic

Hypothetical:
4. Anti-inflammatory
5. Anti-angiogenic
6. Anti-cancer
7. Immunomodulatory
8. Other:
   (a) Mutagenic
   (b) Molecular

Chapter Summary
- Actions of thalidomide

  Proven:
  - Teratogenic
  - Hypnosedative
  - Neurotoxic

  Hypothetical:
  - Anti-inflammatory
  - Anti-angiogenic
  - Anti-cancer
  - Immunomodulatory
  - Other hypotheses
- Conclusions
- References

The first three actions have been proved by many researchers in the past, as described in previous chapters.

The hypothetical actions 4–7 have arisen in recent years in response to 'an urgent need for understanding the mechanism of teratogenicity induced by thalidomide'.[1] This urgent need arose because of the 'recent resurgence of the use of thalidomide for a variety of indications, ranging from the treatment of erythema nodosum leprosum (a complication of lepromatous leprosy) to the treatment of aphthous ulcers and wasting associated with HIV infection.'[1]

Action 8 includes hypotheses that seek to explain thalidomide-induced limb defects in terms of modern developments in molecular biology and genetics.

Anti-inflammatory

Just 3 years after the teratogenic action of thalidomide was recognized, the drug was proposed to have an anti-inflammatory effect through its successful use in treating type II leprosy reaction, also known as ENL (erythema nodosum leprum).[2] This reaction is believed to be due to a humoral immune response whereby groups of painful vasculitic lumps appear. Histologically, there is leucocyte infiltration around the post-capillary venules of the subcutis, producing a focal necrotizing vasculitis.[3] This is associated with severe nerve damage 'through immune attack upon Schwann cells which in lepromatous leprosy are heavily infected by *Mycobacterium leprae*'.[2]

In 1964, Sheskin, a dermatologist and leprologist in Jerusalem, had a patient with ENL and insomnia due to severe neuritic pain.[2] After a few nights' treatment with thalidomide, the patient's pain, fever and nodular swellings regressed, but returned when thalidomide was discontinued. Similar observations were made in two more patients. Thalidomide has subsequently been said to be effective to *relieve pain and reduce the masses in over 90% of type II leprosy reactions.*

This phenomenon opened possibilities of further immunological research, and also stimulated clinical trials of thalidomide in the therapy of other chronic inflammatory diseases.[4] Successful treatment was recorded in Behçet's syndrome and other painful aphthous ulcerations of mucous membranes.

Koch of Vienna has reviewed thalidomide as an anti-inflammatory agent in leprosy, lupus erythematosus, prurigo nodularis, actinic prurigo, aphthous stomatitis and other cutaneous conditions.[5-8] He has also reviewed its role in gastric ulcers and ulcerative colitis. Readers are referred to his comprehensive review.[5]

Anti-angiogenic

Arteries have been seen as a possible target tissue following a publication by D'Amato et al,[9] who looked at the effect of thalidomide on neo-angiogenesis, the formation of new blood vessels. They had developed a model for observing the formation of blood vessels around the cornea on the eyeball of rabbit. They constructed a micropocket in the rabbit's cornea, and into this they inserted a pellet containing basic fibroblast growth factor (bFGF), known to be a potent angiogen. It was bound to sucralfate to provide slow release of the growth factor. Post-operative infection was prevented by erythromycin ointment on the surface of the cornea. This meant that any neovascularization could be assumed as not being due to inflammation, but to stimulation by the bFGF in the pocket. The animals were fed by gavage with daily doses of thalidomide 200 mg/kg for 12 days. A 30–51% inhibition of angiogenesis (median 36%) was detected by second daily slit-lamp examination, to measure vessel length from the limbus.

D'Amato et al[9] concluded that 'thalidomide is an inhibitor of angiogenesis induced by bFGF in the rabbit cornea micropocket assay. The mechanism by which thalidomide inhibits angiogenesis is unknown.'

Their additional claim that the experiment 'sheds light on the mechanism of thalidomide's teratogenicity' was criticized by Neubert and Neubert,[10] toxicologists and pharmacologists from Berlin. They made the following critical points:

1. *On hypothetical vascular lesions as a basis of teratogenicity:*
   There is no vascular pathology in primate offspring:

   'Rhesus and marmoset monkeys with thalidomide-induced malformations show surprisingly few necroses, quite in contrast to abnormalities produced by many other teratogenic agents.'[10]

2. *On the precision and distribution of thalidomide malformations:*

   'It is extremely unlikely that such a broad and common mechanism as angiogenesis would be responsible for such well-defined defects as those induced by thalidomide.'[10]

3. *On the dose levels of thalidomide for anti-angiogenesis:*
   (a) 0.7–3 mg/kg body weight = human sedative/hypnotic dose (average 1 mg/kg)
   (b) 3–7 mg/kg body weight = human anti-inflammatory or immunomodulatory dose
   (c) 200 mg/kg body weight = rabbit anti-angiogenesis in corneal pouch experiments
   The extremely high dose used in these experiments is orders of magnitude greater than human therapeutic dose levels. Neubert and Neubert[10] say that:

   'No relationship can be implied between such discrepant doses. There is no evidence of angiogenic inhibition at human dose levels, and it is misleading to construe any such connection.'[10]

4. *On absence of evidence to support their claim:*

   'Without any evidence of similar effects occurring in embryonic tissue and especially in the developing limb bud, the authors speculated that the anti-angiogenic effect observed in the cornea might be responsible for the teratogenic effect in this class of substances.'[10]

There is no connection between the cornea and the embryo. D'Amato et al[9] suggest that the blood vessels in the embryo are the target. Established facts in human, primate and rabbit experience with thalidomide embryopathy contradict that suggestion.

Anti-cancer

Thalidomide's application as a possible anti-cancer drug was a consequence of the 'anti-angiogenesis hypothesis'. Very high doses were recommended to achieve the theoretical vascular inhibition.

Given the basic flaws in the original experiment and its interpretation, the 'anti-angiogenesis hypothesis' has been been accorded more attention than it deserves. It has been used to argue the case for using thalidomide as an anti-cancer drug, on the basis that many tumours have neovascularity, or abnormal blood vessels feeding them. The theory is that thalidomide might halt the development of new tumour vessels and thus reduce the size of a tumour, on the basis of its proposed 'anti-angiogenic' action. This has led to clinical trials in cancer patients.[11]

But sensory peripheral nerve damage occurred in the 1950–60s with sedative doses, at an average 1 mg/kg body weight. Recommended doses for anti-cancer therapy are orders of magnitude greater than the sedative range, and sensory neuropathy[12–16] in most of these patients was to be a predictable sequel. Sensory neuropathy was not mentioned in the rabbit eyeball experiment, partly because rabbits cannot complain of sensory symptoms, and partly because the experimental focus on the eyeball excluded wider considerations such as the sensory nervous system. Translation of observations on the rabbit corneal pocket to therapeutic use in humans is illogical. It is a leap of faith, not science.

The high doses required for the 'anti-angiogenic' effect did extract a high price from the patients: painful sensory peripheral neuropathy intervened. Individual patients left the trials with pain and paraesthesia in addition to their malignancy.

It is now over 20 years since D'Amato et al[9] launched the anti-angiogenesis hypothesis. Trials of thalidomide in cancer have been reported with varying results. Review articles are now appearing.[11–18] Between 30% and 100% of participants are reported to have peripheral neuropathy. There has been a high rate of patient withdrawal from these studies, and of patient refusal to take the drug. Concerns have been expressed by some clinicians that appropriate diagnostic tests have not been used to establish the presence or absence of sensory neuropathy. Some publications do not treat sensory neuropathy as a parameter to be measured. Others admit that sensory neuropathy has limited the study, and thus the potential therapeutic application of the drug.

So *sensory peripheral neuropathy* acquired during thalidomide treatment has been the limiting factor in therapeutic trials in other chronic inflammatory diseases as well as malignancies. Multiple myeloma has shown the best therapeutic response, but, again, most patients contract sensory peripheral neuropathy from the treatment.

In summary, thalidomide's therapeutic use is limited by its own inherent sensory neurotoxicity. Molecular variants are being sought in an attempt to avoid the neuropathy.

Immunomodulatory

The advent of thalidomide coincided with exponential growth of the science of immunology itself.

An early immunological hypothesis

Hellman et al[19] suggested that if thalidomide inhibited the rejection of transplanted tissue, presumably due to inhibition of normal immunological reactions, it did not deform the fetus, but prevented the spontaneous abortion of an already malformed fetus. On this basis, thalidomide was proposed to have a 'life-promoting' effect on deformed embryos that would not have survived under normal circumstances. If this were true, there should be a very high incidence of dysmelic malformations in all naturally aborted fetuses without thalidomide exposure. This is not the case, for dysmelia is found as rarely in abortuses as it is in normal full-term deliveries. Their hypothesis of an immunological basis for the teratogenic action collapsed before the evidence.

Later immunological hypotheses

Subsequently, many laboratories were engulfed by the exponential growth of immunology (accelerated by the AIDS epidemic in the 1980s). The effect on thalidomide research in laboratories was to redirect efforts into hunting for possible immunological abnormalities. The tissue level was bypassed in favour of tests at the sub-cellular level. The disappointing and inconclusive results of this world-wide immunological research effort was summarized by Zwingenberger and Wnendt[3] of the Grunenthal Centre of Research, Aachen, Germany, in 1996. They reviewed the results of the immunological experiments with thalidomide during three decades. In summary, these experiments have focused upon the lymphatic and immune systems, and the results have been 'disappointing'. These authors note the neuropathic side effects of thalidomide. They also note the fact that *[14]C-labelled thalidomide in mice is taken up in the peripheral nerve trunks, but not in the skin or lymphoid tissues.*

There were problems with the drug and with immunological models for its investigation:

- The main difficulty with the drug was its inherent instability in solution, and rapid hydrolysis into non-teratogenic by-products.
- The main difficulty with the models available for immune-testing was that there was no model of the peripheral nervous system, or, indeed, of any dendritic cell.
- Therefore the standard tests were done on lymphocytes and other haematopoietic cells, which were certainly not targeted by thalidomide in the embryo.

This mismatch between a neurotropic drug and non-neural cell cultures rendered inconclusive the considerable efforts in immunology laboratories to prove thalidomide's alleged properties of immuno-modulation as the basis for its teratogenicity.

Zwingenberger and Wnendt[3] state:

'The organ specificity evident in the teratological alterations caused by thalidomide, and in the response patterns to thalido-mide in clinical use as an immunotherapeutic agent, are not easily explained by pharmacokinetic distribution phenomena. More extensive studies would be required to establish organ specific activation of thalidomide. Yet another possible basis for tissue specificity would be an effect upon intracellular signal transduction pathways operative in some but not all cell types. Both for the nervous and immune systems, such specific signalling pathways are well characterised – as a matter of fact, many of these pathways are shared by the nervous and immune systems. However, this promising area has not been addressed with thalidomide yet.'

They go on to summarize the tests to date, which show no evidence of immunosuppression, and no effect of thalidomide on T-cell populations. There is a doubtful effect of thalidomide on B-cell function (an effect unsupported by recent studies). Thalidomide has no effect on phagocytosis, and there are conflicting reports on its effect on monocytes and granulocytes. Interpretations of experimental results are sometimes *negated by the rapid hydrolysis of thalidomide in solution*, and the probability that the effects relate to some *hydrolytic product* rather than the parent molecule. More complex experiments on the effects of thalidomide on cytokine generation and release (and related genes) are even more difficult to interpret and yield sometimes conflicting results, as do examinations of the Arthus reaction with thalidomide. The thorough review of thalidomide and immunology by Zwingenberger and Wnendt[3] leaves many issues unresolved, ambiva-lent or negated. Many doubts persist and others multiply:

'Given that the inhibition of cytokine synthesis, in particular TNFα [tumour necrosis factor α] (although this was *not* demon-strated by the authors nor by Neubert's team) *may* contribute to an inhibition of angiogenesis, it remains to be determined whether an activity other than immunomodulation is operative in this system.'

They find that thalidomide has no place as an immunosuppressant in solid organ transplants:

'As for chronic graft-vs-host disease, thalidomide is widely used both in multiple drug regimens and, by itself, in long-term maintenance treatment, although controlled studies are lacking.

'There are several conundrums in the study of thalidomide. For instance, there is *no compelling proof for any strictly anti-proliferative activity of thalidomide.*

'In vitro experiments have *never shown signs of cytotoxicity by thalidomide.*

'A molecularly defined common denominator of these activities is not known at present.

'There is *no experimental evidence that thalidomide has an immunosuppressive action.*

'In summary, no single mechanism has been identified yet which could account for the clinical activity of thalidomide. *The molecular target of thalidomide has not been identified.'*

Little or no light was shed upon thalidomide's mode of action.

Subsequent clinical papers in journals of dermatology and other specialties have grappled with the risk of inducing a painful, iatrogenic neuropathy into the lives of patients whose original condition is chronic and not life-threatening.[12,15] The jury is still out on some of these matters.

The inherent difficulties of any research with thalidomide include its instability in solution, as already mentioned. Some research papers have not allowed for this, and therefore unwittingly record results from hydrolytic metabolites rather than the intact drug. Zwingenberger and Wnendt[3] also note that molecular biologists since the 1960s have been constrained by having to use the tissue models already established in that science. They note that, in 1964, Koransky and Ullberg demonstrated ^{14}C-labelled thalidomide uptake in the grey matter of the central nervous system (CNS) and major peripheral nerve trunks, as well as in kidney and liver, but no enhanced radioactivity in skin or lymphoid tissue of adult mice. Thalidomide also damaged sensory peripheral nerves in rabbits,[20] indicating the nervous system as the target organ, as clinically suspected. However, there was no stable laboratory model of ganglion cell culture to enable the conduct of in vitro immunology experiments on peripheral nerves, so existing haematopoietic cells have been employed, despite no known interaction between thalidomide and such cells. This mismatch between materials and methods reflects the state of the art, and the problem may be resolved when appropriate cell cultures become available. At the same time, it means that there are probably other, non-immunological, explanations for the observed phenomena.

The reader is referred to the detailed review of 215 scientific publications by Zwingenberger and Wnendt.[3] Despite analysis of these 215 references, they conclude that no single mechanism has been identified to account for the clinical activity of thalidomide. They do not rule out the possibility of a composite mode of action, which may involve signalling pathways such as exist in nerves and lymphatic tissue, and which they consider a promising area for future research.

Other hypotheses

Genetic mutation

In 1997, there was a news report of a daughter born to a British thalidomide father with the same arm deformities. McBride[21] suggested that thalidomide might be a mutagen that could cause transmission of the malformations to the second generation. Two more British families joined the first. This caused great consternation among the thalidomiders, many of whom had already given birth to normal children. The matter was resolved in a series of letters to the *British Medical Journal*.[22,23] In the early days of medicolegal reviews of the thalidomide children for compensation, it was impossible in doubtful cases to prove that thalidomide had *not* been taken by the mother. The malformations were often consistent with thalidomide embryopathy. The medical assessors in UK decided on a policy to give such a child the benefit of the doubt.[22] Thus a group of children were admitted as thalidomiders and awarded compensation, although there was some doubt about the real cause of their defects. The true diagnosis had to await the next generation, when a few cases declared themselves to be familial/genetic in origin by the birth of their child with similar defects. These were some of the 'look-alikes'. They were not mutations, and thalidomide is not a mutagen.[23]

Molecular

Growth factors from the AER?

A skirmish occurred between Tabin, a geneticist from Boston and a newcomer to thalidomide, and Neubert, Merker and Neubert, veteran toxicologists with 30 years' experience in thalidomide research. The two parties debated the teratogenic action of thalidomide in the scientific correspondence column of *Nature*[24,25] after Tabin launched a new hypothesis related to theoretical growth factors and their supposed origin from the apical ectodermal ridge (AER). He illustrated this idea with a diagram of a malformation that was never recorded in thalidomide embryopathy.[24] He stated that the pharmacological basis for thalidomide's effect remains controversial, presumably unaware of its proven sensory neurotoxicity (Chapters 2 and 4). Instead, he made a vague proposal that it inhibited growth of blood vessels, 'leading to shortening of the long bones'. The German group pointed out that thalidomide acts before the AER is present, and therefore acts medial and deep to the site of the future limb bud.[25] They list several other known factors in relation to thalidomide that are not explained by Tabin's hypothesis, and are possibly unknown to him. Neubert et al propose that thalidomide inhibits cell migration. The argument was left unresolved, but with Neubert et al much closer to the truth, because they argued using facts, not fiction.

Truncation of the limb bud by molecules?

Ever since the early days of the thalidomide epidemic, laboratory scientists have striven to identify its molecular target rather than its target organ. A very large literature has evolved on the possible molecular biology of thalidomide – most of it highly theoretical and unrelated to the realities of the birth defects caused by the drug. In my opinion, any molecular investigations are premature and meaningless unless the target tissue or organ has been identified first. As explained in earlier chapters, the macroscopic target was either never identified, or, if identified, it was not recognized by scientists.

Absence of the target organ is why thalidomide research has come unstuck. Investigation of subcellular targets should *follow* identification of the target tissue or organ, *not precede* that identification. Reversing this logical and systematic approach has converted the search for the pathogenesis of thalidomide into the proverbial hunt for a needle in a haystack. Researchers have sailed into the molecular ocean without a compass. Much money, time and effort has been invested in biochemical and molecular investigations. Hypotheses devised thereby are unrelated to anatomic deformities, and do not help anyone to understand birth defects. The following abstract of Stephens and Fillmore's molecular hypothesis[26] is a prime example, and is quoted verbatim:

'We propose that thalidomide affects the following pathway during limb development: Growth factors (FGF-2 and IGF-1) attach to receptors on limb bud mesenchymal cells and initiate some second messenger system (perhaps SP-1), which activates $\alpha\upsilon$ and $\beta3$ integrin subunit genes. The resulting $\alpha\upsilon\beta3$ integrin proteins stimulate angiogenesis in the developing limb bud. Several steps in this pathway depend on the activation of genes with primary GC promoters (GGGCGG). Thalidomide, or a hydrolysis or metabolic breakdown product, specifically binds to GC promoter sites and inhibits transcription of those genes. Inhibition of the genes interferes with normal angiogenesis, which results in truncation of the limb.'

There are two factual errors embedded in this opacity:

1. Thalidomide did not truncate limbs. Truncation is an excision process transverse to the long axis. Thalidomide subtracted longitudinal, not transverse, bands. Do these authors understand the deformities they say they are researching?
2. Thalidomide did not act in the human limb bud. It acted *before* the limb bud existed when the human records are reconstructed (Figure 13.5). Neubert's group found the same precocious action in subhuman primates; their comments on Tabin's hypothesis also apply to Stephens and Fillmore.

In the absence of a target organ to which subcellular facts can relate, molecular hypotheses read as gibberish.[27] Molecular theories will only be meaningful if derived from studies of that target organ or tissue.

Highly theoretical molecular targets cannot explain any of the following 12 facts of thalidomide's teratogenesis:

1. Action pre-dates limb bud
2. Sensitive period
3. Craniocaudal sequence
4. Bilateral symmetry of 80% of malformations
5. Predominance of upper over lower limb defects
6. Sparing of CNS
7. Longitudinal distribution of bone loss
8. Characteristic shapes of residual bone remnants
9. Dislocations
10. Synostoses
11. Association between skeletal and visceral defects
12. Onset of sensory peripheral neuropathy in middle age

The molecular hypotheses do not address a single one of these 12 fundamental characteristics of thalidomide embryopathy.

The theory of neural crest injury explains all 12.

Only the neural crest theory can explain number 12, a new problem besetting the original thalidomide victims, many of whom began to complain of tingling and numbness in their reduced extremities at middle age. It appears to be a sensory equivalent of post-polio syndrome. No other hypothesis can offer any rationale to explain this. This latest development in the thalidomide saga proves that thalidomide acted upon the neural crest.

Zwingenberger and Wnendt[3] did not find any scientific evidence of anti-inflammatory properties. The anti-inflammatory action may be explained by common sense and simple neurology rather than immunology. If low-dose thalidomide reduces afferent sensory impulses, it will reduce both pain sensation and the paraesthesia of pruritis, the sensation of itching. It is an old maxim in medicine that 'it will never get well if you scratch it'. Reduction of pruritis will reduce the reflex to scratch the skin lesion. Thus secondary inflammation that follows scratching would be reduced. The painful ulcers and pruritis that characterize the dermatological conditions that respond to thalidomide may be responding to a neurotoxic reduction in sensory afferent stimuli.

The anti-cancer action is an intriguing property. The review by Zwingenberger and Wnendt[3] found no proof of any cytotoxic or anti-proliferative action by thalidomide. High doses of the drug have been recommended for cancer therapy. A high incidence of sensory neuropathy has resulted. Is the anti-cancer action related to thalidomide's ability to reduce or stop neurotrophism? If so, is the anti-cancer activity mediated through peripheral sensory nerves and their neurotrophic function? Do peripheral nerves therefore have some role in generating mitoses in cancer? If its anticancer action is not via nerves, does thalidomide target a metabolic pathway in neoplastic mitoses that is similar to the metabolic pathway in sensory nerves responsible for neurotrophic mitoses? Can its anti-trophic action on cancer be separated from its anti-neurotrophic action, so that cancer patients are not further damaged by thalidomide therapy?

Thus four of thalidomide's properties condense into one: teratogenic, hypnosedative, neurotoxic and anti-inflammatory actions are all functions of sensory neurotoxicity.

Conclusion

It is fair to conclude from examining other hypotheses that this drug's *primary action* is to damage sensory nerves. Sensory peripheral neuropathy is *not a side-effect*, as repeatedly stated, but it is the drug's *primary action*. To pretend otherwise is to prefer confusion to clarification.

References

1. Hill B. Characterization of embryopathy risks. In: *Thalidomide: Potential Benefits and Risks. An Open Public Scientific Workshop.* NIH, Bethesda, MD, 9 September 1997. Transcript [on line] p98. http://www.fda.gov/oashi/patrep/nih99.html#hill.

2. Sheskin J. Thalidomide in the treatment of lepra reactions. *Clin Pharmacol Ther* 1965; **6**: 303–306.

3. Zwingenberger K, Wnendt S. Immunomodulation by thalidomide: systematic review of the literature and of unpublished observations. *J Inflamm* 1996; **46**: 177–211.

4. Sheskin J. The treatment of lepra reaction in lepromatous leprosy. *Int J Dermatol* 1980; **19**: 318–322.

5. Koch H. Thalidomide and congeners as anti-inflammatory agents. *Prog Med Chem* 1985; **22**: 166–242.

6. Koch HP. Comments on 'Proposed mechanisms of action in thalidomide embryopathy'. *Teratology* 1990; **41**: 243–4.

7. Koch HP. Die Arenoxid-Hypothese der Thalidomid-Wirkung. Uberlegungen zum molekularen Wirkungsmechanismus des 'klassischen' Teratogens. *Sci Pharm* 1981; **49**: 76–99.

8. Koch HP, Czejka MJ. Evidence for the intercalation of thalidomide into DNA: clue to the molecular mechanism of thalidomide teratogenicity? *Z Naturforsch C* 1986; **41**: 1057–61.

9. D'Amato RJ, Loughnan MS, Flynn E, Folkman J. Thalidomide is an inhibitor of angiogenesis. *Proc Natl Acad Sci USA* 1994; **91**: 4082–5.

10. Neubert R, Neubert D. Peculiarities and possible mode of action of thalidomide. In: Kavlock RJ, Daston GP, eds. *Drug Toxicity in Embryonic Development.* Heidelberg: Springer-Verlag, 1996: 41–119.

11. Singhal S, Mehta J. Thalidomide in cancer. *Biomed Pharmacother* 2002; **56**: 4–12.

12. Wines NY, Cooper AJ, Wines MP. Thalidomide in dermatology. *Australas J Dermatol* 2002; **43**: 229–38.

13. Lafitte E, Revuz J. Thalidomide: an old drug with new clinical applications. *Expert Opin Drug Safety* 2004; **3**: 47–56.

14. Wulff CH, Høyer H, Asboe-Hansen G, Brodthagen H. Development of polyneuropathy during thalidomide therapy. *Br J Dermatol* 1985; **112**: 475–80.

15. Clemmensen OJ, Olsen PZ, Andersen KE. Thalidomide neurotoxicity. *Arch Dermatol* 1984; **120**: 338–341.

16. Isoardo G, Bergui M, Durelli L et al. Thalidomide neuropathy: clinical, electrophysiological and neuroradiological features. *Acta Neurol Scand* 2004: **109**: 188–93.

17. Chaudhry V, Crawford M, Crawford TO et al. Toxic neuropathy in patients with pre-existing neuropathy. *Neurology* 2003; **60**: 337–40.

18. Chaudhry V, Cornblath DR, Corse A et al. Thalidomide-induced neuropathy. *Neurology* 2002; **59**: 1872–5.

19. Hellman K, Duke DI, Tucker DF: Prolongation of skin homograft survival by thalidomide. *BMJ* 1965; **ii**: 687–9.

20. Schwab BW, Arezzo JC, Paldino AM et al. Rabbit sural nerve responses to chronic treatment with thalidomide and supimide. *Muscle Nerve* 1984; **7**: 362–8.

21. McBride WG. Thalidomide may be a mutagen. *BMJ* 1994; **308**: 1635–6

22. Smithells RW. Thalidomide may be a mutagen. *BMJ* 1994; **309**: 477.

23. Kida M. Thalidomide may not be a mutagen. *BMJ* 1994; **309**: 741.

24. Tabin CJ. A developmental model for thalidomide defects. *Nature* 1998; **396**: 322–3.

25. Neubert R, Merker HJ, Neubert D. A developmental model for thalidomide defects. *Nature* 1999; **400**: 419–20.

26. Stephens TD, Fillmore BJ. Hypothesis: Thalidomide embryopathy – proposed mechanism of action. *Teratology* 2000; **61**: 189–95.

27. Wheen F. *How Mumbo-Jumbo Conquered the World: A Short History of Modern Delusions*. London: Harper Perennial, 2004: 88–99.

CHAPTER 31

Conclusion: Beyond thalidomide

'We need Ariadne's thread, cunningly woven from observations from nearly all animals, in order to extricate ourselves from this labyrinth.'
William Harvey in *De Generationes Animalium* (1652)

Research trends in neurology

Thalidomide neuropathy was not forgotten by the neurologists. In their textbooks, thalidomide continued to stand out among known neurotoxins for its initial obtrusive action on the sensory nerves, presenting as painful paraesthesia. Professor PK Thomas, of The National Hospital for Nervous Diseases, Queen Square, London, summarized the normal variability of presentation of toxic neuropathies in 1980 in the conclusion of his chapter 'The peripheral nervous system as a target for toxic substances' in the book *Experimental and Clinical Neurotoxicology*:[1]

'Peripheral neuropathies display a variety of clinical patterns related to selective effects on specific components in the peripheral nervous system. This is reflected in topographical variations in the distribution of the weakness or sensory loss, or in the degree of involvement of the cranial nerves. The different patterns may also depend upon variations in the degree to which particular functional modalities (motor, sensory, or autonomic) are implicated. Some of these are explicable in terms of known pathological effects of the toxins concerned. In others, the mechanism is still obscure. Some may depend upon metabolic peculiarities of particular systems of neurons, making them vulnerable to specific toxic substances and leading to pathological consequences analogous to the genetically determined or metabolically induced system degenerations of the nervous system.

'Autonomic function is not usually affected in marked degree in toxic neuropathies, unless they are especially severe.'

The action of thalidomide on particular subpopulations of neurons within the sensory and autonomic nervous systems remains to be

Chapter Summary
- **Research trends in neurology**
- **Research trends in neurotoxicology**
- **Multidisciplinary research teams**
- **The future of thalidomide research**
- **Scientific predictions**
- **References**

elucidated. This information would enhance our understanding of the origin of birth defects. We have seen in Chapters 18 and 19 that large-diameter axons are eliminated by thalidomide. Does thalidomide injure all neurons of neural crest origin, or just particular subgroups?

Research trends in neurotoxicology

A decade later, fuelled by growing sociopolitical concerns such as pollution, workplace safety and environmental protection, the science of neurotoxicology had budded off from general toxicology. Molecular biology was already probing the neuron's internal mechanisms, some of which were highly sensitive to neurotoxins. In 1994, Herker and Hucho of Berlin edited a textbook *Selective Neurotoxicity*[2] to demonstrate the breadth and depth of this relatively new discipline. They state that:

> 'The toxic substance provides a logical link between the interaction at the molecular level and the tissue damage or functional disorder in the whole animal.'

The chapter by Baumgarten and Zimmerman,[3] on the concept of selective vulnerability of neurons to neurotoxins, is subdivided into 11 sections. Ten metabolic functions are examined, and the 11th section discusses the vulnerability of neurons due to the interaction of toxins with its own cytoskeleton. In neurons, two special cytoskeletal elements – neurotubules and neurofilaments – are important for axonal growth, structural stability and axonal transport.[4] Baumgarten and Zimmermann[3] state that

> 'Neurotubules and neurofilaments are sensitive to a variety of toxins which cause axonal dystrophy or degeneration.'

The quantitative reduction in peripheral axons demonstrated in our thalidomide-exposed rabbit fetuses suggests that thalidomide inhibits axonal growth. Does thalidomide injure the cytoskeleton of the axon? What is its effect on structural stability and axonal transport? And on the fast transport mechanism served by neurotubules?

We know that in adult nerves, thalidomide causes axonal degeneration. Therefore the next logical step in the descent into subcellular structures would be to look at its effect on neurotubules and neurofilaments, the elements that comprise much of the mass/diameter of axons, as well as providing an internal conduction system.[4] The effect of thalidomide on these subcellular elements has apparently not been investigated yet, but that begs to be done, both in adult thalidomide neuropathy and in the rabbit embryopathy, where axonal depletion has already been demonstrated. This next stage of research into thalidomide and limb reduction deformities belongs to the new science of neurotoxicology rather than to teratology.

Multidisciplinary research teams

Cavanagh, of the Institute of Psychiatry, London, in a foreword to the 1994 textbook *Principles of Neurotoxicology*,[5] says that the subject of neurotoxicology must be regarded as part of a number of disciplines, having already developed, unrecognized, as part of scientific progress within several biological disciplines for a long while. At the same time, the newly fledged science of neurotoxicology is more than the sum of its component parts.

> 'Because of the complexity of nervous tissue, it (neurotoxicology) must be a *multidisciplinary* study of the effects of neurotoxic chemicals. It is therefore essential that the physiologist engaged in neurotoxicity must become familiar with the biochemistry and pathology of the neurotoxic problem, and at the same time, the biochemist and morphologist must do likewise. While scientists in different disciplines may not necessarily be steeped in the technology possessed by their colleagues, their experience and learning should be such that they can critically assess the conclusions of their colleagues without those feelings of insecurity that too often overwhelm "trespassers" in another field of study. Neurotoxicology cuts across the artificial divisions and barriers that normally separate academic subjects. In neurotoxicology these barriers need to be broken down if proper judgement about mechanisms, chemical interactions, "risk factors" and other important practical aspects of the subject is to be justly exercised.'

The future of thalidomide research

Teratology needs to heed Cavanagh's advice. Recognition of the neural crest as thalidomide's target organ did not emerge from a teratology laboratory, but from clinical radiology – and not without disparagement from a few teratologists along the way. But in 1997, a scientific committee of the US Food and Drug Administration (FDA) reviewed hypotheses that sought to explain the mode of action of thalidomide, during deliberations prior to licensing the drug for therapeutic use in the USA. This impartial review found that neural crest injury was the best of all the theories reviewed.[6]

At present, the majority of sporadic, non-genetic birth defects within the spectrum of thalidomide embryopathy are concerns of developmental biology, teratology and genetics. Progress will continue to founder pending recognition of the fact that these defects result from neurotoxic injury. As such, these non-genetic birth defects are a neurological disease. The way forward is to adopt a multidisciplinary approach. Further exploration of the theory of neural crest injury is clearly a challenge that suits neurotoxicology. Answers will emerge from future application to the embryo of laboratory methods from neurology, neuropathology and neurotoxicology. Answers will not emerge from indiscriminate sorties among thousands of molecules and chemicals. I predict that many congenital malformations, especially those that are mimicked by thalidomide, will be found to be neuropathies expressed by the embryo as disordered growth in the developmental fields of the damaged nerves: embryonic neuropathy.

Therefore the training of future teratologists and geneticists should include specific education in aspects of neuropathology and neurotoxicology, to introduce some degree of mutual understanding, which is presently lacking. Ideally, the teratology research teams of the future will include neuroscientists such as neurotoxicologists, neurologists and neuropathologists.

Quantitative methods in neuropathology, for example, are used every day in clinical neurology, but these techniques are unknown to most teratologists today. Apart from neuroquantitation techniques, the facts of neurotrophism must be understood by would-be investigators of birth defects. Regeneration biology and neuroscience have much to teach teratology, which lags behind both.

In the ideal multidisciplinary team of future teratology, there would be at least one regeneration biologist. Drugs would be tested on amphibian models before proceeding to higher animals. Interference with amphibian regeneration signals a risk for embryonic neuropathy and malformation in the newborn.

Clinicians who understand the spectrum of human birth defects need to be part of the team of investigators. We clinicians have surrendered much of birth defects research to laboratory scientists. We need to ask ourselves whether it is appropriate, or indeed ethical, for a neuropathological condition to be investigated by non-neuroscientists. This deserves serious debate by medical professionals who look after public health, drug regulation, pregnant women, infants and children. Research into congenital reduction defects is much too complex and important an issue in neonatology, paediatrics, obstetrics and surgery to be left in the hands of neurologically unqualified scientists.

The same clinical and neuroscientific skills need to be available to, or represented on, editorial boards of journals that publish research into birth defects. Review articles should be invited from true experts, not amateurs. An ignorant review dislocates progress in research.

If a multidisciplinary reorganization of research teams in teratology cannot be implemented, the alternative is to transfer investigation of this big group of non-genetic birth defects from teratology to neurotoxicology. At the very least, studies of toxic embryonic neuropathies need to be delegated to those trained in toxicology, neuroscience, neurology and neuropathology. The key researchers *must* understand the processes of normality and disease in the nervous system.

Scientific predictions

A good hypothesis or theory not only inter-relates facts that previously appeared to be unrelated, but also enables new facts to be predicted. Scientific prophesy is fraught with risk, because not all such predictions can or will come true. Within these limitations, several predictions can be suggested on the basis of the neural crest hypothesis.

Molecular and chemical proof may never be obtained

Subcellular proof of the neural crest theory may be difficult, if not impossible, to obtain. Medicine is an empirical science, and many accepted facts are unproven in the strict scientific sense, which demands complete understanding of why a thing is so. Pharmacology is a case in point. The precise chemical action of many drugs has never been demonstrated, yet this does not inhibit their general acceptance or their useful application. It was never shown how thalidomide acted as an anti-emetic, but that did not stop it being marketed. Nor was it proved exactly how it caused sensory peripheral neuropathy at the molecular level, although the clinical symptoms, signs, electrophysiological tests and biopsies were clear evidence that it did so. Nevertheless, the epidemic of sensory peripheral neuropathy in the original thalidomiders as they reached middle age proves that the original damage in the embryo was sensorineural. No other hypothesis can explain this recently recognized phenomenon. One could argue that chemical proof is superfluous in the face of the evidence.

Thalidomide's primary action is neurotoxic (correction of current statements)

Early pharmacologists who investigated thalidomide, such as Williams et al,[7] listed thalidomide's three actions as sedative, neurotoxic and teratogenic. It follows from the neural crest theory that these three actions are one and the same, i.e. action upon the sensory neuron. The difference between sedation (damping down sensory input) and neuropathy (sensory irritation or suppression) is a function of the dose and duration of thalidomide exposure upon the mature peripheral nerves of an adult. The difference between these two actions and its teratogenicity is the immaturity, extreme sensitivity and neurotrophic function of the embryonic precursor of the sensory peripheral nervous system.

Most recent articles about the therapeutic applications of thalidomide have relegated neuropathy to the list of side-effects, and claim that its primary action is anti-angiogenic, immunomodulatory and hypnosedative. Although presented as facts, these claims are theoretical. Any anti-angiogenic action is at very high and neurotoxic dose levels. The immunomodulation is debatable.[8] Thalidomide is still sedative, neurotoxic and teratogenic, as in 1965. No amount of 'spin' can alter these facts.

Functional change precedes histological damage

It can be predicted that subcellular proof of the neural crest theory in animal models may be particularly difficult, because, like many neurotoxins, the drug appears to act primarily by disturbing the function of neurons, their axons or the neural crest. Functional change always predates any detectable structural change. This applies to both adult and embryo. Functional disturbance in sensory nerves is recordable in adult humans, but is difficult to record in animals without language. However, electrophysiology of sural nerves in thalidomide-treated adult rabbits has replicated the early functional changes in human subjects.[9] As far as the embryo is concerned, reduction in mitosis/undifferentiated mesenchymal mass is a critical end-result. Preceding this, the first expression of structural pathology was a quantitative reduction in the embryonic nerves (measured later in the fetus) similar to the findings in adults with thalidomide neuropathy and to those of experiments on limb regeneration.

Regeneration = embryonic morphogenesis: a marriage of two sciences

I would like to see a resolution of the impasse that separates regeneration biology from developmental biology, over the issue of nerves being present in the regenerate blastema but not in the embryonic limb bud.

There are nerves in limb buds. We can no longer accept the dogma that the embryonic limb bud is an autonomous, nerve-free structure. This untruth must be deleted from embryology texts.

What regeneration biologists recognize as the nerve-dependent phase of limb regeneration is equivalent to what Nowack and Lenz called the 'thalidomide-sensitive period' in the human embryo, between 21 and 42 days' gestation. The nerve-dependent, thalidomide-sensitive phase of embryogenesis has been the focus of this book. Perhaps the most important contribution of this whole study is the concept that there is a nerve-dependent period in embryogenesis, previously unrecognized. It follows that exposure of an embryo to any neurotoxic chemical or physical event during this nerve-dependent period runs the risk of birth defects.

In the amphibian regenerate, sensory neurotrophism within the undifferentiated blastema is all-important in securing the later stages of limb formation. So too in the embryo. Sensory neurotrophism in undifferentiated mesenchyme is essential to attain normal limb formation. The two sciences (regeneration and embryogenesis) must now come together on this issue. Their union could catalyse much useful interaction in future research.

The thalidomide-sensitive period = the nerve-dependent phase of embryogenesis: clinical impact

The thalidomide-sensitive period has illuminated the fact of a 'nerve-dependent period' in early embryogenesis. This has significant clinical sequelae.

For pregnant women and their doctors, awareness of a 'nerve-dependent' period from 21 to 42 days' gestation is important, because it defines when, why and what to avoid in early pregnancy. Contact with neurotoxins during the nerve-dependent period of pregnancy carries high risk. Obstetricians and paediatricians will better understand the risks and timing of adverse exposures. Psychiatric patients on constant neurotropic medication may fall pregnant and put the embryo at potential risk. The implications for young women who abuse drugs are obvious. General practitioners also need to know that the nerve-dependent period is very early – just a few days after the missed period – when a patient might present herself for a pregnancy test. All medication and neurotoxic exposures should be checked immediately to minimize risk to her embryo.

A conservative attitude to taking medication in early pregnancy is already widely practised. What is new is an understanding of why, what and when hazards should be avoided.

Late-onset neuropathy in thalidomiders will be recognized as a sensory equivalent of post-polio syndrome

Since turning 40, many thalidomide victims have complained of tingling and numbness in their hands and feet. Some also describe shooting pains. Others describe increasing deafness, tinnitus or deteriorating vision. Many have bad backs that are put down to abnormal physical stresses and strains after years of compensating for short limbs. The Thalidomide Trust in the UK is having these problems investigated by neurologists at present.

The onset at middle age of symptoms of sensory neuropathy is parallel with the experience of people who had poliomyelitis (infantile paralysis) and who suffered a second bout of motor symptoms – weakness, paralysis and wasting of muscles – with onset at middle age. The pathophysiology of post-polio syndrome is twofold.

Firstly, the motor neurons in the anterior horn of the spinal cord were damaged by the poliovirus in infancy, and their population was diminished. Back in infancy, the number of motor axons in their peripheral nerves was less than normal. If the axon number was depleted below a threshold, symptoms appeared – weakness, paralysis and wasting of muscles from infancy and throughout life.

Secondly, there are physiological degenerative processes of aging. At middle age, we all face the onset of degenerative processes, which basically deplete our hair, skin, nerve fibres, etc. In middle-aged people with polio, this second loss of motor fibres on top of an already reduced population provokes another set of symptoms as above – the post-polio syndrome.

Thalidomide attacked the embryo, not the infant. It attacked the sensory, not the motor, nerves. The agent was a chemical, not a virus. But the response in the human body is basically similar. We have shown in rabbits that any thalidomide-exposed nerves have reduced numbers of large nerve fibres, sensory A type. If there is limb deformity, the axon reduction is proportional to the degree of malformation. Axons are deleted. This much we now know.

When the thalidomiders reached middle age, they also sustained the second physiological loss of neurons as normal degenerative processes took hold. In their case, the second reduction of axon numbers may be critical. They experience late-onset sensory symptoms in their reduced limbs because the second drop-out of sensory axons depletes the population of their peripheral nerves, perhaps below the threshold level where symptoms occur.

Normally, our peripheral nerves contain surplus axons in reserve above the threshold number to balance any nerve damage. What neurologists term a 'subclinical neuropathy' is having less than the normal number of nerve fibres, but enough to escape without symptoms, i.e. less than normal but more than the threshold at which symptoms appear. Thalidomiders have coasted along for 45 years with a subclinical neuropathy. At middle age, the additional physiological degeneration of sensory fibres may deplete the axon population to a level below the symptom threshold. A subclinical neuropathy then becomes a clinical (symptomatic) neuropathy. We suspect that this is occurring in the thalidomide cohort at present. They reached the age of 40 between 1998 and 2002. In 2005, 20% of British cases had recorded a recent onset of sensory complaints.

There is a practical aspect in which it is important to recognize the sensory neuropathic basis of their disorder. Medical attendants must understand that these people have neuropathic bones and joints. Therefore they run the risk of poor results from surgery. It is a well-established fact that fractures and surgery in neuropathic bones are slow to heal, or may end in non-union. The thalidomiders who present to doctors with arthritis or skeletal trauma need to be treated conservatively, as neuropathic bones and joints. Surgeons need to be cautious in offering joint replacements and other major procedures.[10] Healing is by no means assured.

Amphibia, cell cultures and seaweed will be used as early modules for teratogenic testing

I predict that newts, axolotls and other amphibia with regenerative ability will assume a role in teratology as models for detection of sensory neurotoxic properties that might cause birth defects. Amphibia provide a cheap and reliable model to test for neurotrophic toxicity in future drugs, and could be used as one module for teratogenicity testing.

It is imperative to accept that the early phase of human embryogenesis (21–42 days' gestation, the 'thalidomide-sensitive period') is *sensory nerve-dependent*. Had this been known before thalidomide was released into the pregnancy market, and had the drug been tested on amphibia,[11] the whole thalidomide disaster might have been averted.

Neurotoxicity would have been revealed in the laboratory by titrating it against neurotrophism in the nerve-dependent phase of amphibian limb regeneration. The paper by Bazzoli et al[11] is a good basic design for adoption in future testing regimes.

Cell cultures of neural crest, if they can be developed, could also be used for drug testing. In theory, this would be a neat way to bypass the biological variables of animal tests in laboratories. But such advances are never simple. Neural crest cells are labile and pleomorphic in culture, volatile, and hard to steer, making it difficult to grow neural lines. Thalidomide is unstable in solution. If neural crest cultures can be stabilized and perfected, we should be able to titrate different concentrations of chemicals directly against target neural crest cells, another testing module.

A cheaper and potentially efficient alternative test would be an adaptation of Boney's experiment with thalidomide and marine red algae.[12] Perhaps this is the closest approximation we will ever have to a dendritic cell model. Any disorder of sporeling morphology should sound teratological alarm bells. Marine red algae appear to simulate axonal outgrowth, and algal cultures could become significant modules in testing drugs for teratogenicity.

Other patterns of malformation may emerge as non-segmental neuropathies

Many of the so-called 'naturally occurring' sporadic malformations with anatomy similar to thalidomide defects still beg an explanation. Those with features of embryonic neuropathy should be considered to be due to sensory neurotoxic insult until proven otherwise. There are many sensory neurotoxins in the environment, but few as strong as thalidomide, and few with its spike action in vivo. Careful case histories of the nerve-dependent period of pregnancy should seek out neurotoxic exposure factors.

The combination of weak neurotoxicity and different pharmacokinetic parameters will conspire to create difficulties in the detection of neurotoxins. Nevertheless, neurotoxins should be sought among the many chemical and physical agents at large and untested in today's environment. The search should not be confined to pharmaceuticals, but to any environmental compounds or physiological disturbances with sensory neurotoxic potential. The weaker the neurotoxicity of any environmental agent, the more difficult will be its detection as a teratogen.

Thalidomide's spike action due to hydrolysis provided comparatively simple pharmacokinetics. This spike action was the reason for its precise assault upon ripe neural crest segments. In the absence of simple hydrolysis, or in the presence of active by-products, different patterns of molecular breakdown and metabolism will cause different anatomical patterns of malformation. Instead of a spike action, the graph of activity versus time might show a plateau of slow disintegration, and/or an increasing curve due to production of one or more active by-products. Such patterns of activity will *not* cause aplasia of *individual* sclerotomes. If the toxicity is prolonged, the reduction tendency will be deletion across a long length of neural crest. The end-result would not be dysmelia, but yet another pattern, if the embryo survived.

The role of molecular biology in this group of birth defects may diminish

What of the current fashion for molecular genetics in research in developmental biology? Would it be missed as far as sporadic birth defects are concerned? Much research has been driven by practical financial realities in recent years. A genetic aspect has been appended to research protocols in order to attract funding from the multi-million-dollar Human Genome Project, and to expand a laboratory's techniques into molecular genetics, considered to be 'à la mode'. Gross anatomy has been virtually abandoned, and, with it, the quest for organ and tissue targets. The result has been to skew research projects in directions that are tangential to clinical problems and often without clinically useful conclusions. These manoeuvres have strewn confusion rather than clarity across the path of birth defects research. Some laboratory research in current teratology has nothing to do with deformed babies.

While the clock cannot be turned back, there is a need to take stock. The bottom line is the infant – not a molecule, a receptor site or a protein sequence. This tends to be forgotten.

A logical freethinker on the sidelines of such research feels like the bystander observing the emperor's new clothes.

The embryo is re-established as our patient

Finally, the neural crest theory has helped to re-establish the embryo as the patient. It shows clearly that the embryo is subject to the same diseases as the adult, although the embryonic form of the disease may be different, or at least not obviously like that in the adult. But the elements of that pathology are present if they are sought. The clinical expression of the disease is simply modified by the stage of maturation of the target cells at the onset of the disease. Such a concept is not new. Attributed to Thomas Browne (1605–82), a contemporary of William Harvey, it was quoted by our Professor of Paediatrics, Sir Lorimer Dods, in the Norman Gregg Oration in Sydney in 1961:[13]

'. . . for we live, move, have a being and are subject to the actions of the elements and malice of diseases in that other world, the truest Microcosm, the Womb of our Mother . . .'

The neural crest emerges from erstwhile obscurity to take its place as a highly vulnerable, extremely important stimulator of embryonic growth, and an easy target for malicious sensory neurotoxins.

References

1. Thomas PK. The peripheral nervous system as a target for toxic substances. In: Spencer P, Schaumberg HH, eds. *Experimental and Clinical Neurotoxicology*. Baltimore: Williams and Wilkins, 1980.

2. Herker H, Hucho F, eds. *Selective Neurotoxicity*. Berlin: Springer-Verlag, 1994.

3. Baumgarten HG, Zimmerman B. Cellular and subcellular targets of neurotoxins: the concept of selective vulnerability. In: Herker H, Hucho F, eds. *Selective Neurotoxicity*. Berlin: Springer-Verlag, 1994.

4. Dyck PJ, Thomas PK. *Peripheral Neuropathy*, 4th edn. Philadelphia: Elsevier Saunders, 2005.

5. Cavanagh J. Foreword to: Chang LW, ed. *Principles of Neurotoxicology*. New York: Marcel Dekker, 1994.

6. Hill B. Characterization of embryopathy risks. In: *Thalidomide: Potential Benefits and Risks. An Open Public Scientific Workshop*. NIH, Bethesda, MD, 9 September 1997. Transcript [on line] p98. http://www.fda.gov/oashi/patrep/nih99.html#hill.

7. Williams RT, Schumacher H, Fabro S, Smith RL. The chemistry and metabolism of thalidomide. In: Robson JM, Sullivan F, Smith RL, eds. *A Symposium on Embryonic Activity of Drugs*. London: Churchill, 1965: 167–93.

8. Zwingenberger K, Wnendt S. Immunomodulation by thalidomide: systematic review of the literature and of unpublished observations. *J Inflamm* 1996; **46**: 177–211.

9. Schwab BW, Arezzo JC, Paldino AM, Flohe L, Mathiessen T, Spencer PS. Rabbit sural nerve responses to chronic treatment with thalidomide and supimide. *Muscle Nerve* 1984; **7**: 362–8.

10. Newman RJ. Shoulder joint replacement for osteoarthrosis in association with thalidomide-induced phocomelia. *Clin Rehab* 1999; **13**: 250–2.

11. Bazzoli AS, Manson J, Scott WJ, Wilson JG. The effects of thalidomide and two analogs on the regenerating forelimb of the newt. *J Embryol Exp Morphol* 1977; **41**: 125–35.

12. Boney AD. Abnormal growth of sporelings of a marine red alga induced by thalidomide. *Nature* 1963; **198**: 1069–9.

13. Dods L. Ourselves Unborn. Norman McAlister Gregg Oration. *Trans Ophthalmol Soc Aust* 1961; **21**: 12–19.

Index

Note: tabulated material is shown by page numbers in italics

ablation of sclerotomes 252–5,
    257–68
  experiments 197–209
algae, utility for neurotrophic
    toxicity testing 407
alimentary tract
  innervation 323
  malformations, as reduction
    deformities 132, 135–6,
    309–13
alkaline phosphatase 31
amelia
  classification/grading 274, 288
  and thalidomide-sensitive
    period *17, 18*
amniotic adhesions, in radial
    aplasia 96
amphibians
  limb regeneration 158–60,
    165–7
  sensitivity to thalidomide
    192–3
  sensory neurotrophism 404
  utility for neurotrophic
    toxicity testing 406–7
  limb-bud mesenchyme,
    presence of axons 172–80
amputation, and denervation
    163–4
anatomical distribution of
    disease in thalidomide
    victims 3–5
'aneurigenic' limb 188–9

animal experimental models
    23–6
  ablation experiments 197–209
  levels of thalidomide post
    ingestion *14*
  limb regeneration 158–67
  search for target tissue 26–7
  see also named animals
anophthalmos 305
anorectal agenesis 70
anorectal malformations 312–13
anotia, and thalidomide-
    sensitive period *17, 18*
anti-angiogenesis hypothesis 52,
    388–9
anti-cancer hypothesis 390,
    396–7
anti-inflammatory hypothesis
    388, 396
aortic coarctation, as a reduction
    deformity 132
aphthous ulcers 52, 53
apical ectodermal ridge (AER)
    394
ARAB bone staining technique
    57–8
arteries, in radial aplasia 95
arthropathy, Charcot's joints
    105–12
atavism 97
Auerbach's plexus, absence 136
auricle, ear malformations
    299–300

Australian series of cases 69–85
autonomic nervous system
    141–2, 151
  craniocaudal segmental order,
    combined sclero- and
    viscerotomes 320
  innervation of specific organs
    323
  viscerotomes (based on
    Netter) 318–20
axillary nerve, in radial aplasia
    96
axon *see* neurons

biliary malformations 311–12
biochemical injuries 27
bladder, ectopic, as a reduction
    deformity 131
bone
  ARAB staining technique
    57–8
  histology 238–41
  pathology 80, 82
    basic patterns,
      generalized/focal/
      random 82
    growth and trabecular
      sructure 104
    melorheostasis 357–60
  referred pain 245–6
  sensory nerve supply 237–44
bone marrow, histology 238
'boomerang' bone 71–2, 252

brachial plexus, in radial aplasia 95
British series of cases 87–90, 296

calcium hydroxyapatite, synthesis 141–2
cardiac *see* heart
case studies, German series, sensory neuropathy 39–40
case studies (diagnostic radiology)
    Australian series 69–85
    British series 87–90
    German series, sclerotome ablation/subtractions 269–78
cats and dogs as experimental models 25
    thalidomide polyneuropathy 49
caudal regression syndrome 328
cervical sclerotomes 258–60, 281–9
    fifth 261–2, 285–9
    seventh and eighth 263, 285–9
    seventh and S1, central and genetic ìsplitî hand/foot 377–8
    sixth 258–60, 281–5
    eighth and S2, femur–fibula–ulna reductions 365–77
    theoretical ablation 258–63
Charcot's joints 105–12
CHARGE syndrome 326
chemotoxicity principles 27–9
chick experimental model 25
    neural crest ablation 197–209
    neural crest theory 326–7
    quail–chick chimera 143–4
chondrification, rat 31
chondromucoid synthesis 141–2
classification 65–6
cleft lip/palate, as a reduction deformity 131, 134–5, 307–8
clinical neurology, examination of patient 44

clinical radiology 57–62
    integration with pathology 59–61
coloboma 304–5
    as a reduction deformity 132
compensation 6–7
congenital dislocation 101–13, *103*
congenital heart disease 320–2
congenital synostosis 115–24, *116*
    definition 115
    embryology 119–22
    incidence and types 115–18
    timing of injury 122–3, 150–5
Cornelia de Lange syndrome 352, 367
cranial embryology 141, 325–6
    head/face skeletal mesenchyme 141
    see also neural crest
cranial and spinal ganglia 119, 140
craniocaudal gradient, neural crest development 147–8, 152–3
craniofacial defects
    not thalidomide-associated 325–7
    thalidomide-associated 325
'crocodile tears' 305, 325
cytoplasm, histochemical mapping 144–5

Darwin, on limb anatomy 164–5
demyelination neuropathies 48
dendritic cell model, utility of algae for axonal outgrowth testing 407
dermatomes *45, 46–7, 248*
    and sclerotomes 247–55
    segmental, limbs (upper/lower) *45, 46–7*
    shared innervation 250–2
    subtraction hypothesis 84–5
dermoid cysts 305
developmental fields
    and neurotomes 318
    tibial and fibular 374–5
diabetic embryopathy 354–7
diabetic neuropathy 355–6
diagnostic process 58

diagnostic radiology 57–62, 69–85
    analysis 77–81
    case studies 69–77, *78–9, 87–90, 89*
    congenital dislocation 101–13
    congenital synostosis 115–24
    discussion 81–5
    integration with pathology 59–61
dimelia 379
distal and transverse reduction defects 380–5
dorsal root ganglion cell 41–2
drug screening procedures, thalidomide impact 19–20
Duane syndrome 305–6, 325
duodenal atresia 70, 310–11
dysmelia, definition 4–5

ear, anatomy and embryology 300–3
ear malformations 299–303, 325
ectromelia
    definition and unsuitability of term 64
    and thalidomide-sensitive period *17, 18*
electron microscopy 145–7
    model limb bud, innervation at 260 and 290 h gestation 170–83
    neurohistopathology 241–2
embryogenesis 119–24
    cranial and spinal ganglia 119
    embryo as patient 408–9
    limb embryogenesis 119–22
    nerve-dependent period 404–5
    new proposal 194
    organizer tissue 123
    symmetry/asymmetry in normal embryos 153–5
    thalidomide as a research tool 189–90
    thalidomide-affected *see* thalidomide embryopathy: *and specific topics*
    timing of injury 122–3, 150–5
embryonic neuropathy, sporadic, due to sensory toxic insult 407–8

enteric neurons 140
epidemic history of thalidomide malformations 1–3, 7–8, 15–16
  sensory peripheral neuropathy 39–40, 52–3
epiphyses
  absence 103
  growth 104
erythema nodosum leprosum 52–4, 388
eye malformations 304–7, 325
  anophthalmos, interpretation by neural crest injury 305
  anotia, and thalidomide-sensitive period *17, 18*
  incomplete expansion as a reduction deformity 132, 136–7

facial mesenchyme, derivation 326
facial nerve palsy 306
Fanconi syndrome 354
femur
  proximal femoral focal deficiency
    of thalidomide embryopathy 290–3, 355
  tibial and fibular developmental fields 375–6
  unrelated to thalidomide 293, 355, 374–6
  in fibular and tibial defects 374–6
femur–fibula–ulna reductions (FFU syndrome) 365–76
fibular developmental field 374–6
fibular reduction 371–3
fifth cervical (etc.) *see* cervical sclerotomes
fish, fin regeneration 165
fluorescence, histochemical mapping 144–5
focal deficiency/necrosis 97–8
foot
  sclerotome maps 248, 250
  sclerotome multiplication 378
  shared innervation 252
  'split'/lobster claw deformity 353, 376–8

fourth and fifth lumbar sclerotomes 264–8
future trends in research 399–409
  importance of neurology qualifications 402
  multidisciplinary approach 400
  order of investigations 58–9
  regeneration and embryonic morphogenesis resolved 404
  scientific predictions 402–4

gastrointestinal atresia, as a reduction deformity 132, 135–6, 309–13
gastrointestinal tract, innervation 323
gastroschisis, as a reduction deformity 131
genetic mutation hypothesis 394
genetics, homeobox genes 277
germ layer theory 142–3
German series of cases
  sclerotome ablation/subtractions 269–78
  sensory neuropathy 39–40
gestational days, vs post-menstrual days 17
glycogen 31
Goya, drawing of tetraphocomelic infant 356

^{3}H-thymidine, labelling neural crest 143–5
hand
  below-elbow amputation (BEA) defects 379–83
  sclerotome maps 248–9
  sclerotome multiplication 378
  shared innervation 251–2
  'split' 377–8
Haversian canals, innervation 239
head, embryology 141, 325–6
head/face skeletal mesenchyme 141
heart
  cardiac malformations 298–9, 354

congenital heart disease 320–2
  diabetic embryopathy 354–7
  innervation 323
  neural crest cells found 326
hemifacial hyperplasia 327
hernia, midline, as a reduction deformity 131
hip dislocation, and thalidomide-sensitive period *17, 18*
Hirschsprung's disease, as failure of migration of nerve cells 136
histochemical mapping of cytoplasm 144–5
history of thalidomide exposure 1–3, 7–8, 15–16
'hockeystick' bone 71–2, 252
Holt–Oram syndrome 322, 354
HOX genes 277
humerus
  and elbow joint reductions 370
  lack of cartilage 284
  in radial aplasia 94, 283
  subtotal aplasia 285
hyperostosis 360
hypotheses (action of thalidomide)
  genetic mutation hypothesis 394
  immunomodulation hypothesis 391–3
  molecular hypothesis 394–5

immunomodulation hypothesis 391–3
intercalary deficiency 285–7
  definition 286
  deletion from classification systems 287

Japan, thalidomide embryopathy 295–6
joints
  congenital dislocation 101–13
  congenital synostosis 115–24
  hip dislocation, and thalidomide-sensitive period *17, 18*
  innervation 240
  pathology 80, 101–24

size/shape of component
  bones 104–5
thalidomide-sensitive period
  17, 18
timing of injury 122–3, 150–5

kidney
  agenesis, as a reduction
    deformity 132, 137
  innervation 323

larynx, innervation 323
legal and insurance issues 6
Lenz, W, evidence for
    prosecution in trial ofDC
    15–19
leprosy, thalidomide treatment
    52–4, 388
ligaments and tendons,
    innervation 239–40
limb-bud
  chick model 32
  'evidence' against nerve
    dependence 187–9, 277,
    278
  evidence for nerve
    dependence 189–90, 278,
    404
  human (37 d) 121
  not a self-differentiating
    system 178
  presence of axons 144, 278
  rabbit model 29–30
    innervation at 260 and 290
      h gestation 170–83
    'self-differentiation' belief 178
    Wolpert on 178
  thalidomide effects
    lack of any action 152, 277,
      395
    neural crest pre limb bud vs
      limb bud stage 151, 190
  truncation? 395
limb-bud mesenchyme
  chick 32
  human (37 d) 121
  rabbit 29–30
limbs (upper/lower)
  anatomy
    Darwin on 164–5
    sclerotomes 245–55
  diagnostic radiology 69–77, *79*

embryogenesis 119–22,
    185–96
  growth, role of sensory
    neurons 127–8
  new concept of reduction
    deformity 130
  reduction deformities 64, 130
  regeneration 158–67, 185–95
    early nerve-dependent
      phase 166–7
    sensitivity to thalidomide
      193–4
  reproduced illustrations of
    Willert and Henkel
    282–92
  sclerotome
    ablation/subtraction
    analysis of case series
      269–78
    theoretical 258–67
  sclerotome maps, upper/lower
    246–50
  segmental dermatomes *45,
    46–7*
  see also specific bones; upper
    limbs
lobster claw deformity 353, 377
lumbar neurotomes,
    malformation sy=s 327–8
lumbar sclerotomes
  case studies (Willert and
    Henkel illustrations)
    289–93
  fourth 289–90
  fourth and fifth 264–8
  theoretical ablation 263–7
  third and fourth 290–2
  third, fourth and fifth 292–3
lung malformations 309

macrodactyly in
    neurofibromatosis 362
malformations (in general)
  internal 295–316
  multiple malformation
    syndromes 327–8
  not due to thalidomide
    325–7, 328
  thalidomide-associated
    327–8
  sequence 18–19
  specific, age of embryo 17–18

sporadic, due to sensory toxic
    insult 407–8
manus valga 366
marsupials, regeneration 165
media and political issues 6
median nerve injury 381–2
Meissner's plexus, absence 136
melorheostosis 357–60
mesenchyme
  absence in radiation-induced
    congenital synostosis 123
  action of thalidomide 191
  chick 32
  deficient mass 191
  developmental capabilities
    142
  facial 326
  head/face skeleton 141
  human limb-bud (37 d) 121
  presence of axons 172–80
  rabbit 29–30
mesoderm, doubts on site of
    thalidomide action 83
mesomelic dwarfism 367
microphthalmos 305
  interpretation by neural crest
    injury 305
midline structures, new concept
    of reduction deformity
    131–2
mitosis
  action of thalidomide? 191–2
  stimulation by neurotrophism
    163, 195
molecular hypothesis 394–5
morphometric studies, rabbit
    model 211–27, 229–36
muscles
  fast/slow, and innervation 166
  in radial aplasia 94–5
myelin sheath
  demyelination 48
  incidence 92–3
  myelination 180–1
  Schwann cells 141, 175

nerves
  in 37 d embryo 120
  cranial and spinal ganglia 119
  injury, and nerve function
    194–5
  in limb-bud mesenchyme 121

in radial aplasia 95–6
neural axis, establishment 141–2
neural crest
  ablation 197–209
    and self-replacement 206
  cells
    axonal outgrowth 149–50
    axonal sprouting 146–7
    axons and dendrites 145–7
    on septum of heart 326
  and cranial embryology 327
  cytoplasmic extensions,
    penetration into
    sclerotomes 181
  development
    chronology of thalidomide
      embryopathy 152
    craniocaudal gradient
      147–8, 152–3
    early 128–9, 140–2
    later 147–50
    trophic activity 128, 130–2,
      157–68
  environment and substrate
    148–9
  first appearance 140, 278
  and hemifacial hyperplasia
    327
  injury 125–56
  markers 142–5
  migration of cells 141–5
  utility for neurotrophic
    toxicity testing 407
neural crest hypothesis 125–6,
  129, 223
  asymmetric defects 327
  chick experimental model
    326–7
neuroanatomy 41–4
neurofibromatosis,
  macrodactyly 362
neurohistopathology
  advances in 241–2
  quantitative changes in rabbit
    model 225
neurology 44–8
  future trends in research
    399–400
  limb segmental dermatomes
    45, *46*–7
neurons 41–2
  axon demonstration 145–6

axon diameter reduction in
  thalidomide embryopathy
  223–6
axonal degeneration 48
axonal sprouting 146–7
axons and dendrites 145–7
axoplasmic flow 42, 161
  ramifications 145
  in regeneration 162–4
  supplying limb deformities vs
    normal limbs 212
  utility of algae for axonal
    outgrowth testing 407
neuropathic arthropathy
  (Charcot's joints) 105–12
  of thalidomide embryopathy
    109–11, *111*
neuropathology 48–54
neurotomes 317–31
  combined sclero- and
    viscerotomes, key to
    segments 320
  concept 317–18
  and developmental fields 318
neurotoxicity principles 397,
  403
  levels of thalidomide post
    ingestion *14*
  sedation/neuropathy/
    teratogenicity = same
    actions 403
  teratogenicity of thalidomide
    13–19
  toxic neuropathies 49
  and triple innervation 251–2
neurotoxicology
  future trends in research 401–2
  malicious neurotoxins 409
neurotrophism (trophic activity
  of sensory neurons) 128,
  130–2, 157–68
  chemical basis 164
  defined 157
  mechanism 160
  mitosis 163
  normal embryogenesis - new
    proposal 194
  other species 164–6
  principles 158
    quantitative/threshold
      factors 160–2
    in regeneration 158–60, 162–4

responsible for limb bud
  development 189–90
neurulation 140
new proposal, embryogenesis
  and neurotrophism 194
non-segmental sensory
  neuropathies 380–5

oesophageal malformation,
  reduction deformity 131,
  309–10
osteogenesis 141–2
oxygen deprivation,
  neurones/other cells 28

pain
  neurological causes 47
  referred 245–6
  see also sensory neuropathy
palate, cleft, as a reduction
  deformity 131, 134–5,
  307–8
Pasteur, chance and the
  prepared mind 61
pectoral and pelvic bones 275
  in amelia 289
  see also joints
perineum, embryology 313
periosteum, innervation 239
peripheral nerves, supplying
  limb deformities vs
  supplying normal limbs 212
peripheral neuropathies 48–56
  axonal degeneration 48
  demyelination 48
  see also sensory peripheral
    neuropathy
peripheral sensory nerves
  anatomy *42*
  and dermatomes, segmental
    origin of thalidomide
    embryopathy 83–4
pharmaceutical industry impact
  of thalidomide 19–20
phocomelia
  definition and unsuitability of
    term 63–4
  Goya's drawing of
    tetraphocomelic infant
    356
  and thalidomide-sensitive
    period *17*, *18*

polydactyly 353–4
popliteal nerve injury 380–3
positional awareness hypothesis 178
post-polio syndrome 405–6
pregnancy, embryogenesis, nerve-dependent period 404–5
pregnancy 404–5
  see also thalidomide-sensitive period
primates
  experimental models 256
  thalidomide-sensitive period, predating appearance of limb buds 189–90
proprioception
  positional awareness hypothesis 178
  property of ectoderm 278
proximal femoral focal deficiency
  of thalidomide embryopathy 290–3, 355
  unrelated to thalidomide 293, 355, 374–6
    histopathology 376
    tibial and fibular developmental fields 374–6
prurigo nodularis 52, 53

rabbit experimental model 24–5, 29–31
  anti-angiogenesis hypothesis 52, 388–9
  innervation of limb buds at 260 and 290 h gestation 170–83
  morphometric studies in tibial aplasia
    sciatic nerve 211–27
    tibial nerve 229–36
  sural nerve electrophysiology 225–6, 404
  thalidomide-sensitive period, predating appearance of limb buds 189–90
radial aplasia 91–113, 133–4, 283
  aetiology 92
  associations 93

clinical features 93
definition and classification 91–2
history 91
  past theories 96–8
  predominance in case series 81
  sclerotome
    ablation/subtraction 252–5
  stages *282*
radial dysmelia 281–9
  reproduced illustrations from Willert and Henkel (1969) 282–92
radial nerve, in radial aplasia 96
radio–ulnar synostosis 283
radiology *see* diagnostic radiology
rat/mouse experimental model 24–5, 31
  mesenchyme absence, radiation-induced congenital synostosis 123
recto–vesical fistula, as a reduction deformity 131
red algae, utility for neurotrophic toxicity testing 407
reduction deformity
  defined 64
  new concept for
    limbs 130
    midline structures 131–2
    tubular structures and solid organs 132–3
regeneration *see* limb regeneration
regeneration blastema 162–4, 185
retinoic acid, teratogenesis 326
Roberts syndrome 322, 352, 355

sacral agenesis 354
sacral sclerotomes 293
SC syndrome 352
scaphoid, in radial aplasia 94
Schwann cells, myelin sheath 141, 175
sciatic nerve (rabbit) in morphometric study 211–27
  axonal diameter reduction 225

total fascicular area reduction 223–4
sclerotomes 245–55, 272
  ablation/subtraction 252–5, 257–68, 269–78
    analysis of case series 269–78
    theoretical 257–64
  defined 247
  disorders other than thalidomide embryopathy 351–64
  limb deficiencies unrelated to thalidomide 365–86
  maps 246–50, 278
  multiplication 378–9
  referred pain 245–6
  sacral S1 and S2 293, 375–6
  see also cervical sclerotomes; lumbar sclerotomes; sacral sclerotomes
scoliosis, ulnar ray defect 369
sedation action of thalidomide 403
segmental sensory neuropathy *see* sensory neuropathy
segmental structures
  combined sclero- and viscerotomes 320
  limb segmental dermatomes *45*, 46–7
  origin of thalidomide embryopathy 83–4
  skeletal defects and related visceral defects *324*
  see also dermatomes; sclerotomes
sensitive period for malformation risk *see* thalidomide-sensitive period
sensory neuroanatomy 41–2
  bone 237–44
sensory neurons
  features 144, 278
  trophic activity 128, 130–2, 157–68
sensory neurotoxicity
  principles 27–9, 397
    sedation/neuropathy/teratogenicity = same actions 403

sensory neuropathy not a side-effect of thalidomide 403
teratogenicity of thalidomide 13–19
toxic neuropathies 49
and triple innervation 251–2
sensory peripheral neuropathy 39–56
equivalence to post-polio syndrome 405–6
first and second epidemics 39–40, 52–3
glove and stocking distribution 383
limb segmental dermatomes *45*, 46–7
location of nerve lesions 45–6
non-segmental neuropathies 379–83
not a 'side-effect' of thalidomide 403
onset in middle age 396
patterns of injury 47–8
result of FDA-approved thalidomide treatment for various conditions 52–4
sixth cranial nerve 98–9, 134
skeletal expressions (other than thalidomide-associated) 51–64
sural nerve degeneration 50–1
thalidomide used as anti-cancer agent 390
sickle cell anaemia 367
sixth cranial nerve, segmental sensory neuropathy 98–9, 134
skeletal defects
related visceral defects *324*
see also bone; *specific regions*
somites, levels 318–20
spina bifida, as a reduction deformity 131, 135
spinal cord transection 47–8
stains and vital dyes 142–3
silver stains fail to reveal distal axons 179
strabismus 304
sural nerve
axonal degeneration human 50–1

rabbit 225–6, 404
Sweden, thalidomide cases 305–6
symmetry/asymmetry 80–1
normal embryos 153
syndactyly 354
synostosis 115–24, *116*
radio-ulnar 283

talocalcaneal synostosis 373
TAR syndrome 352
tear–saliva syndrome 305
teratogenicity of thalidomide 13–19
action on neural crest not limb bud 403–4
future trends in research 401–2
teratogens
and malformations 34
neural crest extirpation 326
research, order of investigations 58–9
terminology 63–5
thalidomide
actions 387–78
evidence 190
on mitosis? 191–2
on neural crest and axons 192
no cytotoxicity in vitro 393
no molecular target known 393
effect on growth of algae 149–50
future trends in research 401–2
hypothetical actions 387–95
metabolism 12–13
pharmacology 11–21, 353
pharmacokinetics in vivo 14–15
safety 11–12
short half-life 12, 151
teratogenicity 13–14, 15–19, 353
structure 12
target organ absence 395–6
see also thalidomide embryopathy; thalidomide victims; thalidomide-sensitive period

thalidomide embryopathy
12 fundamental characteristics 396
absence of vascular lesions 33
anatomical distribution of disease 3–5
bone pathology 80, 82
chronology in relation to neural crest development 152
definition 4–5
differential diagnosis 368
epidemic history 1–3, 7–8, 15–16
impact upon pharmaceutical industry 19–20
Japan 295–6
Lenz' description (1962) 126–7
location of nerve lesions 45–6
nerve supply of deformities 211–27
pathogenesis of damage 61–2
and second generation 65
sequence of skeletal loss, upper/lower limb 271
spectrum of disease 295–8
timing of injury 122–3, 150–5
see also thalidomide-sensitive period
'thalidomide look-alikes' 322–5, 325–7, 328, 351–3
genetic mutation hypothesis 391–3
multiple craniofacial defects 325–7
multiple malformation syndromes 322–5, 328
proximal femoral focal deficiency 293, 355
thalidomide polyneuropathy 39–56
disappears from records 51–2
sural nerve degeneration 50–1
thalidomide-sensitive period 15–18, 122–3, 150–5, 277, 404–5
gestational days *17, 18*
vs post-menstrual days 17

malformation risk
head-to-tail sequence 150–3
predating appearance of
limb buds 189–90
specific malformations
17–18, 122–3, 150–5
neural crest hypothesis 212
neural crest pre limb bud vs
limb bud stage 151, 190
timing of injury 122–3, 150–5
spike action 407–8
thalidomide victims
compensation 6–7
legal and insurance issues 6
media and political issues 6
problems 5
sensory neuropathies in
middle age 405–6
thumb aplasia 94
predominance 81
sclerotome
ablation/subtraction
252–5
thalidomide-sensitive period
17, 18
thumb triphalangism 354
in radial aplasia 94
thalidomide-sensitive period
17, 18
tibial aplasia
morphometric studies (rabbit)
sciatic nerve 211–27
tibial nerve 229–36
sclerotome
ablation/subtraction
252–5
tibial developmental field 374–6

tibial dysmelia 289–94
reproduced illustrations from
Willert and Henkel (1969)
282–92
tibial nerve injury 380–3
timing of injury 122–3, 150–5
gestational days, vs post-
menstrual days 17
spike action of thalidomide
407–8
toxic *see* chemotoxicity
trachea, innervation 323
tracheo-oesophageal fistula, as a
reduction deformity 131,
309–10
transverse reduction defects
379–83
trapezium, in radial aplasia 94
Treacher Collins syndrome 325
trophic activity of sensory
neurons 128, 130–2
see also neurotrophism
truncal neuropathy, and distal
reduction defects 379–83
tubular structures and solid
organs, new concept of
reduction deformity 132–3

UK, cases of thalidomide
embryopathy 296
ulcers
anti-inflammatory action of
thalidomide 388
types 48, 356
ulnar nerve
injury 381–2
in radial aplasia 96

ulnar reduction 365–70
upper limbs
diagnostic radiology 69–77,
78, 284
dysmelia
gross histology 286
'hockeystick' bone 71–2,
252
sclerotome
ablation/subtraction
analysis of case series
269–78
theoretical 258–63
sclerotomes 249
thalidomide-sensitive period
17, 18
see also hand; limbs; radial;
ulnar
urogenital malformations
312–13
urogenital tract, innervation 323

vascular stenosis, as a reduction
deformity 132
vertebrae, innervation 240
vestibular system,
malformations 302–3
visceral defects, related skeletal
defects *324*
viscerotomes
based on Netter 318–20
concept 317–19
vital dyes 142–3

Willert and Henkel, reproduced
illustrations 282–92
wrist joint, in radial aplasia 94

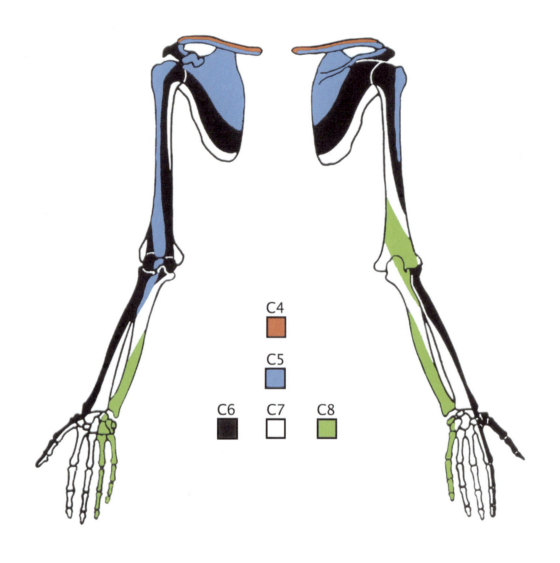

Front and back endpapers: The sclerotome maps. (Reproduced from Inman VT, Saunders JB de C. Referred pain from skeletal structures. *J Nerv Ment Dis* 1944; **99**: 660–7.)